Management
of Head Injuries

Contemporary Neurology Series available:

Fred Plum, M.D., *Editor-in-Chief*
Fletcher H. McDowell, M.D., and J. Richard Baringer, M.D., *Editors*

Management of Head Injuries

BRYAN JENNETT, M.D., F.R.C.S.

GRAHAM TEASDALE, M.R.C.P., F.R.C.S.

Professors of Neurosurgery
University of Glasgow

Directors of the Head Injury Research Programme of the Medical Research Council
Institute of Neurological Sciences
Southern General Hospital
Glasgow, Scotland

 F.A. DAVIS COMPANY, PHILADELPHIA

Library of Congress Cataloging in Publication Data

Jennett, Bryan.
 Management of head injuries.

 (Contemporary neurology series; 20)
 Includes bibliographies and index.
 1. Head—Wounds and injuries. I. Teasdale, Graham, joint
author. II. Title. III. Series.
[DNLM: 1. Head injuries—Therapy. W1 C0769N v. 20 / WE706 J54m]
RD521.J46   617'.51044   80-16785

ISBN 0-8036-5017-5 Hard Cover
ISBN 0-8036-5019-1 Soft Cover

Preface

It is a hard task to treat what is common in a way of your own. —Horace

Head injured patients are so commonplace that they often fail to attract the attention they deserve, as a fascinating natural phenomenon and as a challenge to doctors. The many who are mildly injured pose a logistic problem; failure to solve this results in avoidable mortality and morbidity in the few who develop serious complications. Severe injuries demand intensive investigation and treatment, yet many still die and some survivors are permanently disabled. The scale of the problem is considerable and in developed countries trauma is now by far the commonest cause of brain damage in the young. Many different specialists are involved in the care of these patients, either for different kinds of injury, or at different stages in the management of one patient. Consequently, it is difficult for any one medical discipline to get a coherent view of the problem as a whole. This is what this book endeavors to provide.

We deal practically but we hope thoughtfully with the common problems encountered by the clinician in caring for head injuries. The views that we express are those of the Glasgow Institute and, in particular, our own, but the book deals more with data than with opinion. Wherever possible we offer figures in support of our assertions, drawing on the literature and on the considerable amount of data accumulated in the last decade by ourselves and in other centers across the world. Our aim has not been to catalogue exhaustively the characteristics of the many specific, often rare, complications of head injury but instead to analyze and emphasize the whole sequence of assessment and decision-making which may be called management.

The outburst of information about head injury in the last decade reflects both a perception of the importance of the problem and also the belief that recent developments in investigation and treatment may lead to improved results. Views about head injury are currently changing rapidly and this book can reflect only thinking at the dawn of the 80s. When considering particular types of treatment we have been conscious of the fact that these may change or indeed differ widely from place to place and from time to time. We therefore devote considerable attention to ways and means of analyzing variations in management, using carefully standardized methods for assessing the type and severity of the injury, and the degree of subsequent recovery, in an effort to establish a basis for the critical evaluation of new developments.

Faced with such a broad canvas, stretching from epidemiology and pathology, through intensive investigation and therapy to surgical intervention and on to late effects, we might well have invited colleagues with specialist skills to write some of the chapters. Instead, we asked them to talk to us, and then to read what we had written about what they had told us. In this way we hope that we have presented an account which has the consistency of only two pens, yet the authority of an experience much greater than our own. So many colleagues were willing to respond to our requests for help that they cannot all be named. But Hume Adams and David Graham deserve special thanks for ensuring that our account of pathology was in order and was adequately illustrated. Michael Bond guided us on the chapters on recovery and on mental sequelae, while the late Leslie Stevens provided the CT scans and his successors advice on technical details. Douglas Miller, late of Virginia and happily now returned to Scotland, made valuable comments about pathophysiology, and Iain Ledingham checked that we had not offended too many of the tenets of the Intensive Care Specialist. We also thank our neurosurgical colleagues in Glasgow, in particular Sam Galbraith and John Pickard and also Reinder Braakman, Ted Kurze, and the many other surgeons throughout the world whose comments, criticism, and collaboration have contributed much to our thinking and therefore to this book.

Our wives, Sheila Jennett and Evelyn Teasdale, provided the expertise of their own fields (physiology and neuroradiology), were stern critics of our prose, and tolerated and even encouraged an endeavor which threatened a succession of family vacations. Our thanks to them, and to Sally Brown and Margaret Smith who lost count of the number of drafts they typed, but never their cool or efficiency. The illustrations were mostly produced for teaching in the University and are the work of Mrs. Margaret Murray and her colleagues in the Department of Medical Illustration in the Institute, the quality of whose work we appreciate.

Neurosurgeons and neurologists are uneasy bed fellows on both sides of the Atlantic, but with that ocean between them Fred Plum and Bryan Jennett have enjoyed a fruitful relationship for over 10 years, based on common interests and mutual respect. We are pleased to join the ranks of the series of Black Books, and to be published alongside the Third Edition of *Stupor and Coma,* to which both neurologists and neurosurgeons owe much. Dr. Plum encouraged us to write this book now, rather than postpone it (for ever?) until we had all the answers, and he made several practical suggestions when he read the first draft. We hope therefore that this will be a book for all disciplines, and will help many to understand where their contribution to the evolution of this complex problem fits into the picture as a whole.

Bryan Jennett
Graham Teasdale

Contents

CHAPTER 1

Epidemiology of Head Injury

The descriptive elements of the epidemiology of head injuries are woefully incomplete . . . because no single report includes *all* patients with head injuries (irrespective of severity), within a defined population.

—Kraus, 1978

Head injuries constitute a major health problem in all westernized nations. Rational plans for dealing with this common condition cannot be made nationally, regionally, or in a single hospital unless information is available about the level of risk in different populations, where and when injuries occur, how severe they are, and how often they occur. Several factors account for the relative dearth of reliable statistics about head injury. One is lack of agreement about the definition of a head injury. Another is the variety of sources from which statistics are available, each representing a different population of affected persons. This in turn reflects the wide dispersion of head-injured patients throughout the health care system. Half the fatal cases never reach hospital, while many with milder injuries do not consult a doctor unless complications develop. Even within the hospital, patients with head injuries go to neurosurgeons, accident and general surgeons, rehabilitationists, and pathologists—each of them sees part of the problem, but none of them the whole of it.

WHAT IS A HEAD INJURY?

The International Classification of Diseases (ICD) is the basis of official statistics in most countries, whether of deaths or of hospital admissions. The three-digit "N" code indicates the pathological nature of the injury, but the term "head injury" does not appear. Instead there are ten rubrics (Table 1), which, taken as a group, cover most head injuries. However, there are two limitations to the usefulness of the ICD. One is that the rubrics are not mutually exclusive. For example, intracranial hematoma can be identified only by using a code that excludes those with skull fracture, yet more than 75 percent of hematomas are associated with a fracture. The other limitation is the way in which the system is used by those responsible for coding. Local custom seems to determine this. Some institutions code most injuries as concussion (N850); others prefer "IC injury unspecified" (N854); yet others use "unqualified skull fracture" (N803). Almost certainly this is done without regard to whether or not a fracture was in

1

Table 1. International Classification of Diseases: causes for tabulation of mortality[43]

List B

	EXTERNAL CAUSE OF INJURY	
BE47	Motor vehicle accidents	E810–E823
BE48	All other accidents	{E800–E807 E825–E949
BE49	Suicide and self-inflicted injuries	E950–E959
BE50	All other external causes	E960–E999
	NATURE OF INJURY	
BN47	Fractures, intracranial and internal injuries	{N800–N829 N850–N869

Three-Digit Categories
Fracture of skull, spine and trunk (N800–N809)
N800   Fracture of vault of skull
N801   Fracture of base of skull
N802   Fracture of face bones
N803   Other and unqualified skull fractures
N804   Multiple fractures involving skull or face with other bones
Intracranial injury (excluding those with skull fracture) (N850–N854)
N850   Concussion
N851   Cerebral laceration and contusion
N852   Subarachnoid, subdural and extradural haemorrhage, following injury (without mention of cerebral laceration or contusion)
N853   Other and unspecified intracranial haemorrhage following injury (without mention of cerebral laceration or contusion)
N854   Intracranial injury of other and unspecified nature

fact verified. Nor are the rubrics readily ranked to reflect severity, as recognized by the clinician. It is hoped that the 10th Edition will include a reference to duration of coma—thus recognizing that an injury can be severe without fracture or hematoma.

Clearly there can be no absolute criteria that will define a head injury. It is difficult in many instances to avoid some reference to severity, whether this is defined administratively (how dealt with) or in biological terms. The difficulty of the latter is that scalp, skull, and brain can each be injured, without any involvement of the other. But it is brain damage, actual or potential, that is the key to medical interest in blows to the head, and the term *craniocerebral trauma* is therefore a reasonable synonym for head injury. What matters is the minimal requirement for a patient to be regarded as a "head injury." There is clearly need for something better than "severe enough to cause serious worry" or "associated with cerebral symptoms or signs"—to quote two recent reports. The study of head injuries in Scottish hospitals,[23] which was specifically designed to include cases dealt with by accident/emergency departments but not admitted, evolved an operational definition that has proved practical. This survey included the following cases:

1. Definite history of a blow to the head
2. Laceration of the scalp or forehead
3. Altered consciousness, no matter how brief

Excluded were facial lacerations, fractures of the lower jaw, foreign bodies in the eye, nose, or ear, and epistaxis—unless they were associated with one of the "head injury" features.

SOURCES OF STATISTICS

Deaths

Deaths might be regarded as the most reliable and most readily available data, as these are registered in most countries. However, if only the E code (for external cause) is used, as in mortality data published by the U.S. National Center for Health Statistics or by W.H.O., the location of the injury cannot be determined. This accounts for the lack of information about head injury deaths at a national level in most countries, including the United States. Both the N and the E codes are available for all deaths recorded by the British Registrars General.[35,36] More than half the deaths attributed to head injury occur before the patient can be admitted to hospital; not all cases are autopsied, and few of those that are have detailed dissection of the brain. In both these and hospital deaths, death may be wrongly ascribed to head injury; on the other hand, head injuries may be obscured by a diagnosis of "multiple injury." While most hospital deaths occur in a few days, intensive care now prolongs the lives of some severely injured patients whose eventual death in chronic care or at home may not be registered as due to head injury. In spite of these limitations, annual national death rates provide a useful guide to the prevalence of accidental deaths and their causes, and trends with time can be observed. It can be reasonably assumed that deaths from head injury will change *pari passu* with all accidental deaths.

Hospital Discharge Data

These data are published separately for England and Wales[12] on a 10 percent sample of hospital returns, and for all cases in Scotland.[39] These data include age, social class, duration of stay, and also the type of hospital and the specialty. As the hospital system in Britain is unified under the NHS, these annual reports provide a valuable resource, and analysis of this data for England and Wales up to 1972 has been published.[13]

Informal Clinical Reports

These reports, most often of patients treated by a neurosurgical service, are frequently published. They are obviously selected populations, but the basis of selection is seldom clearly stated—if indeed it is known. Nor is there usually data about the whole population of admitted head injuries from which selection has been made. Some of these reports are limited to cases of a certain severity—with fracture, unconscious, needing operation, and so on. Criteria of severity or of selection vary so much that comparison between such series is difficult, and they seldom provide useful data for epidemiological purposes, except as an indicator of workload in certain departments.

Nonhospitalized Head Injuries

Nonhospitalized patients with head injuries are much more common than those who are admitted to hospital. There are those who die before reaching hospital and the much more numerous cases who are sent home after assessment in accident/emergency departments. No official statistics appear to be available for these

3

latter cases in any country, but specific surveys in Scotland and Canada indicate that they outnumber admissions by four or five to one.[41,27] There are also many patients with minor injuries whose first medical contact is when they come with continuing symptoms of the postconcussional syndrome, or with major intracranial complications. For every patient who develops such complications, major or minor, there must be many who do not, but that number can never be known.

There are certain circumstances in which evidence about a head injury may be purposely minimized or even concealed. Those injured during organized sport are usually anxious not to have limits put on further participation, and injuries associated with assault are also often not declared immediately. Injuries suffered under the influence of alcohol may be unwittingly concealed, with the patient going (or being put) to bed to sleep it off. Ease of access to medical care also influences medical consultation after injury; we have shown that fewer patients from rural areas come to their regional hospital after mild injuries than in large cities.[41] All these factors combine to limit the possibility of making an accurate assessment of the true prevalence of head injuries. For the most part it is possible to count injured patients only when they impinge upon the hospital system, the traffic police, or the coroner.

Planned Surveys

Increasing realization on both sides of the Atlantic, both of the importance of head injuries and of the lack of good data about them, has led to the initiation of a number of formal studies. These are briefly reviewed in order to indicate the extent to which they can be compared or related to each other.

HEAD INJURY CENTERS IN UNITED STATES. In the 1960s a number of centers were funded by NINCDS. It was natural that the neurosurgeons, who were the principal investigators, should have focussed on the small proportion of patients who were severely injured. Most attention was devoted to laboratory-based clinical and experimental investigations of the pathophysiology of the consequences of head injury, but several sizable series of severely injured patients have been reported.[2,6,34]

DATA BANK OF SEVERE INJURIES FROM THREE COUNTRIES. This study began in Glasgow in 1968, then added centers from the Netherlands and the United States. Clinical data was collected prospectively by standardized methods, on consecutive series of patients—but only those severely injured. Over 1500 patients are now on record and data collection continues. There are striking similarities (and a few differences) between this kind of patient in the three countries.[25,26] A multicenter data bank for severe injuries in the United States, using similar methods of assessment, has recently been initiated by NINCDS.

SCOTTISH HEAD INJURY MANAGEMENT STUDY. In 1975 an epidemiological team was established in Glasgow to collect data about head injuries as a whole, to include deaths before hospital, discharges from accident/emergency departments, and all admissions to hospital (the few that go to neurosurgical wards and the much larger numbers that go to primary surgical wards). This latter term was conceived to cover the various kinds of non-neurosurgical wards in which, in most countries outside of North America, the majority of hospitalized head injuries are treated. Reports of a national survey in Scotland for 1974 have already been published.[22,23,31,41] Further data are being collected in Scotland, and also from regions in England where different referral policies prevail for the transfer of patients to neurosurgical units, in order to compare the consequences of alternative organizational approaches to the care of head injuries.

This study is providing a more complete picture of the head injury problem than has hitherto been available. Using it as a reference point, it is possible to extrapolate from the more limited data available for other countries, in order to estimate the scope and scale of the head injury problem there. This requires the assumption that the distribution of injuries of different severity, the proportion admitted to hospital, their duration of stay, and other aspects of care are similar. Already there is evidence that similarities between Western countries are much more marked than differences.

NATIONAL HEAD AND SPINAL CORD INJURY SURVEY. This study, which awaits publication as a supplement in the Journal of Neurosurgery (edited by D. Anderson and R. L. McLaurin), consists of a national probability sample of patients admitted to hospitals in the United States in 1974 after recent central nervous system trauma.

CNS TRAUMA CENTER FEASIBILITY STUDIES. These studies surveyed the incidence of CNS trauma in six centers in the United States for 1978; again it seems likely that most centers confined data collection to hospital admissions. From these, and from the Triangle study, it seems that in the United States, 10 percent CNS trauma is spinal, and 10 percent of patients have both head and spinal injury. An Australian study shows similar proportions.[40]

HOW FREQUENT ARE HEAD INJURIES?

It is clear that this question cannot be answered without specifying whether the denominator is deaths, admissions to hospital, or attenders at emergency rooms. For estimates of general prevalence of head injuries, and of the burden they put on health care resources, it is possible only to use either nationally collected statistics, which are limited in detail and are available only for some countries, or the data from planned surveys.

Head Injury Deaths

Each year in Britain there are 9 deaths from head injury per 10^5 population; they account for 1 percent of all deaths, a quarter of trauma deaths, and almost half of those caused by road accidents (which cause 60 percent of all head injury fatalities). The proportion of deaths that are ascribed to head injury is much higher in young males (Fig. 1). No national statistics are available for head injury deaths in the United States, but an estimate for 1969 indicated more than twice the rate in Britain; preliminary results from the feasibility studies in central Virginia[20] and in San Diego[34] show 24 deaths per 10^5 population (for 1978), again more than twice the British rate. World Health statistical reports record deaths from all accidents and from road accidents for many countries, but do not distinguish head injuries. These show a wide variation between countries (Table 2), but

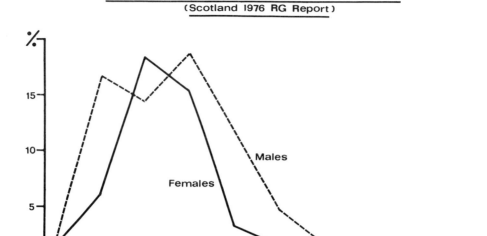

Head Injury Deaths as a Percentage of All Deaths
(Scotland 1976 RG Report)

Figure 1. Percentage of all deaths that are due to head injury at different ages. (From Jennett and associates.[24])

they also show that in most the death rates from accident are either steady or declining (Fig. 2). This is also true for head injuries, to judge from British statistics (Fig. 3).

Head Injury Admissions

Between 200 and 300 per 100,000 of the population are admitted to hospital each year in Britain and the United States, according to various sources available.[20,24,34] These rates are higher for men than women, and for younger than older sections of the population (Table 3). Most of these patients stay for less than 48 hours, and head injuries, therefore, make a smaller contribution to occu-

Table 2. International death statistics (in rank order)[10,32,35,36,43]

Accidents as Percentage of All Deaths		Road Deaths as Percentage of Accidental Deaths		Road Deaths as Rate per 100K Population	
Canada	8	Netherlands	73	West Germany	30
France	7	Australia	56	Canada	30
Australia	6	Italy	53	Australia	29
West Germany	5	Denmark	51	Italy	26
Italy	5	Canada	50	Denmark	24
Denmark	5	West Germany	49	France	24
USA	5	USA	44	Netherlands	22
Japan	5	Japan	43	USA	22
Netherlands	4	England	42	Scotland	16
Sweden	4	Scotland	35	Sweden	15
Scotland	4	Sweden	34	Japan	14
England	3	France	31	England	14

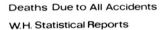

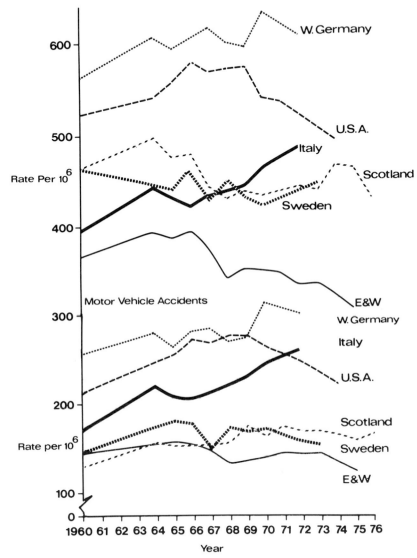

Figure 2. Trends in death rates from all accidents *(above)* and from road accidents *(below)*. E & W = England and Wales. (Based on WHO data, from Jennett and associates.[24])

pied bed days than to admissions.[31] In Scotland 3 percent of all admissions to all acute hospital beds are for head injury, but these account for only 1 percent of bed usage. However, in *surgical* wards they make up 4 percent of occupied bed days. Head injuries account for 30 percent of admissions after accidents.

Since 1963 the number of admissions has increased each year in England and Wales, and in Scotland, but this has been due to more patients going into hospital

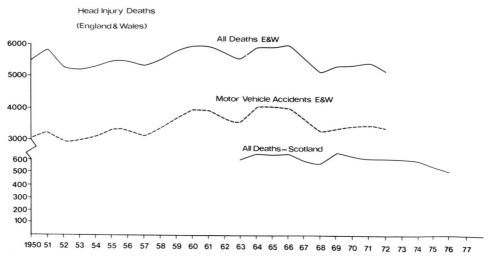

Figure 3. Trends in death rates from head injury in Britain. (From Jennett and associates.[24])

briefly after mild injury; a consequence of this is that case mortality has fallen (Fig. 4). The incidence of more severe injuries in England and Wales reached a peak in the mid sixties, then declined somewhat, and now appears to be steady.[13]

More detailed analysis of patients admitted to hospital is more difficult, because different patient populations are determined according to the local arrangements for the care of head injuries of varying severity. In Europe most neurosurgeons see only the more severe injuries, while in North America they take responsibility for a much greater proportion. This makes for a striking contrast in the features of head injured patients in neurosurgical units in different countries.

Emergency Room Attenders

There are no official statistics available for these patients, but Klonoff and Thompson did a survey in Vancouver in 1969.[27] Their findings for one hospital have been largely confirmed by the more detailed and extensive study of Scottish hospitals for 1974.[41] This study showed an annual attendance rate with head injury (per 100,000 population in Scotland) of 1775; this was more than twice as high in men (2588) as in women (1022). The annual rate for attendance with head injury caused by road accident was 334. Almost double this rate was estimated

Table 3. Accident/emergency department attendance after head injury—annual rate per 100K population in Scotland, 1974[41]

	Males	Females	Total
Aged 15–24	3730	936	2349
Aged 45–54	1420	624	1014
Road accident	422	218	346
Assault	415	95	319
All ages/causes	2588	1022	1775

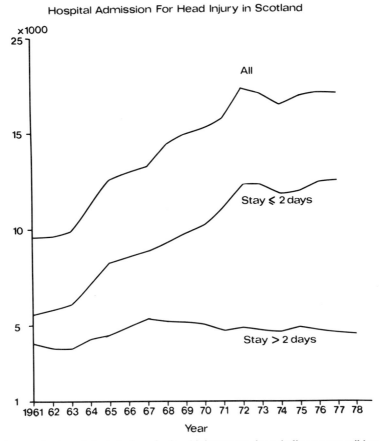

Figure 4. Increasing hospital admissions for head injury were due wholly to more mild cases that stay less than 2 days. (From Jennett and associates.[24])

by Caveness from the NCHS survey in the United States,[7] but the sample was probably too small to be reliable. In the Netherlands a lower rate was recorded, probably because many patients attend general practitioners after minor accidents.[42]

The proportion of attenders who were admitted to hospital was similar in all Scottish hospitals—rather more than 20 percent. The higher attendance and death rates for head injuries in the United States,[20,24,34] coupled with a similar admission rate to Britain (per 100,000 population), suggest that a greater proportion of those attending emergency rooms in the United States are sent home after assessment and treatment.[24]

CAUSES OF HEAD INJURY

There is no uniformity in the use of terms by which cause of injury is classified, and this may account for some discrepancies between reports that cannot be explained by differences in severity. Confusion chiefly arises between descrip-

9

Table 4. Frequency distribution of causes in head injuries of varying severity

Frequency of Each Cause	Severity of Injuries				
	A/E Sent Home[23]	PSW Admission[23]	NSU Admission[23]	Severe Injuries[26]	Deaths[36]
	2735	1181	424	1000	476
Road accidents	13%	34%	38%	58%	56%
Adults (≥15 years)					
Assaults	23%	20%	11%	7%	7%
Alcoholic falls	7%	12%	19%	16%	29%
Work (not road)	12%	7%	9%	7%	4%

A/E = Accident and Emergency
PSW = Primary Surgical Ward
NSU = Neurosurgical Unit

tions of *how* an injury happened, and *where* it occurred. Thus, "road" is a place, but "traffic" suggests movement, while "motor vehicle" may exclude pedestrians and cyclists. Is school equivalent to work, and is informal play deserving of classification as sport? Falls are common, but may be obscured by classification of site of accident, e.g., home or street. What matters is that adequate definitions are given, so that valid comparisons can be made.

Even when definitions are agreed upon, the question "what causes head injuries" is no more readily answered than how frequent the condition is. The causes vary in their distribution with the severity of the injury (Table 4), and with age and sex (Table 5). Local cultural factors also influence the distribution of causes—in Scotland assault is as common as road accident as a cause of injury leading to emergency room attendance of men in the age group 15 to 64 years.

The role of alcohol in the causation of accidents is complex, and it varies between countries and also between injuries of different types and severity. Alcohol was more frequently recorded in patients admitted to hospital than in emergency room attenders sent home; it was more common in the city hospitals than elsewhere (Tables 6 and 7). Men were twice as often affected as women, and more than half male admissions to city hospitals had recently taken alcohol. Certain kinds of injury are frequently associated with alcohol; in Scotland alcohol is more often found in injured pedestrians than in vehicle occupants (Table 8). But the intoxication-associated head injury in Scotland is less often due to road accident than to assault or a fall, incidents that seldom cause serious injury except to the

Table 5. Causes of head injuries attending A/E departments (Scottish study)[41]

	<15 yr 1516	15–64 yr 1826	>65 yr 217	Males 2501	Females 1067
Road accidents	9%	24%	24%	16%	21%
Assault	3%	24%	1%	16%	9%
Falls	16%	13%	28%	14%	14%
Domestic	27%	8%	29%	14%	26%
Sport/leisure	21%	6%	1%	13%	10%
Work/school	4%	12%	2%	10%	4%

Table 6. Percentage with alcohol noted (Scottish adults)[23,31,41]

	A/E Sent Home	PSW Admission	NSU Admission
Male	20%	46%	42%
Female	8%	19%	17%
All	17%	38%	37%

head. Another important effect of alcohol is the confusion it causes in clinical diagnosis after head injury, and this may partly account for alcoholic injuries being associated with a higher mortality and morbidity. However, Galbraith and coworkers have shown that the level of consciousness is not impaired, as evidenced by disorientation, until there is more than 200 mg/100 ml of alcohol, at least in Glasgow subjects.[16] It should be noted that alcoholism is more common in Scotland than in many countries;[29,37] the contribution of alcohol to head injuries may therefore be different elsewhere.

Almost every sport is liable to contribute to a head injury sooner or later. Most head injuries occur accidentally and they are naturally most common in contact sports, but in boxing the aim of the game is to produce head injury. It is difficult to calculate the risk factor, because the numbers engaging in a particular sport are never known accurately, and because many injuries are not reported, probably because players are anxious not to be prevented from playing again. The extent of this was revealed by a questionnaire to 544 rugby football players in the north of England, which revealed that 303 (56%) had suffered concussion associated with post-traumatic amnesia (PTA); the PTA exceeded an hour in 58 players and was more than 5 minutes in 232, yet only 38 patients had been admitted to hospital.[9]

In the Scottish survey 12 percent of new head injuries coming to accident/emergency departments were attributed to sport; under the age of 15 years the rate was double this and over 15 years less than half (Table 9). Sporting injuries constituted 7 percent of admissions to three Scottish neurosurgical units in 1974, and were similar in each; this corresponded closely to the 6 percent calculated for the Cambridge neurosurgical unit in England on the basis of a 12-year census.[17] In this large series of neurosurgical head injuries (over 600 patients), the sports that predominated were horse riding, rugby football (rugger), and association football (soccer). Most injuries were mild, but intracranial hematoma, persisting disability, and post-traumatic epilepsy all occurred and there were occasional deaths. Horse riding was also identified as a frequent cause of concussion in Oxford, where there were 154 riding injuries admitted to one hos-

Table 7. Effect of treatment site on percentage with alcohol noted [23,31,41]

	A/E Attenders	PSW Admissions
City Teaching Hospitals	26%	47%
Hospitals <30 miles from city	20%	23%
Hospitals >30 miles from city	15%	22%
All	22%	38%

Table 8. Effect of cause of injury on percentage with alcohol noted[16,23,31,41]

Cause of Injury	A/E Attenders 2043	PSW Admissions 753	Glasgow City Admissions 918
Assaults	34%	70%	74%
Pedestrians	36%	30%	36%
Vehicle occupants	10%	16%	29%
All road accidents	13%	20%	31%
Falls	53%	80%	—
Other	9%	14%	—

pital over a period of 2 years.[1] Of these 66 percent were concussed: 18 with PTA of more than an hour, 14 with skull fractures.

An important aspect of those sports that frequently cause head injury is that participants may suffer repeated concussion, the effects of which are cumulative. Evidence for this comes from clinical studies on patients with more than one episode,[18] and from the discovery that even mild concussion occasions some organic brain damage, part of which is permanent (p. 39). The questionnaire to rugby footballers revealed that 40 percent had had more than one concussion, and 15 percent three or more head injuries on the field.[9] A recent report of brain damage in five jockeys revealed cases with 10 to 20 head injuries, some of them associated with several hours or days of PTA. One rider had had a skull fracture on 10 separate occasions.[14] There was one fatal case and the brain showed, in addition to the acute damage of the final injury, evidence of extensive Purkinje-cell drop out. The other four jockeys had developed temporal lobe epilepsy and two of them had persisting memory deficits.

What relation these cases in jockeys have to boxer's dementia (p. 39) is uncertain, but they are probably different. Boxers suffer less severe injuries than many of those reported by these jockeys, but before recent regulations were instituted they might sustain as many as 200 to 400 such injuries. This was revealed in a study of 250 men who boxed in Britain between 1929 and 1955 (p. 298).

Table 9. Percentage of head injuries caused by sport[17,22,23,31,41]

	A/E Attenders	PSW Admissions	NSU Admissions
<15 years	23%	31%	19%
≥15 years	5%	4%	2%
Male	13%	14%	6%
Female	10%	13%	9%
All	12%	14%	6%
		Aberdeen NSU	7%
		Dundee NSU	7%
		Cambridge NSU	6%

Type of Injury Sustained as a Basis for Classification

Many reports of head injuries are limited to a certain clinicopathological type, but such classifications are seldom satisfactory, because they are not mutually exclusive. They are also unsatisfactory because they depend partly on how the injury occurred (missile/nonmissile), partly on clinical aspects of severity (concussion/coma or open/closed), and partly on speculative pathology (commotio, contusio, compressio cerebri). Other reports are limited to certain populations or activities, but deal with all kinds of injury in them (e.g., children, adults, military personnel; or road accident, combat injury).

Recent experimental, clinical, and pathological evidence all suggests that concussion caused by blunt trauma is due to acceleration/deceleration forces acting on the brain as a whole (p. 26). Widespread lesions occur in the white matter. The most severely affected patients are deeply unconscious from the moment of impact and frequently do not have a skull fracture, nor are there extensive contusions of the cerebral cortex. If such patients survive they remain vegetative or severely disabled. By contrast, patients with skull fracture and contusions frequently have little or no loss of consciousness, or they have a lucid interval before secondary events develop and produce raised intracranial pressure. This revised view of the clinicopathological correlations is the very opposite of the contusio/commotio concept, which is still popular in continental Europe, and which holds that when unconsciousness is prolonged for more than a few hours, the explanation is contusion. More appropriate terms by which to describe the severity of head injuries are discussed in the final chapter.

In contrast to missile injury, the term "closed" is often used to designate the kind of injury that accounts for most cases seen in civilian life, i.e., blunt or nonmissile injuries. Even if compound depressed fractures of the vault are set aside as "open," because this is clinically obvious, there remain the fractures of the base that are compound into the paranasal or middle ear cavities. While these almost all result from blunt (i.e., closed) kinds of injury, they are undoubtedly *open* injuries from the management point of view. As for missile injuries, what is a missile? Is a hammer or a pair of scissors used in anger, or a stone thrown in play, a missile?

PREVENTIVE MEASURES

Prevention can operate at three stages: forestalling the accident, minimizing the injuries sustained on impact, and ensuring that the risk of subsequent brain damage, consequent to secondary events, is reduced. Much of the rest of this book is about achieving this last objective, which is most specifically focussed in the discussion of avoidable factors in management that contribute to death or persisting brain damage (Chapter 15).

Accident prevention requires the skills of psychologists, sociologists, and politicians to persuade society of the need to make the environment safer for people, but also of the need for people to modify their behavior in relation to known but irremovable hazards. The doctor may help by drawing attention to situations that, in his experience, are associated with injury. There are features of cars and of roads that could be made safer, and architectural follies that make houses a hazard, especially to the young and the old. That fatal industrial accidents are occurring less often in Britain is an index of the effectiveness of safety regulations in an environment where enforcement is more feasible than elsewhere. But road accident deaths are also now contained, and even falling in some countries; this again is almost certainly due to road safety measures rather than to improved medical skills. Three factors have been studied in some detail: speed limits, alcohol levels, and seat belts.

In 1934 Britain introduced (in one Act of Parliament) a speed limit in built-up areas (30 mph or 48 kph), compulsory driving tests, and marked pedestrian crossings. Fatal accidents were reduced by 15 percent and the annual death rate on the road took 30 years to creep back up, by which time traffic had increased fourfold. The speed limits brought in to conserve fuel in the mid seventies provided an experiment that could never have been mounted in order to save lives rather than gasoline; but lives were saved, because the incidence of severe injuries, including head injuries, fell. A detailed statistical analysis of the accident rate on British roads in the period November 1973 to July 1975 showed a highly significant reduction in injuries on motorways, when the speed limit was reduced from 70 mph to 50 mph; the accident rate reverted to its previous level when the speed limit was raised after the oil crisis.[38] The effect of speed restriction is most definite in those accidents that result in death or serious injury. It is widely reported in many countries that open, fast roads may be associated with fewer accidents per vehicle mile run, but when an accident does happen, severe multiple injuries are the rule. The attitude of the public is reflected in the words of the British Minister of Transport, when announcing a relaxation of speed limits: "We want to save life, but we like driving fast. It is dangerous in some respects, but that is life."

The contribution of alcohol to head injuries, and not only in drivers, is so considerable that no one committed to trying to reduce the incidence of traumatic brain damage can afford to ignore it. But it is on the road that the effect of alcohol is most readily assessed.[19] Fifty-three years ago (1927) Norway introduced a legal limit of 30 mg/100 ml for drivers; the level of 80 mg set by Austria in 1961 is that most widely used in Europe, but there are variations from country to country (Table 10). Some have an extra penalty for higher levels (e.g., above 150 mg in Sweden and above 120 mg in France). Statistics on the relationship between drinking and driving have been reviewed recently in a British government report.[11] It estimates that about 10 percent of drivers on the road at high risk times have more than 80 mg/100 ml (the legal limit for the United Kingdom), and that about 10 percent of deaths from serious injuries have resulted from an alcohol-related

Table 10. Legal limits for blood alcohol (per 100 ml)[11]

50 mg	80 mg	100 mg	120–150 mg
Norway	United Kingdom	New Zealand	Ireland
Sweden	Austria	Most USA	S. Africa
Victoria, Australia	Belgium		16 states of
Iceland	Canada		USA
Japan	Denmark		
Netherlands	France		
	W. Germany		
	N. Ireland		
	Switzerland		
	2 states of		
	USA		

14

accident. The risk of an accident is considered to be 10 times increased when the blood alcohol is over 150 mg/100 ml. The effect of introducing a legal limit in Britain in 1967 was to reduce the number of dead drivers (of all ages) with blood alcohol above 80 mg from 25 to 15 percent; it was estimated that 1000 lives were saved in the first year. However, the effect was not lasting and in 1974, 45 percent of dead drivers under the age of 20 years had more than the legal limit of alcohol in the blood. There is now, therefore, pressure for more effective enforcement of the law, in order to reduce the number of drunken drivers on the road. We have already drawn attention to the drunken pedestrian both as the cause of and a victim of road accidents. The proportion of head injured road accident victims with a high blood alcohol is increased by the contribution of pedestrians and also of nondriving vehicle occupants.

The value of protective headgear has been established beyond doubt. Motor-cyclists used to be the road users most vulnerable to head injuries, but since the general use of helmets the head no longer bears the brunt of the injury.[5] Helmets are now becoming the rule for rock climbers and for horse riding; they should be more regularly worn in the construction industry and in engineering, where most head injuries are from falling or swinging objects. It is no accident that it was a neurosurgeon (Sir Hugh Cairns) who campaigned for helmets as regulation equip-ment for British army motorcyclists in World War II, and that it was neurosur-geons who were largely responsible for the pioneering legislation in Australia that required the wearing of seat belts. It is the head that stands to benefit most from the use of personal protective appliances.

It is 20 years since Sweden introduced national standards of seat belts in cars, following the experiments of Colonel Stapp on himself in the United States. In 1970 Victoria (Australia) became the first country to introduce legislation that required front seat occupants of private cars to wear belts.[4] The evidence now is overwhelming that seat belts reduce fatal injuries and severe injuries in survivors, each by a factor of about four times.[3] The most marked reduction is in head-on crashes, particularly single-vehicle accidents. Head injuries caused by frontal impacts against the windshield or dashboard are greatly reduced. Belts also pro-tect against spinal and chest injuries, and against ejection from the car, which is a common mode of death. In the face of all the evidence there can be little doubt about the need for legislation, as it is difficult to persuade people to adopt safety measures. In Britain only 15 percent of front seat passengers were wearing belts in 1971, but by 1976 it had risen to 25 percent following nationwide publicity, which cost £1,5000,000.

It is in defining the value of measures designed to minimize impact injury that the doctor has the most direct contribution to make to the prevention of brain damage outside hospital. Records could be kept more regularly about whether victims of head injury were wearing seat belts or helmets, in order to build up knowledge of their value. By asking patients or relatives about protective mea-sures doctors can demonstrate that they regard these as important, and this in itself is a form of education for the public. Those concerned to promote the wider adoption of preventive measures of such undoubted benefit must feel frustrated by the success of those who claim to be defending individual liberty, and who have not only resisted legislation in some countries, but have even reversed estab-lished laws on motorcycle helmets (in the United States) and on seat-belt wearing (in Switzerland). With these movements afoot, there is no danger that a trauma surgeon will be out of work.

REFERENCES

1. BARBER, H. M.: *Horse-play: survey of accidents with horses*. Br. Med. J. 3:532–534, 1973.
2. BECKER, D. P., MILLER, J. D., WARD, J. D., et al.: *The outcome from severe head injury with early diagnosis and intensive management*. J. Neurosurg. 47:491–502, 1977.
3. Br. Med. J.: *Seat belts: the overwhelming evidence*. 1:593–594, 1977.
4. Br. Med. J.: *Road accidents —seat belts and the safe care*. 2:1695–1698, 1978.
5. Br. Med. J.: *Motorcycle and bicycle accidents*. 1:39–41, 1979.
6. BRUCE, D. A., GENNARELLI, T. A., and LANGFITT, T. W.: *Resuscitation from coma due to head injury*. Crit. Care Med. 6:254–269, 1978.
7. CAVENESS, W. F.: "Incidence of craniocerebral trauma in the United States in 1976, and trend from 1970–1975." In THOMPSON, R. A., and GREEN, J. R. (eds.): *Advances in Neurology*. vol. 22, Raven Press, New York, 1979, pp. 1–3.
8. CLAYTON, A. B.: *Aetiology of traffic accidents*. Health Bull. 4:277, 1972.
9. COOK, J. B.: "The effect of minor head injuries sustained in sport and the post-concussional syndrome." In WALKER, A. E., CAVENESS, W. F., and CRITCHLEY, M. (eds.) Charles C Thomas, Springfield, Illinois, 1969, pp.408–413.
10. *Demographic Year Book (1973 and 1975):* United Nations, Geneva, Switzerland.
11. Department of the Environment: *Drinking and Driving. Report of the Departmental Committee.* Her Majesty's Stationery Office, London, 1976.
12. Department of Health and Social Security (OPCS): *Hospital In-patient Enquiry for England and Wales.* Her Majesty's Stationery Office, London, 1978.
13. FIELD, J. H.: *Epidemiology of head injuries in England and Wales.* Her Majesty's Stationery Office, London, 1976.
14. FOSTER, J. B., LEIGUARDA, R., and TILLEY, P. J. B.: *Brain damage in national hunt jockeys.* Lancet i:981–987, 1976.
15. GALASKO, C. B. S., and EDWARDS, D. H.: *The causes of injuries requiring admission to hospital in the 1970's.* Injury 6:107–112, 1974.
16. GALBRAITH, S., MURRAY, W. R., PATEL, A. R., et al.: *The relationship between alcohol and head injury and its effect on the conscious level.* Br. J. Surg. 63:138–140, 1976.
17. GLEAVE, J.: Personal communication, 1978.
18. GRONWALL, D., and WRIGHTSON, P.: *Cumulative effect of concussion.* Lancet ii:995–997, 1975.
19. HAVARD, J. D. J.: *Alcohol and the driver.* Br. Med. J. 1:1595–1597, 1978.
20. JANE, J.: Personal communication, 1979.
21. JENNETT, B., and CARLIN, J.: *Preventable mortality and morbidity after head injury.* Injury 10: 31–39, 1978.
22. JENNETT, B., MURRAY, A., CARLIN, J., et al.: *Head injuries in three Scottish neurosurgical units.* Brit. Med. J. 2:955-958, 1979.
23. JENNETT, B., MURRAY, A., MACMILLAN, R., et al.: *Head injuries in Scottish hospitals.* Lancet ii:696–698, 1977.
24. JENNETT, B., AND MACMILLAN, R.: *Epidemiology of head injuries.* Br. Med. J. 282:101–104, 1981.
25. JENNETT, B., TEASDALE, G., BRAAKMAN, R., et al.: *Prognosis in series of patients with severe head injury.* Neurosurgery 4:283, 1979.
26. JENNETT, B., TEASDALE, G., GALBRAITH, S., et al.: *Severe head injuries in three countries.* J. Neurol. Neurosurg. Psychiatry 40:291–298, 1977.
27. KLONOFF, H., and THOMPSON, G. B.: *Epidemiology of head injuries in adults.* Can. Med. Assoc. J. 100: 235–241, 1969.
28. KRAUS, J. F.: "Epidemiologic features of head and spinal cord injury." In SCHOENBERG, B. S. (ed.): *Advances in Neurology*. vol. 19. Raven Press, New York, 1978, pp. 261–279.
29. MACRAE, A. K. M., RATCLIFF, R. A. W., and LIDDLE, S. M.: *Alcoholism in Scotland in the 1960's.* Health Bull. 30:16–22, 1972.
30. MCDERMOTT, F. T.: *Control of road trauma epidemic in Australia.* Ann. R. Coll. Surg. Engl. 60:437–450, 1978.

31. MacMillan, R., Strang, I., and Jennett, B.: *Head injuries in primary surgical wards in Scottish hospitals*. Health Bull. 37:75–81, 1979.

32. Maxwell, R.: *Health Care, the Growing Dilemma*. McKinney, New York, 1974.

33. Marshall, L. F., Smith, R. W., and Shapiro, H. M.: *The outcome with aggressive treatment in severe head injuries. Part 1: The significance of intracranial pressure monitoring*. J. Neurosurg. 50:20–25, 1979.

34. Marshall, L. F., et al.: Personal communication.

35. Office of Population Censuses and Surveys: *Mortality Statistics. Review of the Registrar General on Deaths in England and Wales 1976*. Her Majesty's Stationery Office, London, 1977.

36. Registrar General for Scotland: *Annual Report 1975*. Her Majesty's Stationery Office, Edinburgh, 1975.

37. Saunders, W. M., and Kershaw, P. W.: *The prevalence of problem drinking and alcoholism in the West of Scotland*. Br. J. Psychiatry 133:493–499, 1978.

38. Scott, P. P., and Barton, A. J.: *The effects on road accident rates of the fuel shortage of November, 1973 and consequent legislation*. Transport and Road Research Laboratory, Supplementary Report, *236*, 1976.

39. Scottish Home and Health Department: *Scottish Hospital In-patient Statistics (1974)*. Information Services Division of the Common Services Agency, Edinburgh, 1976.

40. Sewell, M., Ring, I., Selecki, B., et al.: *Trauma to the central and peripheral nervous system in New South Wales. Part I. Interim report*. 1979.

41. Strang, I., MacMillan, R., and Jennett, B.: *Head injuries in accident and emergency departments at Scottish hospitals*. Injury 10:154–159, 1978.

42. Van't Hooft: Personal communication, 1979.

43. World Health Organization: *Manual of the International Statistical Classification of Diseases, Injuries and Causes of Death*. 9th revision. Geneva, 1975.

CHAPTER 2

Structural Pathology

So many complex physiopathological processes are initiated intracranially by head trauma that it is often more difficult to relate autopsy findings to the nature of the primary (or impact) damage than after trauma elsewhere in the body. Only some of these secondary events are persistent or severe enough to cause a structural lesion that is recognizable against the background of the primary damage. As a consequence it is sometimes difficult to be certain which lesions are primary and which are secondary and to know how much weight to attribute to each as a cause of death. Only detailed dissection by an experienced neuropathologist is likely to unravel the complexities of this situation. Yet few head injured brains reach such specialist laboratories, and this has limited the growth of knowledge about the pathological substrate of human head injury.

One reason for this is that legal considerations frequently dictate that autopsy examination of the brain after head injury be done by forensic pathologists; and, in order that a report can be written for the coroner without delay, the unfixed brain is often sliced on the spot. In these circumstances attention tends to be focussed on the obvious gross lesions—contusions, lacerations, and hemorrhage. Yet many pathological changes that can shed considerable light upon the nature of severe brain damage are difficult, if not impossible, to recognize on cursory inspection of unfixed brain slices. Even when gross dissection has been delayed, for the 2 to 3 weeks needed for adequate fixation, these lesions may be recognized only by the neuropathologist who knows precisely what he is looking for, and some of them, particularly if death has occurred within 24 to 48 hours of injury, may be discovered only by microscopic examination. Even after the adequately fixed brain has been properly dissected, the mapping of the distribution of the numerous lesions disclosed is a considerable task.

How much valuable information can be revealed by systematic analysis of such brains has been shown by Adams and his colleagues,[1] who have examined large blocks of brain from cerebrum, cerebellum, and brain stem (embedded in celloidin) from a large series of consecutive autopsies. These studies were largely confined to the brains of patients who died in specialized units. However, half the deaths from head injury occur before the victim reaches the hospital, and the bodies go directly to police mortuaries.[7,15] A proportion of those who are rescued by intensive care, but who remain dependent, survive for long periods and eventually die in long-stay institutions, so that their brains seldom reach the neuropathologist's bench.

EXPERIMENTAL HEAD INJURY

These formidable difficulties in securing satisfactory answers to questions about the neuropathology of brain trauma in man have naturally led to attempts to simulate head injuries in the experimental laboratory. The information that has emerged from such experiments that can be directly applied to the practical problem of human head injury has been somewhat limited, but these studies have increased our understanding of how brain damage is produced by mechanical trauma. However, there are many difficulties intrinsic to the problem of experimental head injury: these are briefly reviewed here by way of warning the unwary either of overinterpreting experiments already reported, or of embarking on experiments of their own without due attention to the hard road already trodden by those before them. Four main experimental approaches to head injury can be identified.

Mechanical Components of Skull Injury

Various *in vitro* models have been devised for calculating the kind of stresses created by simulated situations, such as vehicle accidents and falls from different heights. Best known are the human dummies filmed in car frames undergoing head-on collisions at various speeds. These have revealed the kind of forces to which the head is subjected, and the importance of associated stresses to the cervical spine. They have indicated the relative effectiveness of preventive measures such as improved car design, restraining harnesses, and protective helmets. How forces are dissipated once they are applied to the skull has been explored in studies using stress-coat preparations, which can analyze the distribution of forces and explain the lines taken by skull fractures. These various studies have been reviewed by Gurdjian,[11] whose leadership has initiated much of this work over many years.

In the clinical situation, however, it is often difficult to reconstruct the mechanical events involved in the impact injury, because there has often been more than one component. Although the initial blow may have fallen on one part of the skull, it is common for the patient then to fall against something else (often the road or floor), and this may be the more important event. Either one or the other impact may leave a scalp mark or a fracture, and this may mistakenly be regarded as indicating the site of the primary impact; on the other hand, irreversible diffuse brain damage can occur without a blemish on the scalp or a mark on the bone.

Pathophysiological Events Related to Brain Damage

Much of the knowledge that forms the basis of the clinical management of severe head injury has been derived from experiments designed to study separately various consequences of impact injury. These include raised intracranial pressure, reduced cerebral perfusion, cerebral edema, and epileptic seizures — events and processes that are common to many kinds of brain damage (see Chapter 3). Indeed, most have been studied in experiments that do not involve mechanical impact to the head or brain. Having identified the nature of these pathological processes, and what can aggravate or mitigate them, it remains to discover to what extent they actually occur as a consequence of mechanical trauma to the brain. And, if they are a consequence of mechanical trauma, do they follow the

20

same course as when occurring in nontraumatic circumstances and can they be similarly influenced?

Effects of Local Impact on the Brain

It is easier to deliver a standardized injury to part of the brain if the skull is removed and the exposed dura or brain itself is subjected to mechanical impact. Models similar to those devised for spinal cord trauma have been used for determining the immediate local effects on electrical function, on pial circulation and its regulation, on blood-brain barrier function, and on release of active chemical agents such as neurotransmitters and prostaglandins. Such models also allow structural studies by light and electron microscopy.[34]

Effect on the Brain of Impact on the Intact Head

These experiments approach most closely the real life head injury, but the differences between man and other species limit what can be learned. Some of these differences are mechanical, related to the brain bulk or to the internal anatomy of the skull. The forces generated when energy is transmitted to the brain depend in part on the mass of the brain, the weights of which in cat, rhesus monkey, and dog are 7, 8, and 12 percent, respectively, of that of man; even the chimpanzee brain is less than 30 percent of the weight of the human brain. This may account for some of the difficulty experienced in producing in animals pathological lesions that bear a close resemblance to those found in man. Other anatomical differences between species include the angle that the brain stem makes with the cerebral hemispheres above and with the cervical cord below, and the shape and structure of the tentorium, sphenoidal wings, and falx. All these affect the distribution of stresses within the intracranial cavity and will determine the lesions produced by forces imparted to the brain as a whole.

Yet another variable is the thickness of the skull, and the effect that this has on the amount of deformation that can occur locally, as distinct from the transmission of energy to the brain as a whole. In the rhesus monkey with its relatively thin, deformable skull, the energy threshold required for concussion with direct impact is half that for a whiplash-induced acceleration. In the chimpanzee, the two thresholds are the same, i.e., the chimpanzee's thick skull acts to some extent as a helmet, but of course is unable to prevent the generation of rotational forces with acceleration and deceleration injury.[25]

The problem that has largely defeated all attempts at solution is the production of prolonged unconsciousness by head injury in an animal preparation. Historically there has been an interesting interplay between biomechanics and experimental physiology. Much of the original thinking in this field came from Holbourn[12,13] working in Oxford during World War II. He assumed that the behavior of the skull and brain during and after a blow is determined by the physical properties of the skull and brain and by Newton's laws of motion. The brain is incompressible, but lacks rigidity. It is surrounded by the skull, which is not only rigid but has a shape and an irregular internal contour that, together with the dural partitions, determine the distribution of forces acting on the surface of the brain following impact. This probably determines the distribution of surface contusions following impact of the head as a whole.

Apart from this, however, the different components of the brain may be separated by impact and suffer deformation or disruption. Holbourn drew the analogy that the brain behaves as a pack of cards that deformation changes from a rectangular pack to an obliquely angled stack—the so-called shear strain. Movement in a straight line (linear acceleration) produces little relative movement or shear strain between different parts of the brain because the latter is incompressible, and diffuse brain damage is unlikely to result from this type of motion. However, if the head rotates there is great potential for shearing between adjacent parts, because the brain has no rigidity. The amount of brain damage sustained will be related to the rotational acceleration achieved and to the mass of the brain.

Denny-Brown and Russell, also working in Oxford, had demonstrated only a year or so before Holbourn's work that it was much more difficult to produce concussion by hitting an animal's head when it was held fixed, than when it was allowed to move and could develop rotational acceleration.[6] Holbourn's gelatin models demonstrated beautifully the distribution of "lesions" consequent on various kinds of impact; and his predictions were confirmed 20 years later by the studies of Ommaya and Gennarelli on subhuman primates.[23] They suggest that rotational injuries affect the brain in a centripetal sequence, the cortex alone suffering in milder cases, then the diencephalon, and finally the mesencephalon.

This is at variance with a long held view that the immediate loss of consciousness associated with concussion might be related to brain stem damage. In fact, observations on human head injuries confirm that brain stem injury is found only when there is also extensive subcortical and cortical damage; in most cases the brain stem is relatively spared and it is seldom affected alone.[3,21] Ommaya and Gennarelli, using somatosensory evoked potentials, have also demonstrated that interhemispheric corticocortical transfer may be slowed long after recovery of function in the reticular alerting system.[23] This occurs only with rotational injuries.

Holbourn's analysis also explains the clinical observation that the site and degree of damage of the skull bear little or no relation to the distribution and extent of the *diffuse* damage in the brain. Indeed, Adams and coworkers[3] have remarked that skull fractures are infrequent in human cases that have the most marked diffuse damage. Wherever the impact to the head, the lesions are often bilateral and approximately symmetrical and tend to be most marked at the interfaces between tissues that have different physical properties, such as compliance and elasticity (e.g., white matter and gray; brain and blood vessels). While the most readily recognizable shearing lesions are the diffusely distributed tears of nerve fibers in the white matter, the same physical forces can explain some of the more localized lesions—particularly those occurring remote from the site of impact, sometimes termed contrecoup lesions.

When the head as a whole is impacted, certain practical problems also arise, and it can be difficult to devise a reliable and reproducible quantum of damage and to detect its immediate or later effects. The immediate effect of a concussive blow in man is impairment of consciousness, and many of the delayed effects of diffuse damage are psychological in nature. Both of these are difficult to detect in animals. The early effects are obscured by anesthesia, even if this is kept light; their recognition depends on depression of reflexes, such as the corneal, withdrawal, or the pupillary. Alterations in the respiration and cardiovascular function give indirect evidence of brain dysfunction, but these and other intracranial transients must be regarded as accompaniments of concussion rather than direct evidence of the occurrence of brain damage. After recovery it is possible in some circumstances to assess psychological function, particularly if animals have been trained before injury. But the difference in acceleration required to produce minimal concussion and fatal injury is small; even if the severely damaged animal does not die rapidly, it requires skilled nursing to prolong survival, and that is difficult with animals.

HUMAN HEAD INJURY PATHOLOGY

The account of neuropathology of nonmissile head injuries that follows is based on the experience of Adams and Graham in Glasgow. Most of it is based on a consecutive series of 151 autopsied head injuries from the neurosurgical unit. There is clearly a bias in this series towards those in whom the question of surgical management arose; although there are a number who died within the first few hours, very early deaths are under-represented. Reference is made later (p. 42) to the findings in patients who are dead before reaching hospital.

A distinction is made between impact damage and secondary brain damage, because this is a crucial concept for those concerned with management of head injuries; indeed their main objective is to prevent or minimize secondary brain damage. However, recent clinical monitoring techniques, in particular early intracranial pressure measurements and CT scanning, are providing evidence about the rapidity with which secondary intracranial events can occur. Brain swelling, intracranial hematoma, cerebral hypoxia, and ischemia can all develop within an hour or so of injury. Once the interval between injury and death exceeds several hours it is often difficult to decide on clinical grounds whether it is the impact damage or subsequent events that have played the major role in rendering an injury fatal, and even at autopsy it may be difficult to reconstruct the exact sequence of events and to determine the balance between primary and secondary effects.

Impact Damage

Fracture of the Skull

This was found in 80 percent of fatal injuries in a neurosurgical unit, and almost the same incidence was recorded in the severe injuries of the data bank when those with clinical evidence of basal fracture but without x-ray confirmation were included as having a fracture. Those without fracture included an excess of children and also of patients with severe diffuse white matter damage (p. 26). Those who die before reaching hospital very often have severe basal fractures.

Contusions of the Gray Matter

These are the most obvious lesions to the naked eye on the surface of the uncut brain. Cortical contusions affect the crests of the gyri and can be graded according to whether they are superficial or involve the whole depth of the gyrus (Fig. 1). There is usually a degree of bloody extravasation, and this may spread on to the surface as a subpial or subarachnoid hemorrhage. When there are multiple severe contusions these bloody extravasations may coalesce, and it is a matter of doubt in some cases as to when the resulting lesion deserves the label of intracerebral hemorrhage (Fig. 2). With focal damage under the point of impact, and especially if there is a depressed fracture, the brain is sometimes lacerated; again

23

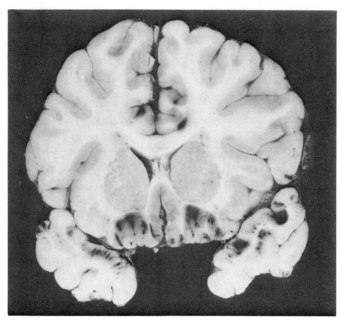

Figure 1. Cortical contusions. Note accentuation of hemorrhage on crests of gyri, with sparing of sulci. Most are in one temporal lobe. (From Adams,[1] with permission.)

there will be varying amounts of parenchymal and surface hemorrhage, which if it reaches a certain degree will justify the label of hematoma.

Focal contusions (and lacerations) occur under the point of impact, if local deformation has been sufficiently severe (e.g., under a depressed fracture). More commonly the contusions are on the undersurface of the temporal and frontal

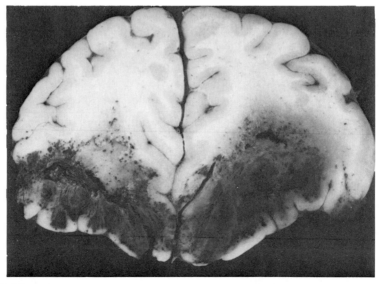

Figure 2. Subfrontal contusions merging into bilateral intracerebral hematoma. (From Adams,[1] with permission.)

24

lobes, and on the anterior poles of the temporal lobes, regardless of the site of impact (Fig. 3). Experimental studies indicate that the distribution is related to the rougher, more irregular inner surface of the skull in these areas, and that occipital blows are more likely to produce contusions than are frontal (or lateral) impacts. Contusions are normally multiple, bilateral but asymmetrical, and can be regarded as surface shear lesions.

A method has been developed by Adams and coworkers[36] for quantifying cerebral contusions at autopsy by ascribing scores for the depth and extent of these lesions. In this way a contusional index can be derived for the brain as a whole, for the right and left cerebral hemispheres, and for each lobe of the brain on each side. This study has confirmed that cerebral contusions are usually more marked in the frontotemporal lobes, wherever the impact has been. In patients with a unilateral fracture of the vault, the contusions are usually more marked on the same side of the brain; while occipital fractures are often associated with frontal contusions, the opposite combination is very unusual. It seems that in fatal head injuries in man it is unusual for the brain damage to be contrecoup to the site of injury (as evidenced by scalp marks and fracture); this contrasts with one report of experimental studies in monkeys.[24] However, bilateral contusions are common in man, and in a series of patients in coma the major location of brain damage was in the cerebral hemisphere opposite a unilateral skull fracture.[16] Comparing CT scan lesions with the site of scalp and skull injury may advance our knowledge of the relationship between brain damage and site of impact.

There is now abundant evidence, both experimental and clinical, that cerebral contusion can be extensive without there being prolonged (or any) loss of consciousness. The significance of contusions lies in the processes of edema, hemorrhage, and swelling that they may initiate, and the consequences of these secondary events (p. 31). These may result in deterioration in the level of consciousness or prolongation of coma that has been caused initially by other mechanisms (p. 91).

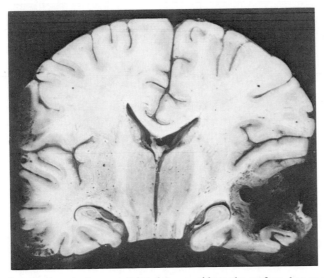

Figure 3. Bilateral cortical contusions, restricted on one side to the surface, but on the other forming an intradural (subdural plus intracerebral) hematoma, or "burst" temporal lobe. (From Adams,[1] with permission.)

25

Diffuse White Matter Lesions

Extensive degeneration in the white matter of brains from patients who had survived for months in the vegetative state was reported from Oxford by Strich in 1956.[30] She proposed that these lesions resulted from tearing of the nerve fibers at the time of impact,[31,33] as had been predicted to happen from the *in vitro* studies of Holbourn[12,13] and the animal experiments of Pudenz and Shelden.[28] While some authors[22,26,27] accepted this explanation, others proposed that these lesions were secondary to necrosis, hemorrhage, and internal herniation,[4] or were due to edema and raised intracranial pressure.[14]

This controversy has now been resolved by careful study of brains from patients who did not have any evidence (at autopsy) of ischemic or hypoxic brain damage, nor of raised intracranial pressure. Adams and colleagues have reported eight such patients who had all the hallmarks of diffuse white matter damage.[3] They found that the features of this lesion were so characteristic that they were able to recognize the same lesion at autopsy also in another 11 patients who did have neuropathological evidence either of raised intracranial pressure or of other secondary intracranial complications (Fig. 4). All these 19 patients had been in coma continuously from the time of impact; not one of them had had a lucid interval after injury, although this phenomenon had been recorded in almost half the other fatal cases in the consecutive series of head injury autopsies. The other clinical feature was the much lower incidence of skull fracture in these patients (32%), as compared with 88 percent for the remaining autopsies; among the eight patients who had only diffuse white matter damage, only one had a skull fracture.

While the pathological features of this lesion can readily be recognized by the neuropathologist who knows what to look for, the brain may look almost normal to the naked eye, when this is the only type of brain damage. There are few, if any, surface contusions, but on coronal slicing there is always a small lesion in the corpus callosum (Fig. 5) and another in or adjacent to the superior cerebellar peduncle (Fig. 6). About half the patients have the latter lesion on both sides, but always larger on one than the other. In the acute stage these lesions are hemorrhagic and there may be blood in the lateral ventricles. But after some weeks they become shrunken scars, which may still have some brown staining and are occasionally cystic. Consistent and characteristic as these two lesions are, they are easily overlooked, especially when the brain is sliced before fixation (Fig. 7). When survival has been for several weeks, there will be dilatation of the ventricles, owing to shrinking of the surrounding, degenerating white matter.

The lesions disclosed by microscopy depend on the duration of survival (Table

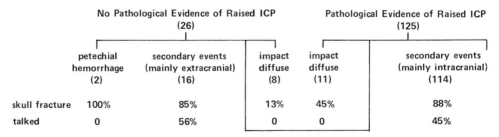

	No Pathological Evidence of Raised ICP (26)			Pathological Evidence of Raised ICP (125)	
	petechial hemorrhage (2)	secondary events (mainly extracranial) (16)	impact diffuse (8)	impact diffuse (11)	secondary events (mainly intracranial) (114)
skull fracture	100%	85%	13%	45%	88%
talked	0	56%	0	0	45%

Figure 4. Features of 151 neurosurgical autopsies. ICP = raised intracranial pressure. (Based on Adams, et al.[3])

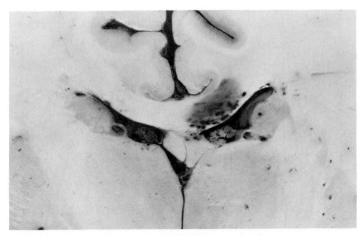

Figure 5. Recent hemorrhagic lesion in corpus callosum. (From Adams et al.,[3] with permission.)

1). In the first 2 weeks numerous retraction balls (Fig. 8) are found; within a few days microglial stars appear, representing small clusters of hypertrophied microglia (Fig. 9). By 2 weeks these are very prominent and are found diffusely through the white matter of the cerebral hemisphere, the cerebellum, and the brain stem; retraction balls are no longer seen after 2 weeks. The lesions of the corpus callosum and superior cerebellar peduncle show either retraction balls or reactive change, according to the time interval since injury. When survival exceeds 6 to 8 weeks, wallerian-type degeneration of white matter can be shown in Marchi preparations; this affects the ascending and descending tracts in the brain stem, and also the white matter of the cerebral hemispheres (Figs. 10, 11, and 12). These various lesions are more frequently seen than formerly because modern methods of resuscitation and intensive care make it possible for such severely injured patients to survive long enough for reactive lesions to develop, and be-

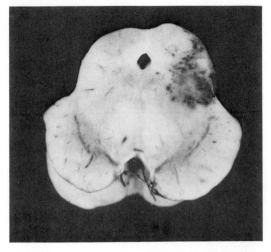

Figure 6. Recent hemorrhagic lesion in superior cerebellar peduncle. (From Adams,[1] with permission.)

27

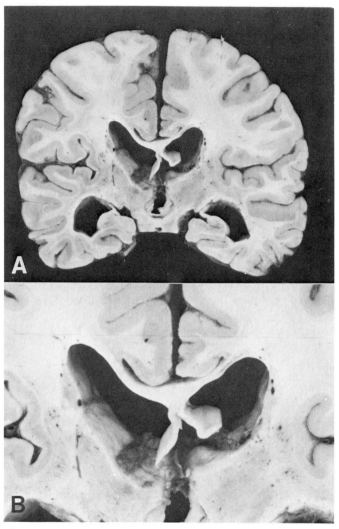

Figure 7. Brain after many months survival in vegetative state. **A,** Ventricular dilatation and absence of contusions. (From Adams,[1] with permission.) **B,** Scar of corpus callosum lesion is evident on close inspection, but by no means obvious. (From Adams et al.,[3] with permission.)

Table 1. Diffuse brain damage of immediate impact type[3]

Survival Time	Pathological Features*	Incidence	
2 days to 2 weeks	retraction balls	8/11	(73%)
3 days to 9 days	moderate microglial stars	5/6	(83%)
2 weeks to 7 months	marked microglial stars	7/7	(100%)
5 weeks or more	long tract degeneration (Marchi positive)	6/7	(86%)

*All patients had lesions in the corpus callosum and the superior cerebellar peduncle.

28

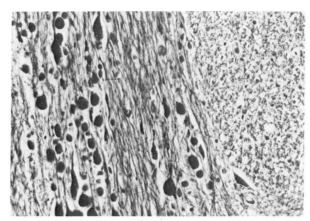

Figure 8. Retraction balls in white matter. Notice that they are evident only in axones that run in one direction, those at right angles being spared; this suggests a mechanical causation. (From Adams et al.,[3] with permission.)

cause some neuropathologists have applied to traumatic cases careful microscopic examination with special stains.

In the early stages after injury these patients are in deep coma with bilateral extensor rigidity of the limbs and usually some autonomic dysfunction. This has often been described by clinicians as indicative of "primary brain stem injury." However, Adams' laboratory did not find a single patient in whom the lesions just described were confined to the brain stem.[3] His group previously expressed doubt as to whether isolated primary brain stem injury was an entity,[21] and work in another laboratory has now confirmed the view that it is not.[35] These conclusions from human neuropathology are in agreement with the hypothesis of Ommaya and Gennarelli,[23] based on their animal experiments: they predicted that primary damage to the rostral brain stem would not occur in isolation, but only as part of a more widespread lesion. Gross disruption of the brain stem, associated with severe fractures of the skull base, is not uncommon in victims of head injury who die before reaching hospital (p. 42), but that does not constitute a *clinical* syndrome.

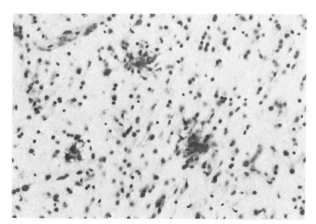

Figure 9. Collections of microglia ("stars") in white matter after survival of some weeks in vegetative state. (From Adams et al.,[3] with permission.)

29

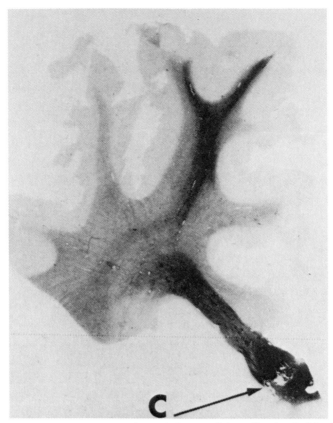

Figure 10. Long tract degeneration, showing a dark area of demyelination in Marchi preparation in subcortical white matter.

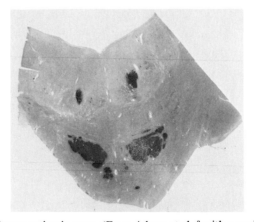

Figure 11. Long tract degeneration in pons. (From Adams et al.,[3] with permission.)

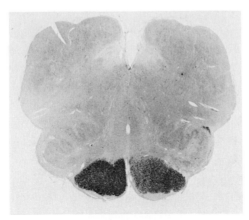

Figure 12. Long tract degeneration in corticospinal tracts in pyramids of medulla. (From Adams et al.,[3] with permission.)

Secondary Brain Damage

It takes time for secondary events to occur and still longer for structural changes to develop in the brain that the pathologist can recognize. How frequently such lesions are found at autopsy will therefore depend on the population studied—particularly on the duration of survival, and on whether the series is unselected, for example, by coming from a neurosurgical unit. Some secondary lesions are obvious, such as intracranial hematoma or meningitis; others, such as evidence of raised intracranial pressure or hypoxic brain damage, can be more difficult to recognize. Yet these two lesions are commonly found in the brains of patients dying in a neurosurgical unit, when these patients are systematically examined. In the Glasgow series of 151 brains, 91 percent had some evidence of ischemic brain damage, 83 percent had pathological evidence of raised intracranial pressure, 79 percent had both lesions, and only 5 percent of brains had no evidence of either kind of secondary brain damage

Raised Intracranial Pressure

Many episodes of raised intracranial pressure produce no structural sequelae, particularly if the pressure has been evenly distributed and the CSF pathways have all been in free communication. The pathologist may find evidence of brain shift, but shift and raised pressure are not synonymous. Recent experimental studies have shown that shift and herniation can develop without there having been a sustained rise of intracranial pressure. This is because spatial compensation (of which brain shift is one component) has enabled an expanding lesion to be accommodated. Such compensation occurs during the early stages of a slowly expanding lesion, such as a tumor, but it hardly applies to the rapidly developing processes that occur after head injury. In these circumstances there is both shift and raised pressure, and this combination produces vascular effects that are the most reliable markers of an episode of raised intracranial pressure. These effects will persist even after pressure has been relieved and shift has been resolved—as may happen when patients survive for a time before reaching the autopsy table— for example, after surgical decompression. In most cases that come to the pa-

31

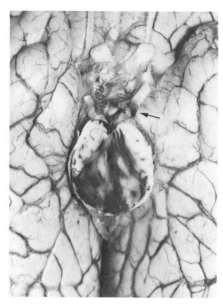

Figure 13. Severe hemorrhage in midbrain secondary to tentorial hernia. Note also focal hemorrhage in left oculomotor nerve (*arrow*). (From Adams,[1] with permission.)

thologist, however, death has occurred in the acute stage and shift will still be evident.

The distribution of brain shift will differ according to whether the brain swelling is primarily in the supratentorial or infratentorial compartment. With raised pressure above the tentorium, which is the most frequent occurrence, the lesions are convolutional flattening, midline shift, tentorial and supracallosal herniae, and some degree of brain stem distortion, hemorrhage, or infarction (Figs. 13 and 14).

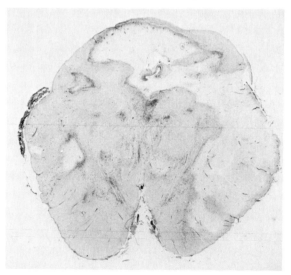

Figure 14. Extensive infarction in midbrain—obvious only after cresyl violet staining of celloidin sections. (From Adams,[1] with permission.)

32

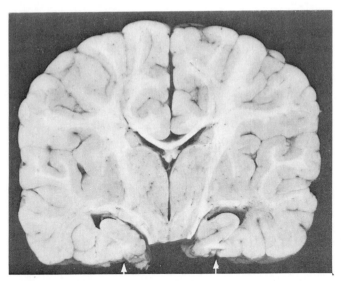

Figure 15. Diffuse post-traumatic edema. Note small ventricles and absence of lateral shift and cortical contusions. Hemorrhage and necrosis (*arrows*) are seen where parahippocampal gyri impinged against tentorial edge during downward herniation. (From Adams,[1] with permission.)

By studying the brains of patients in whom intracranial pressure was measured prior to death, Adams and Graham[2] have established morphological features that are indicative of an episode of high pressure. The most consistent feature is a wedge of tissue necrosis along the line of the tentorial edge in one or both parahippocampal gyri (Figs. 15 and 16); some cases also have pressure necrosis in the

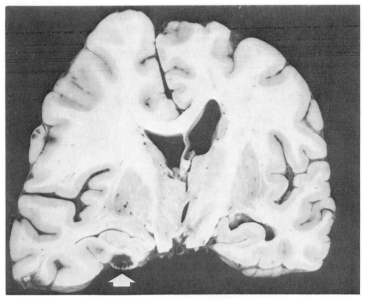

Figure 16. Unilateral edema following evacuation of subdural hematoma. Note minimal cortical contusions, but hemorrhagic pressure necrosis in parahippocampal gyrus ipsilateral to compression (*arrow*).

33

cingulate gyrus and infarction of the medial occipital cortex (calcarine infarction) (Fig. 17). These are the findings when a patient dies in, or shortly after, a crisis of raised intracranial pressure, but they remain as persisting structural markers of previous pressure and shift and will be found even in patients who have survived for months or years after their injury and who do not have shift still present at autopsy. When pressure has been raised because of diffuse supratentorial swelling (e.g., edema or engorgement), without side to side shift, the only lesions may be *bilateral* scars (of previous necrosis) in the parahippocampal gyri. These scars indicate that there has been shift of the brain stem downwards through the tentorial hiatus, but there may be calcarine infarction as well.

Pathological evidence of raised intracranial pressure by these criteria was found in 83 percent of fatal head injuries in the Glasgow series. Some others had evidence of brain shift, but without these features. In 68 percent of those with signs of pressure in this series of autopsies from a neurosurgical unit, an intracranial hematoma had either been evacuated or was found at autopsy.

When raised pressure is due to an expanding lesion in the posterior fossa, the pathological evidence is indentation and necrosis of the cerebellar tonsils, where they have abutted against the rim of the foramen magnum. However, so great is the variation in the normal configuration of the tonsils that tonsillar herniation, without necrosis, is án unreliable sign of raised pressure.

Brain swelling, in addition to or without intracranial hematoma, is common. It may be due to engorgement of cerebral vessels, which seldom leaves any evidence for the pathologist, or to cerebral "edema." Clinicians often refer to "edema" when they mean brain swelling without hematoma; without a CT scan it is not possible clinically to distinguish between engorgement and edema. It is not yet established whether there are appearances on the scan that are sufficiently specific to make this distinction, or that between localized edema and the early stages of infarction. There is need for more studies that compare the CT scan in life with brain slices at autopsy.

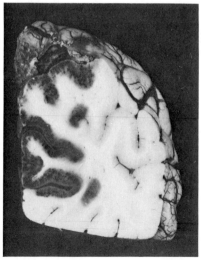

Figure 17. Hemorrhagic infarction in medial occipital cortex caused by tentorial hernia compressing the posterior cerebral artery. (From Adams,[1] with permission.)

34

Experimentalists distinguish between intracellular and extracellular (vasogenic) edema, but for the pathologist dealing with human autopsy material the recognition of cerebral edema of different kinds is less easy. There are certainly some cases, mostly children, whose brains are diffusely swollen, with small ventricles, in the absence of marked contusions or other gross lesions (Fig. 15). More often there is a degree of local edema in relation to lesions such as contusions or hypoxic brain damage. When an acute subdural hematoma has been removed surgically, following an episode of acute compression, the underlying cerebral hemisphere (but not the opposite one) sometimes becomes grossly swollen and edematous, even when there are few or no contusions affecting it (Fig. 16). With such acute edema there is little more to be seen microscopically than pallor of myelin staining.

Intracranial Hematoma

While hematoma is sometimes exposed for the first time at autopsy, the pathologist has more often to deal with the brain after one or more intracranial clots have already been evacuated. Many factors influence the effect that a mass lesion has on brain function; unless shift and internal herniae are marked, pathologists should be cautious in the opinions they express about the size and significance of hematomas disclosed at autopsy. This matter is more fully discussed in Chapter 7.

Ischemic Brain Damage

Certain types of ischemic brain damage have long been recognized: focal infarction in the immediate vicinity of contusions, calcarine infarction from posterior cerebral artery occlusion owing to distortion by transtentorial herniation, and widespread lesions associated with fat embolism. More recently it has been realized that widespread neuronal necrosis and other types of infarction are commonly present in the brain after head injury.[8,9,14]

These lesions, extensive as they are, can often be recognized only after systematic microscopy has been undertaken on the properly fixed brain, particularly when survival has been limited to a few days. In a consecutive series of 151 patients autopsied in a neurosurgical unit, ischemic lesions were found in 91 percent of all cases, a third of whom also had calcarine infarction.[9] Over 85 percent of *affected* brains had lesions in the hippocampus and basal ganglia, and about 50 percent in the cerebral cortex or cerebellum (Table 2). Ischemic lesions were considered significant in 64 percent, and 66 percent of these significant lesions were in the cortex.

Table 2. Frequency of ischemic brain damage (IBD) in different locations (151 cases)[9]

Cortex (other than MOC)*	70	46%
Basal ganglia	119	79%
Hippocampus	122	81%
Cerebellum	67	44%
MOC	50	30%
No IBD	13	9%

*Sixty-four percent of *significant* lesions were cortical (excluding the medial occipital cortex—MOC).

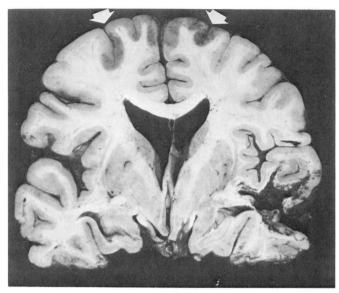

Figure 18. Boundary zone infarcts. Bilateral hemorrhagic lesions between the anterior and middle cerebral arterial territories, associated with "burst temporal" lobe, are shown (*arrows*). (From Adams,[1] with permission.)

Excluding the medial occipital cortex (see Fig. 17), the most common site for lesions in the neocortex was in the boundary zone between adjacent major arterial territories, which were affected in 54 percent of patients with cortical lesions (Figs. 18 and 19).[8] Infarction in the territory of the anterior or middle cerebral artery was found in 27 percent; lesions of this kind were bilateral in almost half the affected brains. Multiple foci of ischemic damage (Fig. 20) were found widely

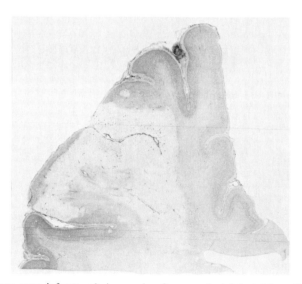

Figure 19. Boundary zone infarct—obvious only after cresyl violet staining of celloidin sections. (From Adams,[1] with permission.)

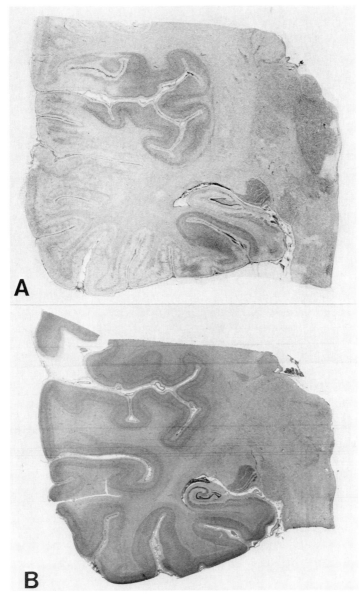

Figure 20. A, Hypoxic brain damage in cerebral cortex stained with cresyl violet. **B,** Normal brain, similarly stained. (From Adams,[1] with permission.)

dispersed throughout the cortex in 14 percent, while 11 percent of brains had diffuse neocortical necrosis of the kind associated with a period of cardiac arrest (Fig. 21). More than 90 percent of the brains with cortical ischemia also had lesions in the basal ganglia and hippocampus, 56 percent had lesions in the cerebellum, and 43 percent in the medial occipital cortex. Ischemic lesions in the medial occipital cortex were found in a third of patients, all of whom also had hypoxic lesions elsewhere in the brain.

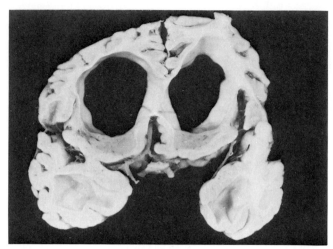

Figure 21. Diffuse neocortical necrosis after several months survival in vegetative state following cardiac arrest.

Many causes can contribute to reduced cerebral oxygenation and can therefore produce hypoxic brain damage. Pathological evidence of tentorial herniation and of raised intracranial pressure was found in the majority of patients in this particular autopsy series; however, they were about twice as frequent in the cases with hypoxic brain damage as in the small number without this finding. The dynamic interaction between many of these factors is described in the next chapter.

Clinical evidence of hypoxemia or of hypotension is always incomplete; not all episodes of hypotension or hypoxemia are observed, nor are those known always recorded. In particular what happens before the patient reaches hospital is seldom known, although hypotension and hypoxia are frequently found within 1 to 2 hours of injury.[20] The relationship of vasospasm on angiography to ischemic brain damage has been reviewed by MacPherson and Graham;[19] with the decline in angiography, data of this kind are unlikely to be available again.

Correlations between such clinical events and the pathological findings of hypoxic brain damage in the Glasgow series are presented in Table 3. More than one of the factors that are likely to affect cerebral oxygenation are commonly found. It does not take a very marked abnormality in any one of the factors that affect cerebral oxygenation for there to be a significant effect on the brain if more than one is contributing—as is often the case. For example, once there is raised intra-

Table 3. Features of cases with and without ischemic brain damage[9]

Feature	Frequency in 138 cases with IBD (%)	Frequency in 13 cases without IBD (%)
Hypoxia	82	31
Raised intracranial pressure	86	46
Intracranial hematoma	66	46
<40 years of age	51	31
Skull fracture	82	69
Associated injury	36	46
Talked after injury	38	46

cranial pressure, or hypoxemia from ventilatory inadequacy, or anemia because of blood loss, the brain will be vulnerable to even modest systemic hypotension. Moreover, the brain may be unable to compensate adequately for these changes because following injury the mechanism of autoregulation may be defective.

Pathological Basis of Late Effects of Head Injury

Residual disability or newly developing complications (e.g., epilepsy or hydrocephalus) may be related to impact damage, to the various early secondary pathological processes already discussed, or to later events such as scarring or adhesions causing traction on parts of the brain or blockage of cerebrospinal fluid pathways. In particular it seems likely that the extensive hypoxic lesions found in the brains of fatal cases occur also in survivors, albeit to a less severe degree; these may contribute significantly to neurological and mental sequelae.

Irreversible Brain Damage

VEGETATIVE STATE (see Ch. 13). This is the outcome in some 5 percent of survivors after severe head injury, now that some patients survive brain damage of a severity that would previously have proved fatal. Some cases prove not to be the result of severe impact damage, but to be a consequence of resuscitation following cardiorespiratory arrest. In the latter event there is extensive neocortical necrosis (Fig. 21), in contrast to the extensive subcortical white matter shearing that characterizes the brains of patients rendered vegetative by impact damage. In either event the effect has been to render the cortex functionally inactive.

POST-TRAUMATIC DEMENTIA—BOXER'S BRAIN. Apart from the effects of hydrocephalus (see below) the only definite syndrome of progressive dementia following head injury is that known as the "punch-drunk" state. This occurs only in victims of repeated, punishing fights, now unlikely to occur because of the stricter control of boxing. The pathological findings are characteristic and have been reviewed by Corsellis and associates,[5] while the clinical features have been described elsewhere.[17] Most of the changes are in deep central structures—corpus callosum, fornices, septum pellucidum, and substantia nigra. These do not conform to the lesions found in naturally occurring dementias (e.g., Alzheimer's disease).

CEREBRAL HEMISPHERE DYSFUNCTION. Hemiplegia, hemianopia, and dysphasia are common sequelae of severe injury. Some patients with these disabilities have had intracranial hematomas removed, in particular from the temporal lobe, and these persisting deficits are not surprising. Judging from the finding of extensive infarction in the distribution of the middle cerebral artery in some fatal cases, and of widespread patchy hypoxic damage in the cortex and basal ganglia in others, it is reasonable to assume that some persisting deficits may derive from ischemic rather than hemorrhagic lesions. On the other hand, it seems unlikely that even extensive cortical contusions commonly produce focal features of this kind; indeed, such lesions are often found in patients known not to have had focal neurological signs soon after injury, but who then developed complications and died. Moreover, widespread contusions are not infrequently found in patients known to have made a good recovery from a head injury (Fig. 22), while shearing lesions are found in mildly concussed patients dying of other causes.[26]

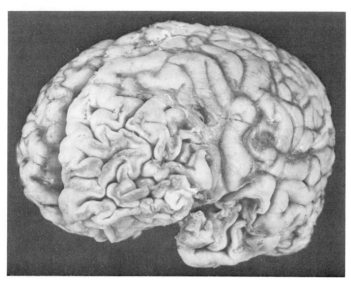

Figure 22. Healed contusions in frontotemporal cortex, many years after injury. (From Adams,[1] with permission.)

Hydrocephalus (see p. 280)

Ex Vacuo. Wherever there has been extensive diffuse brain damage (e.g., lesions causing the vegetative state) there will be hydrocephalus if survival has been long enough. Lesser degrees are seen in patients less severely affected, and enlargement of one horn (particularly the temporal horn) is sometimes seen after a focal lesion such as an intracerebral hematoma.

Obstructive Hydrocephalus. Subarachnoid hemorrhage accompanies many cases of head injury, and adhesions from this may cause blockage in various parts of the CSF circulation, but particularly in the cisterna ambiens. Communicating high pressure hydrocephalus occasionally results and may cause progressive symptoms and require CSF shunting. Occasionally these symptoms occur after mild head injury and investigations reveal evidence of long-standing hydrocephalus, especially that associated with aqueduct stenosis; this suggests that the head injury has acted as a precipitating factor in making the hydrocephalus clinically evident—perhaps owing to the spill of blood or an episode of brain swelling.

Normal Pressure Hydrocephalus. This ill-understood condition is increasingly recognized, and in some cases trauma appears to have been the precipitating agent. What mechanism is involved remains uncertain.

Post-traumatic Epilepsy

Much was made 40 or 50 years ago of the characteristics of the scars produced by missile injuries in relation to subsequent epilepsy, and it was suggested that there was a time factor needed for these scars to "mature" into an epileptogenic state. It now seems more likely that whether or not epilepsy occurs depends more on the extent of the cortical damage and on the inherent susceptibility of the individual patient. In the case of depressed fracture it seems likely that the degree of impact damage is what matters, not whether or not bone depression remains. Recent studies suggest, however, that not only the amount of local cortical damage but also the extent of diffuse damage (reflected in duration of PTA) may also matter—both factors being required to produce a potentially epileptogenic situation (p. 284). The frequency of temporal lobe epilepsy after nonmissile head injuries corresponds with the high incidence of cortical contusions in these lobes and of disruption owing to intradural hematomas in this situation.

Cause of Death and Time to Death

That a patient dies *with* certain lesions does not necessarily mean that he died *of* them. In describing pathological findings and cause of death there is need for the same care in making comparisons as was discussed in Chapter 1 for head injury statistics in general. Comparisons may be invalid if the denominator is not the same (many reports are limited to road accidents, or to hospital deaths, or to deaths in neurosurgical units). Inevitably most of the detailed neuropathological data comes from specialized units; the pathological findings in such deaths may be different from those reported from a city mortuary, which deals only with deaths at the scene.

TIME TO DEATH. National statistics in Britain show that 60 percent of English[7] and 50 percent of Scottish deaths attributed to head injury occurred before admission to hospital. Detailed study of 254 road accident victims in one English area[29] showed that those with head injury less often died within the first 4 hours (or in the first half hour) than did those considered at autopsy not to have a brain lesion. A possible reason for there being fewer early deaths among head injuries from road accidents (than would be expected from the proportion of all head injuries who die before reaching hospital) is that road accident victims are usually transported to hospital without delay.

Combining evidence from various sources, it seems that about 70 percent of head injury deaths occur within 24 hours, over 80 percent by a week, and over 90 percent within a month. But of deaths occurring in patients who survive the first 6 hours, almost 20 percent are delayed for more than a month, probably because modern intensive care permits the survival (for a time) of some severely damaged patients who would previously have died soon after injury.

CAUSE OF DEATH. It is not customary to record the *cause* of death, as distinct from the findings at autopsy, even in institutions that carry out informal reviews of deaths at which opinions are expressed about the probable cause of death. Pathologists are usually reluctant to be drawn into such discussions, rightly recognizing that their evidence represents a static scenario at the end of a complex and dynamic drama.

However, in the collaborative severe head injury study clinicians were asked to allocate 5 points between four main categories of cause. In 79 percent of cases 3 or more points were given to one cause, which was then regarded as the major cause of death. About a third of almost 400 deaths were ascribed to primary brain damage and more than half to expanding intracranial lesions. Only 8 percent of cases were considered to have died from an extracranial complication.

Primary brain damage was more often judged to have been the cause of death in patients under 45 years of age; an expanding intracranial lesion was common in older patients, according with the higher incidence of intradural hematomas as age increases (p. 159). Extracranial complications, as the major cause of death, were no more often recorded in the older than the younger patients. Deaths after the first week were more often due to secondary expanding intracranial lesions.

The analyses in the above paragraphs are of deaths in a neurosurgical unit. The autopsy reports of 102 cases who died before reaching hospital from two British cities have been scrutinized.[15] These revealed that more than two thirds had multiple injuries; in 13 percent there was a cervical cord injury. More than half of the head injuries involved severe fractures of the skull base, and in a third of all cases the pons or medulla was lacerated. In 15 percent the whole brain was disrupted.

REFERENCES

1. ADAMS, J. H.: "The neuropathology of head injuries." In Vinken, P. J., and Bruyn, G. W. (eds.): *Handbook of Clinical Neurology.* vol. 23. North-Holland Publishing Co., Amsterdam, 1975, pp. 35–65.

2. ADAMS, J. H., AND GRAHAM, D. I.: *The relationship between ventricular fluid pressure and the neuropathology of raised intracranial pressure.* Neuropathol. Appl. Neurobiol. 2:323–332, 1976.

3. ADAMS, J. H., MITCHELL, D. E., GRAHAM, D. I., ET AL.: *Diffuse brain damage of immediate impact type.* Brain 100:489–502, 1977.

4. ADAMS, R. D.: In Walker, A. E., Caveness, W. F., and Critchley, M. (eds.): *The Late Effects of Head Injury.* Charles C Thomas, Springfield, 1969, pp. 524–526.

5. CORSELLIS, J. A. N., BRUTON, C. J., AND FREEMAN-BROWNE, D.: *The aftermath of boxing.* Psychol. Med. 3:270–303, 1973.

6. DENNY-BROWN, D., AND RUSSELL, W. R.: *Experimental cerebral concussion.* Brain 64:93–164, 1941.

7. FIELD, J. H.: *Epidemiology of head injuries in England and Wales.* Her Majesty's Stationery Office, London, 1975.

8. GRAHAM, D. I., AND ADAMS, J. H.: *Ischemic brain damage in fatal head injuries.* Lancet i:265–266, 1971.

9. GRAHAM, D. I., ADAMS, J. H., AND DOYLE, D.: *Ischemic brain damage in fatal non-missile head injuries.* J. Neurol. Sci. 39:213–234, 1978.

10. GRONWALL, D., AND WRIGHTSON, P.: *Cumulative effect of concussion.* Lancet ii:995–997, 1975.

11. GURDJIAN, E. S.: *Impact Head Injury. Mechanistics, Clinical and Preventive Correlations.* Charles C Thomas, Springfield, 1975.

12. HOLBOURN, A. H. S.: *Mechanics of head injuries.* Lancet ii:438–441, 1943.

13. HOLBOURN, A. H. S.: *The mechanics of brain injuries.* Br. Med. Bull. 3:147–149, 1945.

14. JELLINGER, K., AND SEITELBERGER, G.: *Protracted post-traumatic encephalopathy: pathology, pathogenesis and clinical implications.* J. Neurol. Sci. 10:51–94, 1970.

15. JENNETT, B., AND CARLIN, J.: *Preventable mortality and morbidity after head injury.* Injury 10:154–159, 1978.

16. JENNETT, B., TEASDALE, G., GALBRAITH, S., ET AL.: *Severe head injuries in three countries.* J. Neurol. Neurosurg. Psychiatry 40:291–298, 1977.

17. LANCET: *Boxing brains.* ii:1064–1065, 1973.

18. LANCET: *Preventing secondary brain damage after head injury.* ii:1189–1190, 1978.

19. MACPHERSON, P., AND GRAHAM, D.I.: *Correlations between angiographic findings and the ischemia of head injury.* J. Neurol. Neurosurg. Psychiatry 41:122–127, 1978.

20. MILLER, J. D., SWEET, R. C., NARAYAN, R., ET AL.: *Early insults to the injured brain.* J.A.M.A. 240:439–442, 1978.

21. MITCHELL, D. E., AND ADAMS, J. H.: *Primary focal impact damage to the brainstem in blunt head injuries: does it exist?* Lancet ii:215–218, 1973.

22. NEVIN, N. C.: *Neuropathological changes in the white matter following head injury.* J. Neuropathol. Exp. Neurol. 26:77–84, 1967.

23. OMMAYA, A. K., AND GENNARELLI, T. A.: *Cerebral concussion and traumatic unconsciousness: correlations of experimental and clinical observations on blunt head injuries.* Brain 97:633–654, 1974.

24. OMMAYA, A. K., GRUBB, R. L., AND NAUMANN, R. A.: *Coup and contre-coup injury: observa-*

tions on the mechanics of visible brain injuries in the rhesus monkey. J. Neurosurg. 35:503–516, 1971.

25. OMMAYA, A. K., AND HIRSCH, A. E.: *Tolerances for cerebral concussion from head impact and whiplash in primates.* J. Biochem. 4:13–21, 1971.

26. OPPENHEIMER, D. R.: *Microscopic lesions in the brain following head injury.* J. Neurol. Neurosurg. Psychiatry 31:299–306, 1968.

27. PEERLESS, S. J., AND REWCASTLE, N. B.: *Shear injuries of the brain.* Can. Med. Assoc. J. 98:577–582, 1967.

28. PUDENZ, R. H., AND SHELDEN, C. H.: *The lucite calcarium—a method for direct observation of the brain. II. Cranial trauma and brain movement.* J. Neurosurg. 3:487–505, 1946.

29. SEVITT, S.: *Fatal road accidents in Birmingham: times to death and their causes.* Injury 4:281–293, 1973.

30. STRICH, S. J.: *Diffuse degeneration of the cerebral white matter in severe dementia following head injury.* J. Neurol. Neurosurg. Psychiatry 19: 163–185, 1956.

31. STRICH, S. J.: *Shearing of nerve fibres as a cause of brain damage due to head injury.* Lancet ii:443–448, 1961.

32. STRICH, S. J.: "The pathology of brain damage due to blunt head injuries." In Walker, A. E., Caveness, W. F., and Critchley, M. (eds.): *The Late Effects of Head Injury.* Charles C Thomas, Springfield, 1969, pp. 501–524.

33. STRICH, S. J.: *Lesions in the cerebral hemispheres after blunt head injury.* J. Clin. Pathol. 23 (suppl. 4):154–165, 1970.

34. SULLIVAN, H. G., MARTINEZ, J., BECKER, D. P., ET AL.: *Fluid percussion model of mechanical brain injury in the cat.* J. Neurosurg. 45:520–534, 1976.

35. TURAZZI, S., AND BRICOLO, A.: *Acute pontine syndromes following head injury.* Lancet ii:62–64, 1977.

36. ADAMS, J. H., SCOTT, GRACE, ET AL.: *The contusion index. A quantitative approach to cerebral contusions in head injury.* Neuropathol. Appl. Neurobiol. 6:319–324, 1980.

CHAPTER 3

Dynamic Pathology

The damage to the brain in head injuries that are seen by the pathologist is only the ultimate consequence of a variety of dynamic processes. The brain is such a functionally refined organ, and its function so sensitive to changes in its milieu, that many significant biological events can occur that leave little trace for the pathologist to find, even when he makes the fullest use of modern neuropathological techniques. However, the same processes that can leave their mark as permanent structural damage when they have been sufficiently severe and persistent are responsible also for reversible functional disturbances. Whatever the nature of the initial event, in the final analysis most brain damage is probably the result of tissue hypoxia or ischemia. Adequate cerebral oxygenation depends upon the interaction of several factors, many of which are at least potentially under the control of the clinician. It is therefore of considerable practical importance to understand the various factors that are involved in maintaining oxygen supply to the brain and the way in which these may be affected by head injury.

The account that follows deals with the reactions of the normal brain to systemic changes, such as variations in arterial blood pressure and blood gases, and with the effects of brain damage, whether they be edema, infarction, contusion, or hemorrhage. As explained in the previous chapter these processes are all liable to be precipitated by head injury, although one or the other may predominate in one brain, or in different parts of the same brain. The pathophysiological mechanisms described below apply to a wide range of conditions that cause acute brain damage and are not specific to head injury. However, in the context of multiple injury, or when head injury is associated with chest complications, the combination of local brain damage with systemic abnormalities (e.g., in blood pressure, serum electrolytes, and blood gases) makes the brain particularly vulnerable.

CEREBRAL ENERGY SUPPLY

The normal brain has a high, surprisingly stable overall metabolic rate, and its oxygen requirements are extremely large (see Siesjo[64] for a comprehensive review of brain energy metabolism). Most of the energy derived from metabolism is expended in maintaining the membrane potentials and electrochemical gradients of the neurons, and in the neurochemical processes responsible for synaptic transmission. A continuous supply of energy is important also in the maintenance of the integrity of intracellular organelles and membranes. If energy supply fails completely, the ensuing events are rapid and dramatic: neuronal function fails after a matter of seconds and permanent structural damage occurs within minutes.

Energy Production and Utilization within the Brain

Energy is produced in the brain almost entirely from the oxidative metabolism of glucose. The pattern of energy flow within the brain is summarized in Figure 1.

The size of the continuous metabolic demand of the brain is reflected in its enormous consumption of oxygen. Although the brain accounts for only 2 percent of the adult body weight, its consumption of 45 to 50 ml/min oxygen represents 20 percent of the whole body's oxygen expenditure. Cerebral glucose consumption (60 mg/min) is even higher—a quarter of the total for the whole body. This high rate of glucose utilization reflects the brain's inability to make use of the more complex substrates that are available to other tissues.

Oxidative metabolism of glucose yields energy in the form of high energy phosphate bonds. The most important of these is adenosine triphosphate (ATP), formed from the combination of adenosine diphosphate (ADP) and inorganic phosphate (Pi). Complete metabolism of one molecule of glucose produces 38 molecules of ATP:

$$1 \text{ glucose} + 6O_2 + 38 \text{ ADP} + 38 \text{ Pi} \rightarrow 6CO_2 + 44H_2O + 38 \text{ ATP}$$

The energy status of any part of the brain is reflected by its content of high energy phosphate; the overall energy charge within the adenosine nucleotide pool is reflected in the formula described by Atkinson:[3]

$$\text{Energy Charge Potential} = \frac{\text{ATP} + 0.5 \text{ ADP}}{\text{ATP} + \text{ADP} + \text{AMP}}$$

As well as the adenosine pool being the source of energy, the "energy charge potential" may be an important factor in controlling a cell's rate of metabolism: the rate of turnover of ATP is normally coupled to the rate of oxygen consumption; furthermore, the level of energy production is coupled to the functional activity of the cell. Thus oxygen is used up in proportion to the work being done: increasing function results in increasing oxygen requirements; decreasing function reduces demands.

The brain's ability to store glucose is very limited and its store of oxygen is sufficient for only a few seconds' needs; therefore an incessant supply of both is essential for the continuing function of the brain. Three factors govern the deliv-

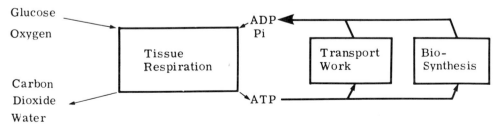

Figure 1. Energy metabolism in the brain. (Modified from MacMillan and Siesjo.[37])

ery of metabolic substrates to the brain: those factors that determine their concentration in the blood; the rate of cerebral blood flow; and, for glucose at least, the rate of its facilitated diffusion across the blood-brain barrier. After head injury the brain is more likely to suffer from a lack of oxygen than a shortage of glucose. Oxygen supply to the tissues may be restricted as a result of a fall in the blood oxygen content (hypoxemia) or because of impaired tissue perfusion (ischemia), which in turn may be diffuse or focal; often there is a combination of both factors.

Tissue hypoxia is said to exist when the supply of oxygen is so low that metabolism changes predominantly to an incomplete anaerobic form in which glucose is only partially oxidized to lactic acid, with the release of only 5 percent of the energy resulting from its complete oxidative metabolism:

$$1 \text{ glucose } + 2 \text{ ADP } + \text{ Pi} \rightarrow 2 \text{ lactate } + 2 \text{ ATP}$$

There are some alternative means of production of small amounts of ATP, but the maximum anaerobic yield of ATP, even if glucose were continually available, would supply less than half of the brain's energy requirements.

Cerebral tissue hypoxia is characterized by a fall in the levels of ATP and other high energy phosphates in the brain. However, this is usually preceded by other evidence of oxygen lack, such as a shift in the redox state of the coenzymes of the electron transport system, which are responsible for linking hydrogen release with oxygen. For example, in the case of the nicotinamide nucleotides, the ratio of the reduced form (NADH) is increased at the expense of the oxidized form (NAD^+) (Fig. 2).

An accumulation of lactate accompanies the reduction of the electron transport system; lactate is formed when pyruvate (derived from glycolysis of glucose) is reduced:

$$\text{Pyruvate } + \text{ NADH } + \text{ H}^+ \rightarrow \text{lactate } + \text{ NAD}^+$$

It has been proposed that the lactate/pyruvate ratio in the brain or the CSF may provide an indication of tissue hypoxia. However, metabolite concentrations in the CSF may not reflect the levels in cerebral interstitial fluid, a relatively more dynamic medium. Moreover, the ratio can be increased purely as a result of acidosis, and without a knowledge of brain tissue pH it is not possible to draw other than very broad parallels between a lactate/pyruvate ratio and tissue hypoxia, particularly that degree of hypoxia necessary to produce structural brain damage.

The determination of amounts of ATP, ADP, and AMP in the brain or of the $NADH/NAD^+$ ratio involves either sampling the brain or exposing its surface for fluorescence studies. These techniques have proved useful in experimental studies

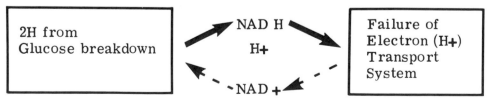

Figure 2. Nicotinamide nucleotides in cerebral hypoxia: increase in NADH relative to NAD^+.

47

in animals, but clinicians have had to seek less direct indices of brain oxygenation and energy utilization. Jugular venous oxygen levels have been measured in the hope of their reflecting cerebral tissue PO_2 levels; determination of the arterial-jugular venous oxygen difference, coupled with measurement of cerebral blood flow, provides an estimate of overall cerebral oxygen consumption. Even these simple measures are, to some degree, invasive; but their major defect is that they are subject to great limitations in interpretation. They provide only gross overall measurements, whereas most often the brain is disordered in a focal or multifocal, patchy manner, even by "insults" that appear to be uniform.

Cerebral blood flow and metabolism can now be mapped in three dimensions using recently developed techniques, but the methods are expensive and elaborate and available in only a few centers. Despite their potential, no principles relevant to the care of the head injured patient have as yet emerged from their use, beyond what had been learned previously about the interactions between cerebral function and oxygen supply.

Effect of Increased Cerebral Activity on Energy Metabolism

Because of the close coupling between function and energy flow, increased activity of the brain is accompanied by an increase in oxygen demand. This is well demonstrated in an epileptic attack, when the cerebral metabolic rate is increased by up to three times above normal. If the effects of the fit upon respiration and cardiac function are controlled, the oxygen supply to the tissues keeps pace with the demand. Blood flow and oxygen extraction are both increased and there is only slight energy depletion. Physiological focal increases in brain activity have similar effects upon local metabolism;[66] here the call for an increased oxygen supply can be met by an increased local blood flow (p. 52). However, during such states of increased neural activity the brain is more than normally susceptible to any interference with its oxygen supply, and the respiratory and cardiovascular insufficiency, which may accompany an epileptic fit, can result in brain hypoxia.

Effect of Tissue Hypoxia on Brain
Metabolism and Function

This topic has created considerable controversy, although some general principles have emerged from recent studies. These are shown in Tables 1 and 2, which relate to hypoxia resulting either from a fall in arterial oxygen or from a cessation of cerebral blood flow.

Hypoxemia

If the level of O_2 in arterial blood is lowered progressively, metabolism and function are affected only when PaO_2 falls below 50 mm Hg (Table 1). There is some correlation between jugular venous PO_2 and the adequacy of brain oxygenation, but even when there is apparently an overall oxygen deprivation, there may be a considerable dissociation between the cerebral venous PO_2 and the energy state of the brain. The reasons that the brain's function begins to fail are still unclear. One of the surprising facts to have emerged from recent work is that brain mitochondria are able to maintain energy production during very extreme hypoxia, far below the levels at which electrical activity fails.[37,64] This then cannot

Table 1. Effects of hypoxemia on cerebral metabolism and function

Arterial PO$_2$ mm Hg	Cerebral Venous PO$_2$ mm Hg	Biochemical Events	Functional Disorders
<50 mm Hg	<35 mm Hg	*Increased* glycolysis and lactate production; *normal* high energy phosphates; *decreased* neurotransmitters	Impaired learning; minor EEG change
<35 mm Hg	<25 mm Hg	*Pronounced* lactate production; *still normal* energy charge	Psychological testing abnormal; altered behavior; impaired judgment
<20–25 mm Hg	<10–15 mm Hg	*Decreased* ATP and energy charge; *increased* NADH/NAD$^+$ ratio	Loss of consciousness; EEG slowed →absent
<5–10 mm Hg	Tissue PO$_2$ <2 mm Hg	Mitochondrial function impaired; permanent damage to some neurons	Death from cardiovascular failure

be due to an overall cessation of energy supply. Other events have to be invoked: there may be very focal metabolic defects in only a few neurons or even in only one part of a cell such as the synaptic area; it may be that it is the metabolism of neurotransmitters that is critically affected, for this seems to be sensitive to relatively mild hypoxia.[15]

Ischemia

When there is systemic hypoxia, blood flow to the brain increases, and the increased flow, at least initially, maintains oxygen delivery. If blood flow stops completely, not only do substrates become depleted, but waste products accumulate. The situation is more complex than in asphyxia or hypoxemia, but it is still possible to see a progressive sequence of functional and metabolic events, in this case related to the duration of ischemia (Table 2).

Recovery after Cerebral Hypoxia

It has long been thought that complete anoxia of 3 to 4 minutes damaged the brain irreparably. However, it has become clear recently that one of the limiting factors in the brain's recovery from anoxia is a failure of the cardiovascular system; if disturbances of cardiac output are prevented the brain can tolerate several minutes of ischemia and still regain some function. In experiments where the ischemia has been limited to the brain, and circulatory disorders prevented, Hossman and colleagues [21] have found that cerebral energy state and metabolism can recover to a great extent, after even an hour of total ischemia. Some evidence of neuronal activity also returns. But the significance of recovery of *some* function as observed in animals can be questioned, and it is far from clear whether the period of ischemia after which normal function and behavior can be expected to

49

Table 2. Effects of complete ischemia on the brain

Duration of Ischemia	Biochemical Changes	Functional Changes
0–20 seconds	*Decreased* $CMRO_2$; *increased* NADH/NAD^+ ratio	Consciousness lost; EEG slows, then ceases
1–5 minutes	*Depleted* ATP and energy charge; *increased* lactate, H^+, and extracellular K^+; cellular swelling and Na^+ entry	Brain stem reflexes lost; pupils unreactive; pyramidal response lost
5–15 minutes	*Decreased* protein synthesis; *increased* cyclic AMP, GABA; some aminoacids and FFA	Some cells irreversibly damaged
>60 minutes	Energy metabolism ceases; protein metabolism stops; biochemical changes still largely reversible	Widespread neuronal damage but some cells may still regain some function; vascular reflow impaired

return is any longer than a few minutes (unless special techniques to protect the brain are employed—see below).

If the cerebral circulation has been at a standstill for some time it can be difficult to re-establish flow to some parts of the brain. Hopes that this "no reflow" phenomenon might be the critical factor in limiting tolerance to ischemia, and that it might be susceptible to treatment, have not been fulfilled; careful studies by, among others, Levy and colleagues[32] have shown that permanent neuronal damage can become established before impairment of microcirculatory reflow appears. "No reflow" may therefore be an accompaniment rather than the cause of ischemic brain damage.

Brain Protection: Promotion of Recovery after Hypoxia

An effective and safe means of increasing the brain's tolerance to ischemia or injury could be of immense benefit in a variety of circumstances. A number of ways of protecting the brain against the effects of hypoxia have been proposed at different times. Most are based upon inducing a depression of cerebral function; because of the close coupling between function and metabolism, energy requirements are then reduced and the effects of hypoxia can be postponed.

The oldest method is *hypothermia,* used intermittently in different aspects of neurosurgery for 30 years. When the body's temperature is reduced from 37°C to 22°C, cerebral oxygen consumption declines to 40 percent of normal level. This is accompanied by a comparable fall in the level of cerebral blood flow required.[17] With more extreme hypothermia (e.g., 16°C) cardiac arrest can be tolerated for up to 30 minutes.[18] However, although cerebral blood flow falls with hypothermia, any further fall, in response to external stresses, may be just as damaging as if it occurred at normothermia. Major systemic complications have limited the use of profound hypothermia; moderate hypothermia alone has not been found useful in head injury.

BARBITURATES. Anesthetics, such as barbiturates, depress energy utilization and result in a high energy state in the normal brain. There is now clear evidence from studies on animals that the previous administration of barbiturates can protect brain metabolism when oxygen supply is restricted;[53] cerebral function is also protected.[20,42,60] When given before the insult their protective effects probably depend upon reducing cerebral metabolism, but barbiturates are still of benefit even when given shortly after an episode of ischemia, although the mechanism of their effect at this stage is unclear [50,53] Even during ischemia there may be a distinction between the amount of energy spared by the depression of cortical function induced by barbiturates and the level of energy that is required to maintain basic brain cell viability.[29]

Other ways in which barbiturates may protect the brain have been suggested. In oxygen lack the coenzymes of electron transport systems (p. 47) are freed from "control" and, in their reduced state, can initiate pathological "free radical" reactions that damage the lipids of the membranes of brain cells. Barbiturates may regain control of these free radical reactions and retard the peroxidation of the lipids.[8,12] Steroids have been thought to have similar beneficial effect.[7]

It is not clear by what mechanism barbiturates might promote recovery after head injury, as distinct from protecting a previously normal brain against the effects of an ischemic episode of finite, limited duration. Barbiturates can reduce acutely raised intracranial pressure in head injured patients and their effect may be additive with mild hypothermia and hyperventilation.[63] They probably reduce intracranial pressure by reducing cerebral blood volume (p. 60). A preliminary trial of barbiturate treatment of severe head injuries with raised intracranial pressure (ICP) has suggested that outcome may be improved.[41] Assessment of this claim awaits the results of more extensive studies.

Hopefully, some pharmacological means of ameliorating the effects of head injury will emerge, but it is already evident that this is likely to depend upon treatment commencing very soon after injury and that very large dosages of drugs may be necessary. The levels of barbiturates currently being used would, by themselves, produce very deep coma. Because of the depression of respiration, ventilatory support is inevitable and marked hypotension can also occur; intensive care is essential. At present it remains unclear which patients should receive these drugs, how much should be given, for how long, and even whether real benefits will follow their use.

CEREBRAL BLOOD FLOW

The brain receives about 15 percent of the entire cardiac output. This represents a flow of about 800 ml/min of blood through the brain as a whole. The level of cerebral blood flow is normally closely regulated and adapted to local metabolic needs, but the precise mechanisms responsible for this coupling, and for many other aspects of the control of the cerebral circulation, are still controversial.

In the last 30 years it has been possible to measure total cerebral blood flow in man. For about half of that time perfusion has been measurable on a regional, two-dimensional basis. Recently, methods for measuring cerebral blood flow in three dimensions in life have been developed. Over the years a fairly clear picture of the various factors that affect cerebral blood flow has emerged. Knowledge of the various factors and their effects upon cerebral blood flow are essential as a step to understanding how they might be altered after head injury, but it is important to realize that what applies to the normal brain may not be true for the damaged brain.

51

Factors Affecting Cerebral Blood Flow

Regional Differences

The rate of perfusion of different parts of the brain varies. The normal level of cerebral blood flow is about 50 ml/100 g/min of perfused brain as a whole. The level of flow within the gray matter (80–100 ml/100 g/min) is much higher than that in white matter (20–25 ml/100 g/min). This reflects the greater metabolic activity and greater vascularity of gray matter. The level of flow varies between different parts of the cerebral cortex. In man, flow is high in the frontal lobes and can be increased markedly in some areas by physiological stimulation during measurements, e.g., the occipital cortex during photic stimulation, or the motor cortex during contralateral arm exercises. Anesthesia reduces these variations, but its overall effect upon CBF and its regulation depends upon the individual agent and on the depth of anesthesia (p. 56).

Metabolism

Regional variations in blood flow in relation to the function of the brain reflect the close relationship between cerebral metabolism and blood flow. The blood flow of the brain as a whole can vary between wide extremes, depending upon whether function, and therefore metabolism, has been pathologically increased or decreased (Fig. 3). It is unclear by what mechanism flow and metabolism are coupled. Indeed it is this question that is the greatest challenge still facing those who study the physiology of the cerebral circulation. Changes in tissue H^+ concentration in the extracellular fluid have been strongly favored by Lassen,[28] but this possibility has been denied recently.[31] Adenosine, potassium, calcium, and prostaglandins have each been proposed as important agents; probably more than one factor is involved.[6]

Chemical Factors

OXYGEN. Moderate changes in arterial oxygen have little effect upon the cerebral vessels. When arterial PO_2 is below 50 mm Hg, a distinct increase in cerebral blood flow takes place; at a PaO_2 of 30 mm Hg, cerebral blood flow is more than doubled (Fig. 4A). Again the mechanism responsible for the vasodilatation is controversial.

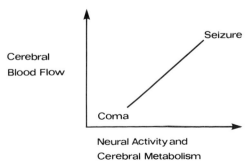

Figure 3. Schematic illustration of the interrelationships between cerebral activity, metabolism, and cerebral blood flow.

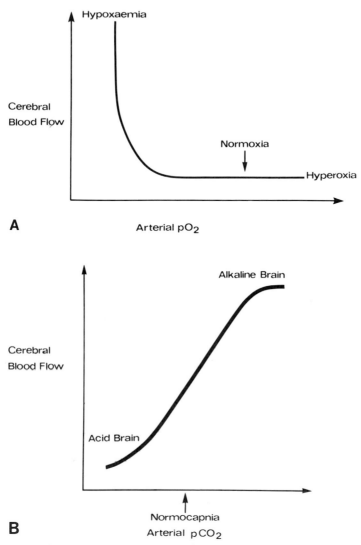

Figure 4. Chemical influences upon cerebral blood flow: **A,** arterial oxygen level; **B,** arterial carbon dioxide level.

Raising PaO_2 above normal causes only slight changes in cerebral blood flow; breathing 100 percent O_2 reduces CBF by about 10 percent. Under hyperbaric conditions (100% oxygen/2 atmospheres) arterial PaO_2 can be increased to 800 to 1200 mm Hg; CBF then falls by 20 to 25 percent. At even higher levels of PaO_2 CBF is reduced only transiently and it has been suggested that vasoconstriction is then being balanced by vasodilatation owing to the toxic effects of hyperoxia.

CARBON DIOXIDE. Variations in arterial $PaCO_2$ can cause profound changes in cerebral blood flow because CO_2 is a very potent stimulus to cerebral vasodilatation. Cerebral blood flow doubles when $PaCO_2$ is increased from 40 to 80 mm Hg and halves when $PaCO_2$ drops to 20 mm Hg (Fig. 4B). Below 20 mm Hg, $PaCO_2$ changes have little further effect on cerebral blood flow, probably because the

53

flow is so low that tissue hypoxia is occurring. However, there is little evidence that hypocapnic vasoconstriction can result in hypoxia to a degree that results in structural brain damage.[18]

The more rapid the change in CO_2 the more marked the response of the cerebral vessels; after a few hours the cerebral vessels seem to adapt to persisting CO_2 changes. The pH of the CSF and cerebral blood flow then return towards normal levels. The exact mechanism responsible for the normal responsiveness of cerebral vessels to CO_2 is still controversial. What is clear is that the capacity of the cerebral circulation to respond to either hypoxia or CO_2 changes may be profoundly altered in a variety of pathological situations. Cerebral blood flow may fail to increase during hypoxia and hypercapnia and, when there is a focal disorder, an increase in $PaCO_2$ may even lead to a reduction in local perfusion (blood flow in the surrounding normal brain is increased at the expense of a fall in flow to the affected area, the so-called "steal").

pH. The cerebral vessels are very sensitive to alterations in the pH of the extracerebral fluid of the brain. Acid solutions cause dilatation, and alkaline solutions constriction. In contrast, alterations in intravascular pH do not affect cerebral blood flow, provided that CO_2 does not change and the blood-brain barrier is intact. Thus, with a metabolic acidosis or alkalosis, CBF is unaffected.

Pressure Regulation

ARTERIAL PRESSURE. It was previously believed that cerebral blood flow depended passively on arterial blood pressure. It is now known that this is true only for damaged brain and that the normal brain has an extremely well-developed capacity to maintain a constant flow despite wide changes in arterial pressure. The mechanism probably resides in the cerebral vessels themselves and may be largely myogenic; when pressure is reduced, dilatation occurs; increases in pressure induce vasoconstriction. These reactions can hold blood flow relatively constant when mean arterial pressure is reduced by hemorrhage to about 60 mm Hg. At lower arterial pressures, although vasodilatation is not exhausted, this mechanism is no longer sufficient to prevent blood flow from falling (Fig. 5). During acute, extreme rises in blood pressure over 160 mm Hg, vasoconstriction fails and the cerebral vessels become distended; cerebral blood flow increases and there may be a patchy breakdown of the blood-brain barrier with foci of cerebral edema.[36]

The maintenance of flow in response to pressure changes has been termed autoregulation, because the autonomic nervous system does not seem to be an essential factor in the response. Nevertheless, activity in autonomic nerves does influence the *range* of pressure over which the regulatory response is effective. Blocking the vasoconstrictive activity in the sympathetic nerves shifts the lower limit, below which regulation fails, to even lower levels of blood pressure, around 30 to 35 mm Hg. Sympathetic blockade also reduces to around 130 mm Hg the upper limit at which "breakthrough" takes place, but stimulating the sympathetic nerves increases the capacity of the brain to adapt to rises in arterial pressure.

Autoregulation is probably not an "all-or-nothing" phenomenon; it may best be regarded as being present to greater or lesser degrees, and it may be affected only locally. Any factor which alters the ability of the cerebral vessels to constrict or dilate interferes with autoregulation (Fig. 5). It can be impaired or even abolished by a wide variety of insults, such as ischemia, hypoxia, hypercapnia, and brain

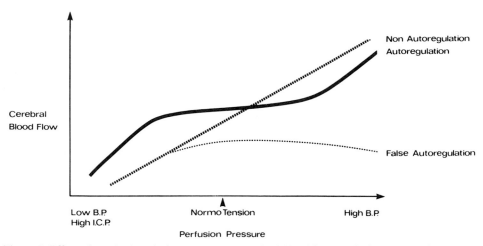

Figure 5. Effect of cerebral perfusion pressure on cerebral blood flow. Perfusion pressure is low when either blood pressure is low or intracranial pressure is high. A high perfusion pressure exists when blood pressure is high, providing that intracranial pressure does not also increase. Autoregulatory "pattern" of blood flow in the normal brain is shown as solid line. Impaired autoregulation characteristic of damaged brain is shown as interrupted lines.

trauma; and it seems to be much more easily disturbed than the responsiveness of the vessels to CO_2.

INTRACRANIAL PRESSURE. The rate of blood flow through the brain depends upon two factors: the pressure difference between its arteries and veins, and the resistance of the intervening vessels. The first defines the cerebral perfusion pressure, the latter the cerebrovascular resistance. The pressure inside the cerebral veins is practically the same as the intracranial pressure in almost all situations, so that the cerebral perfusion pressure (CPP) is commonly regarded as being the difference between the arterial pressure (SAP) and intracranial pressure (ICP):

$$CPP = SAP - ICP$$

The interactions between ICP and CBF are complex: a primary increase in cerebral blood flow, consequent upon vasodilatation, can increase intracranial pressure; in other circumstances an increase in intracranial pressure will reduce cerebral perfusion pressure. Small changes in intracranial pressure are compensated for by changes in cerebrovascular resistance in the same way as the cerebral vessels accommodate to changes in arterial pressure. Indeed, it has been suggested that the stimulus to autoregulation is a change in the transmural pressure differential between arterial, on the luminal surface, and intracranial, on the adventitial surface. A critical point is reached when the intracranial pressure is within about 40 mm Hg of the arterial pressure, after which CBF falls as perfusion pressure further decreases (Fig. 5).

Without knowledge of the blood pressure, the exact level of ICP, which corresponds to the critical point at which cerebral blood flows begins to fall, cannot be predicted. A rise in arterial pressure is a common response in experimental animals, but is generally thought to occur only as a terminal agonal event in people. This systemic pressure response can maintain perfusion pressure until quite high levels of intracranial pressure are reached. Conversely, a critical reduction in perfusion pressure may be reached at much lower levels of intracranial pressure if arterial pressure has been reduced, e.g., as a result of hemorrhage or administration of drugs.

When autoregulation is impaired and ICP is increased, blood flow falls at an early stage[46] (Fig. 5). In this circumstance an increase in arterial pressure is not always beneficial; sometimes it is accompanied by a parallel increase in intracranial pressure so that there is no net effect upon perfusion pressure. Even when perfusion pressure is increased, blood flow in damaged brain may fail to show any increase from a low level; this is sometimes termed "false autoregulation."[45]

After a head injury efforts should be directed to keeping the cerebral perfusion pressure in the normal range. Because of the complexity of their interactions, it is not possible to predict to what extent measures that alter either arterial pressure or intracranial pressure will be reflected in a given change in cerebral perfusion pressure; neither can it be predicted, should this be affected, to what degree cerebral blood flow may be influenced.

Drugs and the Cerebral Circulation

Drugs, particularly those used in anesthesia, may affect cerebral blood flow in a number of ways: by direct dilatation or constriction of the cerebral vessels; by altering cerebral function and so influencing blood flow secondarily; and by affecting either blood pressure or respiration and thus affecting the cerebral circulation indirectly, e.g., by the rise in CO_2 that occurs as a consequence of respiratory depression. The cerebral effects of a pharmacological agent are dependent upon its ability to cross the blood-brain barrier and to gain access to the extracellular fluid of the brain and its blood vessels. Biogenic amines and prostaglandins, which do not cross the barrier, normally have little effect upon cerebral blood flow; if the blood-brain barrier is disrupted, however, as commonly occurs under pathological conditions, they can cause profound changes in cerebral blood flow and metabolism.[10,35,54,55]

ANESTHETIC AGENTS. Anesthetic drugs that affect the cerebral circulation can be divided broadly into those that cause vasoconstriction and those that cause dilatation.[65]

Cerebral Vasoconstriction. When vasoconstriction occurs it is usually secondary to reduction in cerebral metabolism. This is a characteristic effect of most anesthetic drugs that are given intravenously, e.g., sodium thiopentone and Althesin (alphaxolone + alphadione). Ketamine is the one exception to this rule, because it is a cerebral stimulant and so vasodilates.

Cerebral Vasodilatation. All currently available inhalational anesthetics dilate cerebral vessels. The extent of this effect varies and any changes in cerebral blood flow also depend upon the extent of the drug's additional effects upon the metabolism. Nitrous oxide produces a moderate vasodilatation, but its overall effects are still the subject of controversy; Wollman and colleagues[70] reported a reduction of cerebral metabolism, Theye and Michenfelder[69] a slight increase.

When there is already an intracranial space-occupying lesion, inhalational agents that are potent vasodilators can increase intracranial pressure to a dangerous extent. Even if hyperventilation is used to bring about hypocapnic vasoconstriction, halothane[16] still produces this effect; even nitrous oxide is not entirely free from this risk. These drugs also dilate systemic vessels and can cause systemic arterial pressure to fall, further compromising cerebral perfusion.

NARCOTICS AND NEUROLEPTICS. Opiate analgesics, e.g., morphine and pethidine, reduce cerebral metabolism. Cerebral blood flow would be lowered were this effect not countered by the cerebral vasodilatation that is induced by the hypercapnia resulting from the concomitant respiratory depression. Fentanyl, by itself, has little effect upon the cerebral circulation; commonly it is given with droperidol, and cerebral blood flow and metabolism are reduced by 50 percent. The reductions resulting from a combination of phenoperidine and droperidol are not so profound. Diazepam can also reduce cerebral blood flow and metabolism.

MUSCLE RELAXANTS. Curare and nondepolarizing relaxants such as pancuronium have either no effect upon the cerebral circulation or they produce, at the most, a mild vasodilatation. Curare may have effects upon systemic arterial pressure and so indirectly affect cerebral blood flow; this is less likely with pancuronium. Suxamethonium probably has no direct effect upon the cerebral circulation, but its administration is accompanied initially by a transient increase in central venous pressure; this is reflected in a brief rise in intracranial pressure.

Effects of Reduced Cerebral Blood Flow

There is much evidence, including clinical studies, that there is a close correlation between reduced levels of cerebral blood flow and disordered cerebral function: either a decline in overall mental performance or a focal neurological lesion. But it is difficult in most clinical studies to unravel the sequence of events leading to a reduction in cerebral blood flow; indeed an observed reduction in flow seems often to reflect a primary decrease in function that has then reduced the requirements for energy supply. Studies performed during carotid artery surgery in man, and in a variety of situations in experimental animals, have provided evidence about the effects that a primary reduction in cerebral blood flow has on neural function.

When cerebral blood flow is reduced, a progressive sequence of events, related to the level of cerebral blood flow, can be demonstrated. Initially, electrical function and metabolism continue but become disordered. The levels of CBF at which impaired function has been detected have varied in different reports, probably reflecting variations in the different measures of function that have been employed. The response of the cerebral cortex to an electrical stimulus applied directly to its surface alters almost as soon as CBF begins to fall,[68] as does cerebral metabolic rate.[5] EEG slowing during carotid clamping has been observed when blood flow is reduced by as little as 12 percent.[30] In contrast, somatosensory cortical responses, evoked by stimulating peripheral nerves, tend to be unaffected until cerebral blood flow has fallen considerably.[4]

The change from an impairment of function to a complete failure of electrical activity followed by a loss of cell homeostasis occurs at certain "critical" reductions in blood flow, and about these there is considerable agreement. Complete failure of the somatosensory evoked response and direct cortical response occurs when blood flow is reduced to about 30 to 35 percent of normal values. This corresponds with rates of blood flow in the cerebral cortex of 15 to 25 ml/100 g/min. Failure of electrical activity is not due to the development of an extracellular acidosis nor to a depolarization of the cells by the leakage of potassium into the extracellular fluid; failure to maintain ionic equilibrium occurs only when blood flow has fallen to about half the level at which electrical function fails.[1] Even then, the rise in extracellular potassium may be reversible if cerebral blood

57

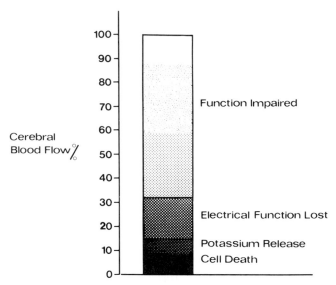

Figure 6. Effect of reduced cerebral blood flow on cerebral function and cellular homeostasis. (Modified from Astrup et al.[1])

flow is restored; cell death becomes inevitable only at even lower levels of blood flow (Fig. 6). It is quite clear that, at least in the short term, ischemic neurological dysfunction can be reversed by restoring blood flow.

INTRACRANIAL PRESSURE

After head injury, intracranial pressure (ICP) frequently becomes elevated for a variety of reasons. Whatever the primary disturbance, the consequence of increased intracranial pressure is often impaired cerebral perfusion, which results in ischemic brain damage. When there is a focal expanding lesion, whether an intracranial hematoma or localized brain swelling, there will also be distortion and shift of the brain. Yet, at the same time that the brain is deforming, compensatory mechanisms may dissipate the pressure effects so that there is not a consistent relationship between shift and raised intracranial pressure. Indeed, it is often unclear whether a patient is suffering mainly from the effects of brain shift or from an overall impairment of cerebral perfusion caused by raised intracranial pressure; commonly both factors are present.

Raised Intracranial Pressure

When an intracranial space-occupying lesion expands there is initially only a slight increase in intracranial pressure; eventually, a dramatic increase in intracranial pressure ensues (Fig. 7). The concept of this progression from a phase of "compensation" for the presence of the lesion to one of "decompensation" has been recognized for many years.[25] Four stages of evolution were described by Duret a century ago,[9] and Langfitt and his colleagues made an experimental analogue of these.[27] During the first stage, spatial compensation, there is only a minimal increase in intracranial pressure. Decompensation occurs in three successive phases. Initially intracranial pressure rises, even in response to small

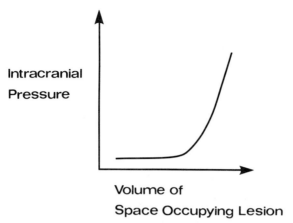

Intracranial Pressure

Volume of

Space Occupying Lesion

Figure 7. Changes in intracranial pressure as an intracranial lesion progressively increases in size. Initial phase of compensation is followed by an exponentially increasing pressure.

additions to the space-occupying lesion. Subsequently, spontaneous waves of intracranial pressure occur, cerebral function becomes impaired, and the cerebral circulation is unresponsive to physiological stimuli (cerebral vasomotor paralysis). In the final phase these changes become irreversible.

The brain can be characterized as a "wobbling lump of fat enclosed inside a rigid box, buoyed up by the cerebrospinal fluid"; it lacks rigidity but is incompressible. The latter quality accounts for the sequence of events leading to raised intracranial pressure.

Seventy-five percent of the brain is water, although only a small proportion of this is extracellular fluid. The brain takes up 80 percent of the space inside the skull, the remainder being occupied by cerebrospinal fluid and by blood in the cerebral arteries and veins (Fig. 8). Because they are largely fluid, the intracranial contents are incompressible. Since the work of Monro[47] and Kellie[23] it has been recognized that the rigidity of the adult skull means that the total intracranial volume is always the same and that a rise in intracranial pressure depends upon the balance achieved between any process tending to add to the intracranial volume and compensatory reductions in cranial constituents. The precise biophysical explanation for the sequence of events and for determining the level of intracranial pressure is still a matter for debate, 150 years after the original Monro/Kellie doctrine was proposed.

The initial and probably the major change, following the expansion of a space-occupying intracranial lesion, is a reduction in the volume of the cerebrospinal fluid inside the skull; this occurs mainly by expression of CSF from the skull into the distensible spinal dura sac. The effectiveness of compensation is reduced if the egress of CSF from the skull is impeded or if there are factors promoting a relative increase in either brain water or blood volume. On the other hand, compensation is increased by removal of CSF and by reductions in the volume of either the extracellular fluid (ECF) or the cerebral blood volume.

A block to the flow of CSF can develop in the final stages of brain shift and herniation, or as a complication of a hematoma in the posterior fossa. If this happens acutely the volume of CSF may be little above normal, yet intracranial pressure may rise dramatically. The removal of even small volumes of CSF can reduce an elevated ICP, but this is usually effective for only a period of minutes.

59

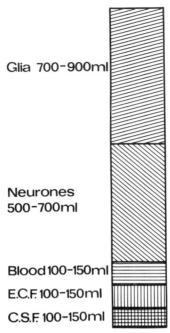

Figure 8. Approximate volumes of normal intracranial contents. (From Jennett,[72] with permission.)

The exaggerated effect on ICP of exchanging small volumes of CSF is made use of in the volume/pressure test (p. 62).

The accumulation of ECF as part of the edema that develops around contusions and lacerations may contribute to brain swelling and to a rise in ICP. Whether traumatic brain edema is susceptible to therapy is a debated point, and the effect of osmotic agents such as mannitol is believed to be the removal of fluid from nonedematous areas, where the blood-brain barrier is still intact.

The most readily induced changes that affect intracranial compensation are in the cerebral blood volume, which can be increased by vasodilatory stimuli such as hypercapnia, hypoxia, and hyperthermia or be reduced (at least for a period) by the vasoconstrictive effects of hypocapnia and hypothermia.

Intracranial pressure is most reliably recorded from the cerebrospinal fluid spaces; with the exception of certain extreme situations, to which we will return later, the CSF pressure reflects the pressure throughout the intracranial space. Under stable, normal conditions the cerebrospinal fluid pressure is determined by two factors: the relationship between the rate of formation of CSF and the resistance to its outflow from the CSF spaces into the cerebral veins; and an additional component representing the pressure in the dural venous sinuses (equivalent to the opening pressure of the drainage system).

CSF pressure = (formation rate × outflow resistance) + venous pressure

The formation of CSF is a complex process, in part being a simple filtration from plasma but in part an active process of transport that requires energy and that is independent of pressure effects. The rate of formation of CSF is fairly constant over quite wide ranges of CSF pressure but probably does taper off at

60

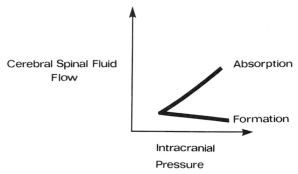

Figure 9. Effect of intracranial pressure on the rates of formation and absorption of cerebral spinal fluid. Formation is unchanged or slightly reduced at high intracranial pressure; absorption increases as pressure rises.

very high levels. CSF absorption is largely dependent upon the difference in pressure between the CSF and the large venous sinuses, the rate of absorption increasing as the differential pressure increases (Fig. 9).

Reducing the rate of CSF formation and so reducing its volume might be one means of reducing an elevated ICP. In itself an increased intracranial pressure might be expected to promote increased CSF absorption, but there is some evidence that, in the presence of an intracranial expanding lesion, there is an increased resistance to the flow of CSF.[40] Also, in many circumstances the increased intracranial pressure is transmitted to the intracranial veins.

Intracranial Elastance

This property determines what the CSF volume will be at that CSF pressure at which production and absorption of CSF are in equilibrium. The main factor determining the level of intracranial pressure and the capacity to compensate for further changes in the volume of a space-occupying lesion seems to be the elastic properties of the walls of the CSF spaces.[67] The more rigid these are (i.e., the "tighter" the brain), the smaller the CSF equilibrium volume, the higher the intracranial pressure, and the greater the increase in intracranial pressure resulting from any additional volume stress. The more "compliant" the walls of the CSF space, the greater the equilibrium volume, the lower the intracranial pressure, and the better the system's ability to adapt to changes.

The elastic properties of the walls of the CSF spaces depend upon interaction between several structures: the spinal dural sac (which is easily distensible); the intracranial vessels (the veins collapsible, the arteries and arterioles more rigid); the brain tissues; and the rigid dura and calvarium. The interactions between these components and any new pathological lesion determine what is termed the cerebrospinal fluid "elastance." Elastance is the inverse of compliance and is defined as the change in intracranial pressure resulting from any unit change in cerebrospinal fluid volume. Estimates of CSF elastance can be obtained by observing the change in pressure in response to a very small injection of fluid. A high elastance is "bad," i.e., there is a relatively large rise in ICP for injection of a given small volume.

As the size of an experimental intracranial lesion is progressively increased, the instantaneous pressure change in response to adding or withdrawing the same

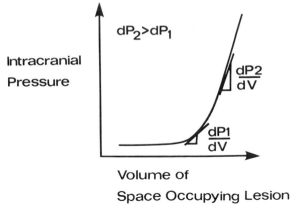

Figure 10. Intracranial pressure responses to unit volume change (elastance) at different points on the space-occupying lesion volume/pressure curve (see Fig. 7). The increase in pressure produced by the addition of the same unit of volume is greater (dP_2) in the "decompensated" state.

small volume becomes progressively greater.[43] The relationship between the volume of the lesion and the persisting level of intracranial pressure was illustrated previously (see Fig. 7). Figure 10 illustrates the relatively small increase in intracranial pressure for the sudden addition of a small volume on the horizontal, compensated part of the curve, compared with the much larger increase in pressure occurring when the same volume is added on the steep part of the curve. The occurrence of progressive increases in the elastance as a space-occupying lesion expands has been confirmed in a number of clinical and experimental studies.[34,67] Clinicians usually refer to estimates of elastance as the "volume/pressure response."

Measurements of elastance have been held to offer a way of predicting what will happen to intracranial pressure if the volume of a space-occupying lesion changes, and also the likely response to treatment directed towards enhancement of intracranial compensation (p. 239). Intracranial elastance is affected by a variety of factors (Table 3). Those tending to add volume to one of the intracranial compartments, whether blood, CSF, or ECF, or to increase the rigidity of the walls of the CSF spaces, increase elastance and have adverse effects upon intracranial compensation. Those that decrease elastance reduce the pressure change that occurs in response to a unit volume change and so increase intracranial compensation.

CLINICAL EFFECTS OF INCREASED INTRACRANIAL PRESSURE AND SPACE-OCCUPYING LESIONS

The relation between the level of intracranial pressure and the clinical state of the patient is far from direct. In some circumstances intracranial pressure may

Table 3. Factors affecting intracranial elastance

Increased Elastance	Decreased Elastance
Hypercapnia (any degree)	Hypocapnia (any degree)
Hypoxia ($PaO_2 < 50$ mm Hg)	Hyperoxia (PaO_2 1000–1500 mm Hg)
REM sleep	Hypothermia
Volatile anesthetic agents	Barbiturates
Nitrous oxide	Neuroleptanalgesia

rise to 100 mm Hg without any evidence of neurological deterioration, particularly in patients without expanding intracranial lesions in whom the high pressure is produced by diffuse processes, without distortion of the brain, as in benign intracranial hypertension. At the other extreme some head injury patients whose brain is irrecoverably damaged show no evidence that their intracranial pressure was ever high (p. 26).

Raised intracranial pressure cannot therefore by itself provide an adequate explanation for impairment of brain function, and the association between raised pressure and functional impairment is a result of either or both of two mechanisms: the effect of intracranial pressure upon cerebral blood flow or the relationship between raised intracranial pressure and brain shift.

The effects of raised intracranial pressure upon cerebral blood flow and of changes in the latter upon cerebral function have been dealt with previously (p. 57). In experiments in baboons we have confirmed that an increase in intracranial pressure, even as high as 80 mm Hg, has no effect upon the electrical function of the cerebral cortex, provided that cerebral blood flow is maintained.[68] The ability of the healthy brain to autoregulate its blood flow to account for changes in intracranial pressure has been described (p. 541), but in the head injured patient, it is important to realize that the same processes that lead to an increase in intracranial pressure are likely, at the same time, also to impair autoregulation. Moreover, a period of raised intracranial pressure may itself disturb autoregulation so that, should any further episodes ensue, these will now be against a background of impaired autoregulation. Repeated elevations of intracranial pressure are cumulative insults to the brain, even though pressure returns to normal in between.

The disparity between levels of intracranial pressure in patients with focal space-occupying lesions, and the occurrence of often dramatic episodes of deterioration, emphasizes the importance of the second mechanism: brain shift.

Brain Shift and Herniation

The brain's lack of rigidity allows considerable mechanical distortion to develop around intracranial expanding lesions, and this deformity can occur remarkably quickly with a rapidly expanding lesion. Deformity tends to be most marked, however, when a lesion has been expanding very slowly and there has been time for considerable compensation to occur. Brain shifts conform to a number of fairly predictable patterns, each associated with characteristic clinical signs, and these have been described by Plum and Posner.[56] These various patterns depend largely upon the site of the expanding lesion.

Supratentorial Expanding Lesions

When there is an expanding lesion above the tentorium, the cerebral hemispheres and brain stem are displaced downwards, towards and through the gap (hiatus) in the tentorium cerebelli (tentorial or uncal hernia). If the lesion is unilateral, the brain may be displaced from one side to another; the falx cerebri distorts, but to a considerably lesser extent than the brain, and the cingulate gyrus is distorted around its lower margin (subfalcine or supracallosal hernia) (Fig. 11). Displacement of the contents of the posterior fossa downwards through the foramen magnum (cerebellar cone, foraminal impaction, tonsillar hernia) may

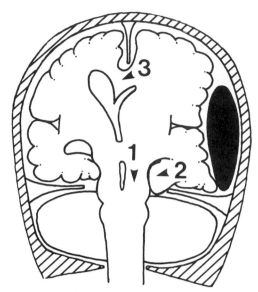

Figure 11. Shift with a unilateral supratentorial hematoma:
   1. Downward displacement of brain stem
   2. Herniation of uncus of temporal lobe into tentorial hiatus
   3. Herniation of cingulate gyrus below falx cerebri
Note also shift of the ventricles, compression of the ventricle on the same side as the clot, and dilatation on the opposite side.

occur as a sequel to a supratentorial expanding process, but it also happens at a relatively early stage in the evolution of a posterior fossa mass lesion.

CENTRAL TENTORIAL HERNIATION. When the supratentorial lesion is in the midline, either frontally or occipitally, or when there are bilateral lesions or a diffuse swelling of the brain, the herniation through the tentorium is symmetrical (central tentorial herniation). The midbrain and diencephalon are displaced downwards into the posterior fossa. Minor degrees of this kind of displacement may be difficult to detect at postmortem. Major degrees are associated with pressure necrosis of the posterior parts of the hippocampal gyri, with distortion and angulation of one or both oculomotor nerves and with compression of the posterior cerebral artery. Severe distortion of this artery can produce an infarct within its territory of supply (the medial occipital cortex—see p. 34). Infarction can also occur within the mammillary bodies and the pituitary, from stretching and distortion of the small vessels that supply these structures.

The clinical effects of central herniation reflect dysfunction within the upper brain stem and diencephalon. Consciousness is progressively impaired; eye movements are disturbed, with a loss of upward movements and release of vestibulo-ocular reflexes from cortical suppression; and motor responses on both sides of the body become progressively more abnormal (Fig. 12).

It may be the buckling and distortion of the midbrain and diencephalon that is responsible for the clinical events. Another theory is that when the brain stem shifts downwards, the basilar artery does not: the perforating branches from the basilar artery to the brain stem then become stretched and narrowed and the blood supply to the brain stem is impaired; venous obstruction may also play a part. To the pathologist the principal histological abnormality is an ischemic

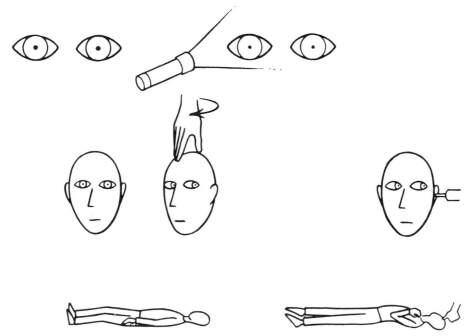

Figure 12. Clinical signs with central tentorial hernia. Pupils are small, but a slight reaction to light is present. There are active, conjugate doll's eye movements and tonic conjugate vestibular/ocular (caloric) reflexes. Symmetrical abnormal motor responses are present, initially flexor in the arms. (Modified from Plum and Posner.[56])

infarction in the midbrain, adjacent to the midline. Hemorrhages are more evident to the naked eye, but are probably the result of bleeding into the previously infarcted area in a patient who has survived some time, often after the compressing lesion has been removed.

LATERAL TRANSTENTORIAL HERNIATION. When the expanding lesion is towards one side of the cranial cavity, particularly if it is in the temporal lobe or middle cranial fossa, the brain is shifted sideways as well as downwards. The medial part of the temporal lobe (the uncus) is displaced towards the midline and over the free edge of the tentorium falx cerebelli. In this circumstance the distortion of the third cranial nerve and posterior cerebral artery occurs first on the side adjacent to the herniating uncus (Fig. 13). This is responsible for the characteristic clinical features of this variety of herniation (Fig. 14): early involvement of the third nerve on the same side as the expanding lesion causes dilatation of the pupil, loss of the light reflex (Fig. 15), ptosis, and eventually lateral deviation of the eye (owing to the unopposed action of the sixth cranial nerve). If the lesion expands at a relatively slow rate, pupillary changes can develop well in advance of impairment of consciousness. As herniation progresses the midbrain becomes narrowed from side to side and its border opposite the expanding lesion may be compressed against the free edge of the tentorium (Kernohan's notch). Focal infarction in this site can produce hemiplegia on the same side of the body as the expanding lesion; this is then a "false localizing" sign.

It is in their initial stages that the two kinds of tentorial herniation are most distinctive; both forms eventually produce dysfunction bilaterally in the midbrain

65

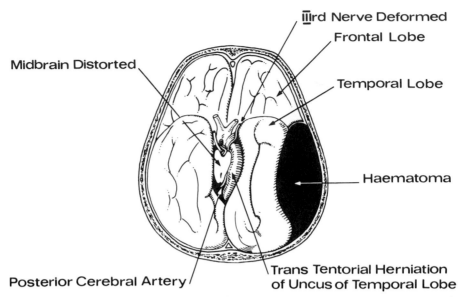

IIIrd Nerve Deformed

Frontal Lobe

Midbrain Distorted

Temporal Lobe

Haematoma

Posterior Cerebral Artery

Trans Tentorial Herniation
of Uncus of Temporal Lobe

Figure 13. Lateral tentorial herniation. A view of the undersurface of the cerebrum shows the distortion produced by a hematoma in the right temporal region. (Modified from Jennett.[72])

and then involve lower levels in the brain stem. In the brains of fatal cases, pathologists are accustomed to finding a combination of both types of hernia.

TONSILLAR HERNIA. The cerebellum and brain stem are forced downwards towards and through the foramen magnum. The medulla becomes compressed and the perfusion of the whole brain stem is in peril; the end result of unrelieved brain compression is respiratory arrest.

Infratentorial Lesions

With a lesion in the posterior fossa the brain stem may be compressed directly or as a consequence of tonsillar herniation. Disturbances of respiration can appear at an early stage without there having been clinical warning in the form of changes in consciousness or motor signs. Upward herniation through the tentorial hiatus rarely occurs after head injury, but might do so if acute hydrocephalus, caused by a clot in the posterior fossa, was relieved by ventricular drainage and the hematoma was not soon evacuated.

A Critical Rate of Compression?

It is a well-known clinical observation that slowly growing tumors can achieve greater size before giving rise to noticeable effects than more rapidly expanding lesions. Indeed there is a lack of any consistent relationship between the size of an intracranial mass and intracranial pressure, brain shift, and herniation. Because of the several dynamic processes that interact to determine the response to an expanding lesion, apparent inconsistencies are not surprising.

In studies in monkeys, Nakatani and Ommaya[48] showed that, below a certain rate of expansion, the inflation of an extradural balloon provoked little rise in intracranial pressure and no rise in systemic blood pressure before the pupils

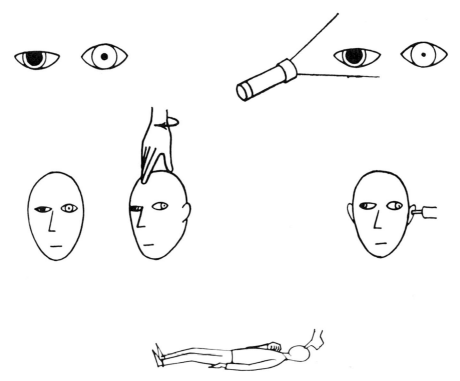

Figure 14. Clinical signs with lateral tentorial hernia resulting from a right supratentorial hematoma. The right pupil is dilated and un-reacting; there is ptosis and loss of medial movement in the right eye. Motor responses are abnormal on the left side. (Modified from Plum and Posner.[56]).

became dilated and EEG activity was lost. With faster rates of inflation, ICP did rise, a systemic pressure response occurred, and yet evidence of "terminal" brain compression was delayed and appeared only at greater balloon volumes than with the slow rates of compression. Extrapolating their results to man, they estimated that if a space-occupying lesion expanded at a rate below 0.3 ml/min, systemic blood pressure would not rise and a critical level of brain compression would be reached when the volume of the lesion reached 70 cc (5% of intracranial volume). In cats, Sullivan and his colleagues[67] expanded an extradural balloon at a rate roughly five times greater than the "critical" rate of Nakatani and Ommaya,[48] but usually saw a systemic pressure response only *after* pupillary dilatation had occurred. In this study the CSF pressure/volume relationships changed from the so-called "compensated" phase to one of rapidly worsening elastance when the balloon volume was 6 percent of estimated total intracranial volume; by the time of pupillary dilatation the balloon volume had increased to 10 percent.

Few precise clinical observations have been made in this field. In one study[13] the age of the patient was shown to be important in determining the extent of the effects resulting from a chronic subdural hematoma. Older patients, presumably having cerebral atrophy and thus a greater displaceable CSF volume, tolerated larger collections than younger patients.

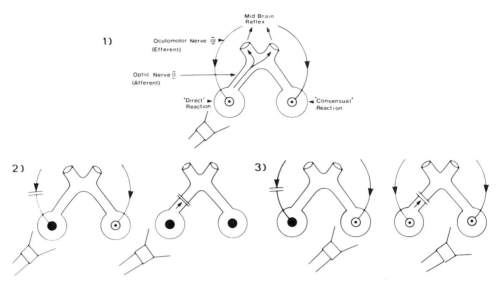

Figure 15. Pupillary light reflex. 1. Normal reflex pathways and reaction of pupils to light shone into the right eye. 2. Responses to light shone into the right eye in the presence of right oculomotor (third) nerve lesion (left) and right optic nerve lesion (right). 3. Responses to light shone into the left eye in the presence of right oculomotor (third) nerve lesion (left) and right optic nerve lesion (right). Direct and consensual responses are absent in the right eye with a third nerve lesion; consensual response is maintained with right optic nerve lesion.

Transmission of Increased Intracranial Pressure

When the CSF spaces are in free communication, the pressure measured at any one point will accurately reflect the level throughout the whole system. Being fluid, CSF will not support a pressure difference between two points unless there is either a substantial resistance between them or a complete block in the continuity of the spaces. Brain shift may produce just this situation. In tentorial herniation the aqueduct is narrowed and the cisterna ambiens around the brain stem and upper surface of the cerebellum is compressed and obliterated. When this has occurred there may be substantial differences between the pressure in the supratentorial compartment and that in the posterior fossa or spinal canal, where pressure can be falling while supratentorial pressure rises. Similarly, when there is coning at the foramen magnum, there is a pressure difference between the posterior fossa and the spinal canal.

When the CSF spaces are not in free communication, withdrawing fluid from one compartment may precipitate herniation. For this reason a lumbar puncture should never be performed in a head injured patient, unless meningitis is suspected and an expanding lesion has been excluded or is considered unlikely. Herniation may also be precipitated by any factor that makes the brain "tighter" (p. 62). For example, in animals with experimental expanding lesions, the vasodilatation resulting from the administration of halothane or CO_2 causes an increase in pressure gradients between supratentorial and infratentorial compartments, and this may be accompanied by pupillary dilatation even though the volume of the expanding lesion is remaining constant.[11,44]

Although there is clear evidence that pressure gradients can develop between major intracranial compartments, the possibility that the brain tissues can support differential pressures is more controversial. These differences have always been considered to be likely and to be responsible for initiating brain shift and herniation. It is now clear that there may be differences in the pressure of the brain tissues at different sites, with higher pressures close to an expanding lesion, but the magnitude of these pressure differences is not more than about 5 mm Hg. In stable conditions tissue gradients are likely to be dissipated and the pressure in the ventricular CSF can be taken as a reasonable representation of the pressure within the brain—at least within the same compartment of the skull.

BRAIN WATER AND EDEMA

The use of the term edema to cover all varieties of cerebral swelling may be correct on etymological grounds (*oidema,* Greek "swelling"), but it is becoming increasingly important to differentiate swelling caused by expansion of cerebral blood volume (engorgement) from that caused by an increase in brain water. In current usage, edema refers to an increase in tissue fluid content that results in an increase in tissue volume.

The brain has a high water content: 80 percent in normal gray matter and 70 percent in the white matter, where the fat content is higher. The majority of brain water is intracellular, but the extracellular fluid volume of the brain may make up as much as 10 percent of the intracranial space. Brain water is derived from the blood and ultimately returns to it. In the normal situation this is largely by re-entry at the venous end of the capillaries (Fig. 16). Relatively little brain water passes through the alternate pathway, via the CSF, but this route may be more important when edema is present.

Two different forms of cerebral edema are recognized: vasogenic and cyto-toxic.[24] In vasogenic edema the abnormality is thought to lie in the walls of the cerebral vessels, which allow outflow of fluid into the extracellular space.[57] This form of edema largely affects the white matter and may be the most common kind of edema encountered after head injury. Cytotoxic edema is a result of damage to the vitality of brain cells and the fluid is found within swollen neurons and glia in the gray matter.

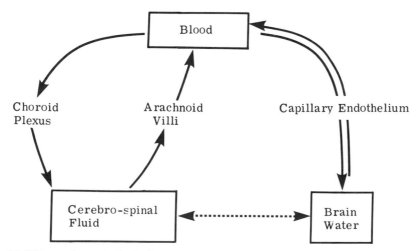

Figure 16. Water exchange in the brain.

The endothelial cells of the cerebral vessels normally prevent the passage of large molecules from the vascular space to the extracellular fluid. These cells are responsible for the blood-brain barrier, and their characteristic ultrastructural features are tight junctions between adjacent cells, no pores or fenestrations, and, in normal conditions, almost no vesicular transport. In vasogenic edema, large molecules, such as protein, are able to pass through the barrier, along with electrolytes and fluid. This may be due to an opening of the junctions between adjacent endothelial cells, but recent studies have suggested that there may be increased vesicular transport across the endothelial cells, from intravascular space to extracellular fluid. Whatever mechanism is responsible, the arterial pressure provides a driving force so that increasing arterial pressure can lead to an increase in edema. Conversely, if arterial pressure is lowered the development of edema is retarded.[58]

When the source of vasogenic edema is a local lesion within the brain, fluid passes away from the involved area into regions where barriers are still intact. In part the process of dissipation of edema is a simple diffusion, but it is now clear that there is also a bulk flow of the fluid, under the influence of tissue pressure gradients. The fluid flows through widened extracellular spaces, towards the ventricles, and this may result in a substantial portion of the edema being cleared from the brain into the CSF.[59]

After head injury edema is usually found focally, releated to contusions and hematomas; occasionally it may be more generalized throughout one or both hemispheres. The mechanisms responsible for the deleterious effects of brain edema are still controversial. One is a rise in intracranial pressure, either the overall level or local tissue pressure levels, which then reduces blood flow. However, cerebral blood flow may be reduced even before intracranial pressure rises.[39] Changes in intracellular ionic equilibrium, e.g., an increase in sodium and decrease in potassium, may be important in impairing the electrical excitability of the neurons and glia, and any changes in blood flow may be secondary to this.

DYNAMIC INTERACTIONS

The many factors that influence cerebral energy metabolism, cerebral blood flow, intracranial pressure, and the degree of shift of the brain are but the individual components in an overall pattern of interaction (Fig. 17). It is the net effect of these various interactions that determines the extent and pattern of dysfunction and damage within the brain. Also many of the consequences of brain damage, such as impaired cardiorespiratory function, altered cerebrovascular reactivity, and the development of cerebral edema, have effects that can "feed back" and accelerate the cycle of events leading to deterioration.

Measurement of the individual factors contributing to the interactions summarized in Figure 17 gives at best only an incomplete view of events in the brain after head injury. Yet in clinical circumstances it is rarely possible to observe more than one or two factors at a time and then usually on an intermittent basis only. The methods that have been employed and their results are discussed as each form of investigation is described in Chapter 6. Experimental studies have been limited by the difficulty of producing an appropriate animal model of human closed head injury (p. 21), but it seems likely that an injury sufficient to produce "concussion" can have profound, if transient, effects upon cerebral function and blood flow.

In a model of cerebral concussion in rats, Nilsson and Nordstrom[52] have shown

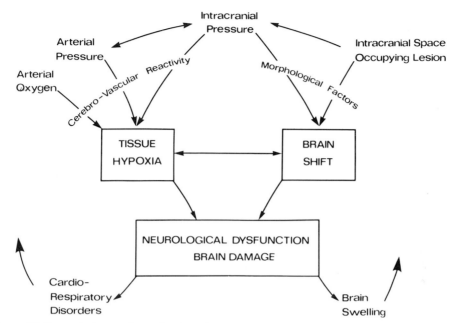

Figure 17. Dynamic interactions after head injury. Several pathological processes can interact and lead to brain damage.

that the immediate effects of impact include an increase in cerebral blood flow by about 50 percent; blood pressure and intracranial pressure also increase. The rise in blood flow cannot be explained wholly by disturbance of autoregulation and changes in perfusion pressure, for there is a fall in cerebrovascular resistance by 20 to 40 percent. It seems likely that the increase in blood flow, at least in part, is an adjustment to an increased rate of cerebral metabolism.[51,52] These experiments suggest therefore that the immediate effect of concussion is an excitation caused by a sudden depolarization of neurons, perhaps because of sudden release of neurotransmitters or because of mechanical effects upon neural membranes. Some other studies have, in contrast, suggested that the effect of concussion is to reduce cerebral electricity activity.[14]

In Nilsson's experiments the increase in blood flow was transient: 2 minutes after concussion, flow had fallen to about half of control values. This appeared to be due to vasoconstriction, for cerebral metabolic rate was still high and energy supply became inadequate. This would render the brain vulnerable to any impairment of respiratory function or cerebral perfusion and may be a critical phase in the development of hypoxic brain damage. Kontos and his colleagues,[26] using the fluid percussion model of cerebral concussion developed by Rinder and colleagues,[33] have also shown transient increases in blood pressure, and also dilatation and impaired reactivity of the pial blood vessels. Using the same model Miller and colleagues found impairment of the cerebral vascular response to carbon dioxide.[61]

The impact/acceleration model used by Nilsson and the fluid percussion model of Rinder both result in a pattern of brain damage maximum in the brain stem. Cerebral blood flow, metabolic rate, and cerebrovascular reactivity have been found to be impaired in many studies where localized lesions have been made in the brain stem by stereotaxic methods.[62] However, in some reports, although the lesions have produced severe neurological abnormality, the animals have shown no immediate change in cerebral blood flow and metabolism.[19]

Subarachnoid hemorrhage is a prominent feature of both the impact and the fluid percussion models of head injury. The possibility that vasospasm may contribute to ischemic brain damage is supported by the correlation between angiographic vasospasm and ischemic brain damage in fatal human head injuries.[38]

If diffuse impact injuries are most appropriately represented by a centripetal sequence of disruptive effects, as suggested by Ommaya (p. 22), brain stem effects will be found with only the most severe degrees of trauma. The relevance of models in which brain stem damage appears to be a major component in even mild injuries might then be questioned. However, trauma to the surface of the brain has long been recognized as an extremely potent way of impairing local cerebrovascular reactivity. Progression from a phase of arterial dilatation with increased blood flow to one of venous dilatation and stasis with reduced blood flow occurs over a period of an hour following direct trauma to the cerebral cortex.

CONCLUSION

After head injury the brain can be damaged by anoxic/metabolic disorders, by structural disruption and distortion, and, very often, by a combination of these pathological processes. The various basic mechanisms likely to be involved are now fairly well understood. Unfortunately, what is true for the normal brain may not apply after a head injury; moreover, the events observed in the experimentally injured animal are not necessarily those taking place in the brain of a head injured patient.

The interactions between normal and disordered cerebral mechanisms, and between intracranial and extracranial factors, can be complex. This sometimes can make it difficult to identify the primary problem in a particular clinical situation, but also means that the correction of any abnormality can have diverse beneficial effects. The aim in management of a head injury is to maintain, by the application of the principles described in this chapter, the intracranial milieu as near normal as possible. If this can be achieved, the risks of secondary brain damage will be minimized and the optimum circumstances will be provided for recovery from any damage that has already occurred.

REFERENCES

1. ASTRUP, J., SYMON, L., BRANSTON, N. M., ET AL.: *Cortical evoked potentials and extracellular K^+ and H^+ at critical levels of brain ischaemia.* Stroke 8:51–57, 1977.

2. ATKINSON, D. E.: *The energy charge of the adenylate pool as a regulatory parameter. Interaction with feedback modifiers.* Biochemistry 7:4030–4034, 1968.

3. BERING, E.A.: *Effects of profound hypothermia and circulatory arrest in cerebral oxygen metabolism and CSF electrolyte composition in dogs.* J. Neurosurg. 40:199–205, 1974.

4. BRANSTON, N. M., SYMON, L., CROCKARD, H. A., ET AL.: Relationship between the cortical evoked potential and focal cortical blood flow following acute middle cerebral artery occlusion in the baboon. Exp. Neurol. 45:195–208, 1974.

5. BRUCE, D. A., SCHUTZ, H., VAPALAHTI, M., ET AL.: *Pitfalls in the interpretation of xenon CBF studies in head-injured patients.* In Langfitt, T. W., McHenry, L. C., Reivich, M., et al. (eds.): *Cerebral Circulation and Metabolism.* Springer-Verlag, Berlin, 1975, pp. 406–408.

6. CAMERON, I. R.: *The chemical control of the cerebral circulation*. Clin. Sci. Molec. Med. 52:549–554, 1977.

7. DEMOPOULOS, H. B., MILVY, P., KAKAM, S., ET AL.: "Molecular aspects of membrane structure in cerebral oedema." In Schuermann, K., and Reulen, H. J. (eds.): *Steroids and Brain Edema*. Springer-Verlag, Berlin, 1972, pp. 29–39.

8. DEMOPOULOS, H. B., FLAMM, E. S., SELIQMAN, E., ET AL.: "Antioxidant effects of barbiturates in model membranes undergoing free radical damage. In Ingvar, D. H., and Lassen, N. A. (eds.): *Cerebral Function, Metabolism, and Circulation*. Munksgaard, Copenhagen, 1979, pp. 7.12–7.13.

9. DURET, H.: *Etudes experimentales et clinique sur les traumatismes cerebraux*. Paris, 1878.

10. EDVINSSON, L., AND MacKENZIE, E. T.: *Amine mechanisms in the cerebral circulation*. Pharmacol. Rev. 28:275–348, 1977.

11. FITCH, W., AND McDOWALL, D. G.: *Effect of halothane on intracranial pressure gradients in the presence of intracranial space occupying lesions*. Br. J. Anaesth. 43:904, 1971.

12. FLAMM, E. S., DEMOPOULOS, H. B., SELIQMAN, M. L., ET AL.: "Possible molecular mechanisms of the barbiturate-mediated protection in the regional cerebral ischaemia." In Ingvar, D. H., and Lassen, N. A., (eds.): *Cerebral Function, Metabolism and Circulation*. Munksgaard, Copenhagen, 1977, pp. 7.10–7.11.

13. FOGELHOLM, R., HEISKANEN, O., AND WALTIMO, O.: *Chronic subdural haematoma in adults. Influence of patient's age on symptoms, signs and thickness of haematoma*. J. Neurosurg. 42:43–46, 1975.

14. FOLTZ, E. L., JENKER, F. L., AND WARD, A. A.: *Experimental cerebral concussion*. J. Neurosurg. 10:342–352, 1953.

15. GIBSON, G. E., AND BLASS, J. P.: *Impaired synthesis of acetylcholine in brain accompanying mild hypoxia and ischaemia*. J. Neurochem. 27:37–42, 1976.

16. GORDON, E.: "The action of drugs on the intracranial contents." In Boulton, T., Bryce-Smith, R., Sykes, M., et al. (eds.): *Progress in Anaesthesiology*. Excerpta Medica Foundation, Amsterdam, 1970, pp. 60–68.

17. HAGERDAL, M., HARP, J., NILSSON, L., ET AL.: *The effect of induced hypothermia upon oxygen consumption in the rat brain*. J. Neurochem. 24:311–316, 1975.

18. HARP, J. R., AND WOLLMAN, H.: *Cerebral metabolic effects of hyperventilation and deliberate hypotension*. Br. J. Anaesth. 45:256–262, 1973.

19. HASS, W. K.: "Cerebral blood flow and metabolism after experimental brainstem trauma." In McLaurin, R. L. (ed.): *Head Injuries: Second Chicago Symposium on Neural Trauma*. Grune and Stratton, New York, 1975, pp. 209–211.

20. HOFF, J., SMITH, A. L., HANKINSON, H. L., ET AL.: *Barbiturate protection from cerebral infarction in primates*. Stroke 6:28–33, 1975.

21. HOSSMAN, K. A., AND KLEIHUES, P.: *Reversibility of brain damage*. Arch. Neurol. 29:375–382, 1973.

22. JENNETT, W. B., BARKER, J., FITCH, W., ET AL.: *Effects of anaesthesia on intracranial pressure in patients with space occupying lesions*. Lancet i:61, 1969.

23. KELLIE, G.: *The kind of appearances observed in the dissection of two or three individuals presumed to have perished in the storm of the 3rd and whose bodies were discovered in the vicinity of Leith on the morning of the 4th November 1821, with some reference to the pathology of the brain*. Trans. Med. Chi. Soc. Edin. 1:84–169, 1824.

24. KLATZO, I.: *Neuropathological aspects of brain oedema*. J. Neuropathol. Exp. Neurol. 24:1, 1967.

25. KOCHER, T.: *Hirnerschuttering, Hirndruck and Chirurgische Eingriffe bein Hirnsrkrankungen*. Nothnagel's Specialle Pathologie u Therapie 9:92, 1901.

26. KONTOS, H. A., WEI, E. P., NAVARI, R. M., ET AL.: *Responses of cerebral arteries and arterioles to acute hypotension and hypertension*. Am. J. Physiol. 234:H371-H383, 1978.

27. LANGFITT, T. W.: *Increased intracranial pressure*. Clin. Neurosurg. 16:436, 1969.

28. LASSEN, N. A.: *Brain extracellular pH: main factor controlling cerebral blood flow*. Scand. J. Clin. Lab. Invest. 22:247, 1968.

29. LASSEN, N. A., AND CHRISTENSEN, M. S.: *Physiology of cerebral blood flow*. Br. J. Anaesth. 48:719–734, 1976.

30. LEECH, P. J., MILLER, J. D., FITCH, W., ET AL.: *Cerebral blood flow, internal carotid artery*

pressure and the EEG as a guide to the safety of carotid ligation. J. Neurol. Neurosurg. Psychiatry 37:854–862, 1974.

31. LENINGER-FOLLERT, E., URBANICS, R., HARBIG, K., ET AL.: "The behaviour of local pH NADH-fluorescence during and after direct activation of the brain cortex." In Ingvar, D. H., and Lassen, N. A. (eds.): *Cerebral Function, Metabolism and Circulation.* Munksgaard, Copenhagen, 1977, pp. 11.6–11.7

32. LEVY, D. E., BRIERLEY, J. B., SILVERMAN, D. G., ET AL.: *Brief hypoxia-ischaemia initially damages cerebral neurons.* Arch. Neurol. 32:450–456, 1975.

33. LINDGREN, S., AND RINDER, L.: *Production and distribution of intracranial and intraspinal pressure changes at sudden extradural fluid volume input in rabbits.* Acta Physiol. Scand. 76:340–351, 1959.

34. LOFGREN, J., AND ZWETNOW, N. N.: *Influence of a supratentorial expanding mass on intracranial pressure-volume relationships.* Acta Neurol. Scand. 49:599–612, 1973.

35. MACKENZIE, E. T., MCCULLOCH, J., O'KEANE, M., ET AL.: *Cerebral circulation and norepinephrine: relevance of blood brain barrier.* Am. J. Physiol. 231: 483–488, 1976.

36. MACKENZIE, E. T., STRANDGAARD, S., GRAHAM, D. I., ET AL.: *Effects of acutely induced hypertension in cats on pial arteriolar caliber, local cerebral blood flow and the blood brain barrier.* Circ. Res. 39:33–41, 1976.

37. MACMILLAN, V., AND SIESJO, B. K.: "Cerebral energy metabolism." In Critchley, M., O'Leary, J. L., and Jennett, W. B. (eds.): *Scientific Foundations of Neurology.* Heinemann, London, 1972, pp. 21–32.

38. MACPHERSON, P., AND GRAHAM, D. I.: *Correlation between angiographic findings and the ischaemia of head injury.* J. Neurol. Neurosurg. Psychiatry 41:122–127, 1978.

39. MARMAROU, A., POLL, W., SHAPIRO, K., ET AL.: "The influence of brain tissue pressure upon local cerebral blood flow in vasogenic oedema." In Beks, J. W., Bosch, and Brock, M. (eds.): *Intracranial Pressure, III.* Springer-Verlag, Berlin, 1976, pp. 10–12.

40. MARMAROU, A., SHAPIRO, K., AND SHULMAN, K.: "Isolation of factors leading to sustained elevations of the ICP." In Beks, J. W., Bosch, and Brock, M. (eds.): *Intracranial Pressure, III.* Springer-Verlag, Berlin, 1976, pp. 33–36.

41. MARSHALL, L. F., SMITH, R. W., AND SHAPIRO, H. M.: *The outcome with aggressive treatment in severe head injuries. II. Acute and chronic barbiturate administration in the management of head injury.* J. Neurosurg. 50:26–30, 1979.

42. MICHENFELDER, J. D., MILDE, J. H., AND SUNDT, T. M., JR.: *Cerebral protection by barbiturate anaesthesia.* Arch. Neurol. 33:345–350, 1976.

43. MILLER, J. D.: *Volume and pressure in the craniospinal axis.* Clin. Neurosurg. 22:76–105, 1975.

44. MILLER, J. D.: "Effects of hypercapnia on pupillary size, ICP and cerebral venous PO_2 during experimental brain compression." In Lundberg, Ponten, and Brock (eds.): *Intracranial Pressure, II.* Springer-Verlag, Berlin, 1975, pp. 444–446.

45. MILLER, J. D., GARIBI, J., NORTH, J. B., ET AL.: *Effects of increased arterial pressure on blood flow in the damaged brain.* J. Neurol. Neurosurg. Psychiatry. 38:657–665, 1975.

46. MILLER, J. D., STANEK, A., AND LANGFITT, T. W.: *Concepts of cerebral perfusion pressure and vascular compression during intracranial hypertension.* Prog. Brain Res. 35:411–432, 1971.

47. MONRO, A.: *Observations on the Structure and Functions of the Nervous System.* Creech and Johnson, Edinburgh. 1783, pp. 5–6.

48. NAKATANI, S., AND OMMAYA, A. K.: "A critical rate of cerebral compression." In Brock, M., and Dietz, H. (eds.): *Intracranial Pressure, II.* Springer-Verlag, Berlin. 1972, pp. 144–148.

49. NEMOTO, E. M.: *Pathogenesis of cerebral ischaemia-anoxia.* Crit. Care Med. 6:203–214, 1978.

50. NEMOTO, E. M., KOFKE, W. A., KESSLER, P., ET AL.: "Studies on the pathogenesis of ischaemic brain damage and the mechanism of its amelioration by thiopental." In Ingvar, D. H., and Lassen, N. A. (eds.): *Cerebral Function, Metabolism and Circulation.* Munksgaard, Copenhagen, 1977, pp. 7.2–7.3.

51. NILSSON, B., AND NORDSTROM, C. H.: *Rate of cerebral energy consumption in concussive head injury in the rat.* J. Neurosurg. 47:274–281, 1977.

52. NILSSON, B., AND NORDSTROM, C. H.: *Experimental head injury in the rat. Part 3: cerebral blood flow and oxygen consumption after concussive impact acceleration.* J. Neurosurg. 47:262–273, 1977.

53. NORDSTROM, C. H., CALDERINI, G., REHNCRONA, S., ET AL.: "Effects of phenobarbital anaesthesia on post-ischaemic cerebral blood flow and oxygen consumption in the rat." In Ingvar, D. H., and Lassen, N. A. (eds.): *Cerebral Function, Metabolism and Circulation*. Munksgaard, Copenhagen, 1977, pp. 7.6–7.7

54. PICKARD, J. D., DURITY, F., WELSH, F. A., ET AL.: *Opening of the blood brain barrier: value in pharmacological studies on the cerebral circulation*. Brain Res. 122:170–176, 1977.

55. PICKARD, J. D., MACDONELL, L. A., MACKENZIE, E. T., ET AL.: *Prostaglandin-induced effects in the primate cerebral circulation*. Eur. J. Pharmacol. 43:343–351, 1977.

56. PLUM, F., AND POSNER, J. B.: *Stupor and Coma*. ed. 3. F. A. Davis, Philadelphia, 1980.

57. RAPOPORT, S. J.: *Blood Brain Barrier in Physiology and Medicine*. Raven Press, New York, 1977.

58. REULEN, H. J.: *Vasogenic brain oedema. New aspects in its formation, resolution and therapy*. Br. J. Anaesth. 48:741, 1976.

59. REULEN, H. J., GRAHAM, R., FENSKE, A., ET AL.: "The role of tissue pressure and bulk flow on the formation and resolution of cold induced oedema." In Pappius, H., and Feindel, W. (eds.): *Formation and Resolution of Brain Oedema*. Springer-Verlag, Berlin, 1976.

60. SAFAR, P., BLEYAERT, A., NEMOTO, E. M., ET AL.: *Resuscitation after global brain ischaemia-anoxia*. Crit. Care Med. 6:215–227, 1978.

61. SAUNDERS, M., MILLER, J. D., STABLEIN, D., ET AL.: *The effects of graded experimental trauma on cerebral blood flow and responsiveness to CO_2*. J. Neurosurg. 51:18–26, 1979.

62. SHALIT, M. N., REINMUTH, O. M., SHIMAJYO, S., ET AL.: *Carbon dioxide and cerebral circulatory control. III. The effects of brainstem lesions*. Arch. Neurol. 17:342–353, 1967.

63. SHAPIRO, H. M., WYTE, S. R., AND LOESER, J.: *Barbiturate-augmented hypothermia for reduction of persistent intracranial hypertension*. J. Neurosurg. 40:90–100, 1974.

64. SIESJO, B. K.: *Brain Energy Metabolism*. Wiley & Sons, New York, 1978.

65. SMITH, A. L., AND WOLLMAN, H.: *Cerebral blood flow and metabolism: effects of anaesthetic drugs and techniques*. Anaesthesiology 36:378–400, 1972.

66. SOKOLOFF, L.: *Relation between physiological function and energy metabolism in the central nervous system*. J. Neurochem. 29:13–26, 1977.

67. SULLIVAN, H. G., MILLER, J. D., BECKER, D. P., ET AL.: *The physiological basis of intracranial pressure change with progressive epidural brain compression*. J. Neurosurg. 47:532–550, 1977.

68. TEASDALE, G., ROWAN, J. O., TURNER, J. W., ET AL.: "Cerebral perfusion failure and cortical electrical activity." In Ingvar, D. H., and Lassen, N. A. (eds.): *Cerebral Function, Metabolism and Circulation*. Munksgaard, Copenhagen, 1977, pp. 23.14–23.15.

69. THEYE, R. A., AND MICHENFELDER, J. D.: *The effect of nitrous oxide on canine cerebral metabolism*. Anaesthesiology 29:1119–1124, 1968.

70. WOLLMAN, H., ALEXANDER, S. C., COHEN, P. J., ET AL.: *Cerebral circulation during general anaesthesia and hyperventilation in man: thiopental induction to nitrous oxide and tubocurarine*. Anaesthesiology 26:329, 1965.

71. YATSU, F. M., DIAMOND, I., GRAZIANO, C., ET AL.: *Experimental brain ischaemia; protection from irreversible damage with a rapid-acting barbiturate (methohexital)*. Stroke 3:726–732, 1972.

72. JENNETT, W. B.: *Introduction to Neurosurgery*. ed. 3. Year Book Medical Publishers, Chicago, 1977.

CHAPTER 4

Assessment of Impaired Consciousness

The most consistent characteristic of the brain damage that results from acceleration/deceleration trauma is altered consciousness. Half a century ago Symonds suggested that the duration of unconsciousness might be used as a measure of the degree of cerebral damage after closed head injuries.[30] Subsequent studies have confirmed that the degree and duration of coma does indeed provide a reliable guide to the severity of the *diffuse* brain damage sustained. However, *local* injury can be extensive and can cause focal neurological dysfunction, without there being any loss of consciousness; the most obvious example is when there is a compound depressed fracture.

Assessment of the level of consciousness is not only important as an index of severity of brain damage; repeated measures of the state of responsiveness also form the basis of monitoring the recently head injured patient. Change in the degree of impairment of consciousness is usually the best indicator of either improvement in the overall function of the brain, whether occurring naturally or as the result of treatment, or development of an intracranial complication. Continuous monitoring for this purpose depends largely on nurses and junior doctors, who change frequently during each 24-hour period. It is therefore necessary to have a system that is consistent when used by different observers and that can be recorded and displayed in such a way that different personnel can immediately recognize not only the patient's present state but also how this relates to his condition over the last few hours or days. These repeated observations will be more restricted than the initial physical examination, which subserves a diagnostic rather than a monitoring purpose.

GLASGOW SCALE

This practical scale was designed to meet the above-mentioned requirements.[13,32,33] It has been shown that nurses and general surgeons can be as consistent as neurosurgeons when using the scale, which is also relatively resistant to differences in language of the observers.[34] Moreover, it enables degrees and types of coma to be defined in descriptive terms, without reference to supposed anatomical sites of dysfunction or to levels that depend on the concurrence of certain degrees of responsiveness with other features (such as pupil reactions or abnormalities of respiration). Three features are independently observed: eye opening, motor response, and verbal performance (Table 1).

Table 1. Glasgow "Coma" Scale

Eye Opening		
spontaneous	E	4
to speech		3
to pain		2
nil		1
Best motor response		
obeys	M	6
localizes		5
withdraws		4
abnormal flexion		3
extensor response		2
nil		1
Verbal response		
orientated	V	5
confused conversation		4
inappropriate words		3
incomprehensible sounds		2
nil		1

Coma score (E + M + V) = 3 to 15

Eye Opening

The eyes may open spontaneously, or only when the patient is spoken to (not necessarily on command to open his eyes), or when he is given a painful stimulus, or not at all. Taking account of eye opening is vital when distinguishing coma from other unresponsive states, which becomes important after the first few days (p. 85).

Motor Response

The motor response in limbs is tested in patients who do not obey commands by two standardized stimuli: pressure on the nail bed using a pencil and supraorbital pressure. If the hand moves above the chin towards the supraorbital stimulus, the response is recorded as localizing. Patients who respond only by flexor withdrawal (without localizing) represent the next level of response. Abnormal or spastic flexion is scored if there is preceding extension movement in either arm or leg at the time of examination, or if there are two of the following responses: stereotyped flexion posture, extreme wrist flexion, abduction of the upper arm, or flexion of the fingers over the thumb. If there is doubt about this response, it should be recorded as flexor withdrawal. Nurses and nonspecialist doctors are sometimes in doubt about recognizing abnormal flexion, and for this reason abnormal flexion is omitted from some bedside charts used by nurses (Fig. 1). The next response is extension (at the elbow), and the lowest level of response is no motor movement at all.

The upper limbs show a greater range of responses than the lower and are usually the basis for assessing the motor response. A focal lesion causing hemiplegia will sometimes result in an extensor response on that side; on this scale it is the limb with the least abnormal response that is used to categorize the "best motor response." In the event that more than one type of response is observed in one limb during the course of the single examination, it is the *best* response that

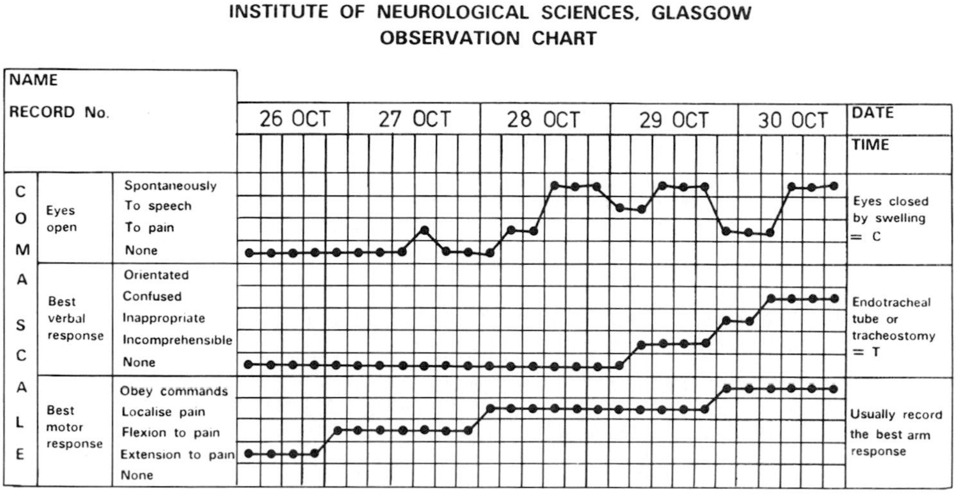

INSTITUTE OF NEUROLOGICAL SCIENCES, GLASGOW
OBSERVATION CHART

NAME								
RECORD No.		26 OCT	27 OCT	28 OCT	29 OCT	30 OCT	DATE	
							TIME	
C O M	Eyes open	Spontaneously / To speech / To pain / None					Eyes closed by swelling = C	
A S C	Best verbal response	Orientated / Confused / Inappropriate / Incomprehensible / None					Endotracheal tube or tracheostomy = T	
A L E	Best motor response	Obey commands / Localise pain / Flexion to pain / Extension to pain / None					Usually record the best arm response	

Figure 1. Coma chartlet.

is recorded. The pattern of response in all four limbs, which may be indicative of local brain damage, is of diagnostic and prognostic significance and should be recorded separately from this assessment of the responsiveness of the brain as a whole (p. 81). In recording the *best* motor response at any time it might be considered that significant abnormal movements would be overlooked, but with frequent assessment it will usually be found that the best response is better on some occasions than on others. This enables a picture of the response over a period of time to be drawn; this is best done by displaying the responsiveness of the patient on a chart (Fig. 1). Variations in responsiveness may be summarized by rating the best and the worst levels of the best motor response over a succession of periods of time. As explained later, it is the *best* response that correlates more closely with outcome and is therefore the more reliable marker of severity (Chapter 14).

Notice that this system avoids the use of words such as decerebrate, decorticate, and purposeful, when describing movements in the limbs, and no reference is made to tone. We have shown in observer-error trials that using such terms, which depend upon interpretation rather than on description of what is observed, incurs a greater degree of inter-observer variation than when the motor response is recorded by the terms of the Glasgow scale.

Verbal Performance

Speech is classified as normal, oriented conversation; confused conversation; inappropriate words (not in the form of exchange); grunts, groans, and incomprehensible conversation (sounds); or no vocalization at all. The capacity to speak even a few words indicates a high level of brain functioning, in comparison with coma or other unresponsive states. The converse is not true, however, and it is a limitation of some classifications that too much reliance is placed on the absence of speech. Verbal response may be impossible because of the presence of an endotracheal tube, and young children or patients who have only a foreign tongue may remain silent when other aspects of behavior betray a higher level of responsiveness. Such absence of speech also occasionally occurs when there is total aphasia. One of the advantages of this coma scale is that it allows responsiveness to be assessed even when some information is missing.

Definition of Coma

Unless coma is defined, its duration cannot be determined. In practice it is a word loosely used, and its scope is often stretched by adjectival qualifications — light coma, semi-coma, deep coma, and so on. For some, coma begins when speech is no longer observed; others would include in light coma patients who are talking and sensibly responsive but who are simply drowsy. Stupor is often used for altered alertness in patients who speak, and it may also be subdivided into light, semi, or deep.

The Head Injury Committee of the World Federation of Neurosurgical Societies has defined coma (or unconsciousness) as "an unrousable, unresponsive state, regardless of duration; eyes continuously closed."[9] This definition implies that there is no motor response to command and no speech. But the considerable range of motor activity in the limbs that can occur in response to painful stimuli in patients in coma is an indication of responsiveness, as are pupil reactions and eye reflex movements; even the patient who is "brain dead" may be responsive at a spinal level. It is therefore misleading to define coma as an "unresponsive state."

We have defined coma as "not obeying commands, not uttering words, and not opening the eyes." This definition of coma has been used as a criterion in the International Data Bank study and has proved to be acceptable and practical in several clinics in different countries. In practice this definition corresponds closely to that proposed by the Head Injury Committee mentioned above,[9] but it is a rigorous definition of coma in that if a patient does not meet any one of the three components he is regarded as not in coma. This excludes some patients who would be in coma by definitions based on inability *either* to obey commands or to speak, but not both. In over 2000 early observations on patients in coma after severe head injuries, we observed 4 percent who did not speak but who could obey commands, and another 4 percent who uttered words but did not obey. Among patients who could neither obey nor speak, 16 percent opened their eyes and were therefore judged not to have been in coma by our definition.[13] This can be of importance when comparing outcome in series of cases of supposedly similar severity on the basis of coma and its duration. Eye opening as part of the definition ensures that coma is distinguished from other forms of reduced responsiveness (p. 85).

Coma Score (or Sum)

The overall responsiveness can be expressed by giving each response on each component of this scale a number higher by one than the less responsive grade below it (Table 1). If these are summed, a score is obtained, which ranges from 3 (least responsive) to 15. When patients are in deep coma they will usually be intubated and a verbal score cannot be given. However, analysis of the coma scores in 1000 patients in the Data Bank indicates that in the first day or so after head injury, coma sums of 3, 4, 5, and 6 reflect the best motor response, and from this alone an estimate of the coma score can be made (Table 1). After the first few days, however, the eyes may open, and even in patients who neither obey nor speak one response score may be made up of different combinations. The coma score correlates closely with outcome, as do the grades of response on each component of the scale (Chapter 14). In the range from 3 to 15 there is not a point that discriminates absolutely between patients in coma (by our definition) and those who are more responsive than this. However, all combinations that sum to 7 or less define coma, as do 53 percent of those totalling 8; thus 90 percent of all observations summing to 8 or less, and none of those that add up to 9 or more, define coma.

Other Aspects of Coma

Plum and Posner's classic text, *Diagnosis of Stupor and Coma,*[24] proposed that the determination of the cause and of the site of the lesions associated with these states should be based on the pattern of changes in five physiological functions: state of consciousness, pupillary reaction, eye movements, ocular reflexes, motor responses, and breathing patterns. The coma scale described above deals only with state of consciousness, and alone it does not adequately describe brain dysfunction in the comatose patient. Each of these other functions may, however, be disordered by reason of local brain damage rather than from brain dysfunction as a whole, and in some circumstances the correlation between these abnormalities and the depth of coma may not be very close. On the other hand, they frequently provide useful clues to local damage, in particular to the development of tentorial herniation. These other aspects of coma are recorded on the same chart as the coma scale in this Institute (Fig. 2).

Motor Response Pattern

In distinction to the *best* motor response in any limb, which is recorded on the coma scale, it is important to take account of all four limbs. Hemiplegia is noted, and whether abnormal flexion or extensor limb responses are unilateral or bilateral. Development of focal signs may indicate that a local intracranial complication has occurred, in particular hematoma, infarction, or brain shift. Prognosis is progressively less favorable when there is abnormal flexion, extensor response, or motor unreactivity; bilateral abnormalities are worse than unilateral. However, no marked difference is observed in the outcome of groups of patients who have hemiplegia, with weakness as distinct from abnormal responses, and those who have normal, symmetrical motor activity. This emphasizes yet again the different significance that attaches to focal brain damage, as distinct from dysfunction that affects the brain more widely.

Pupil Reaction and Size

Great emphasis is traditionally placed on pupil function in the assessment and monitoring of recently head injured patients. Yet the interpretation of the findings can be difficult because pupil size and responses are sensitive to a range of different influences. Like motor responses, abnormalities may reflect local tissue damage (in the globe or in the nerves involved in the reflex activity of the iris), or they may indicate the functional state of the brain stem as a whole and be related to the depth of coma. However, it is important to realize that bilateral local damage to peripheral structures may on occasion cause nonreacting pupils, which may be

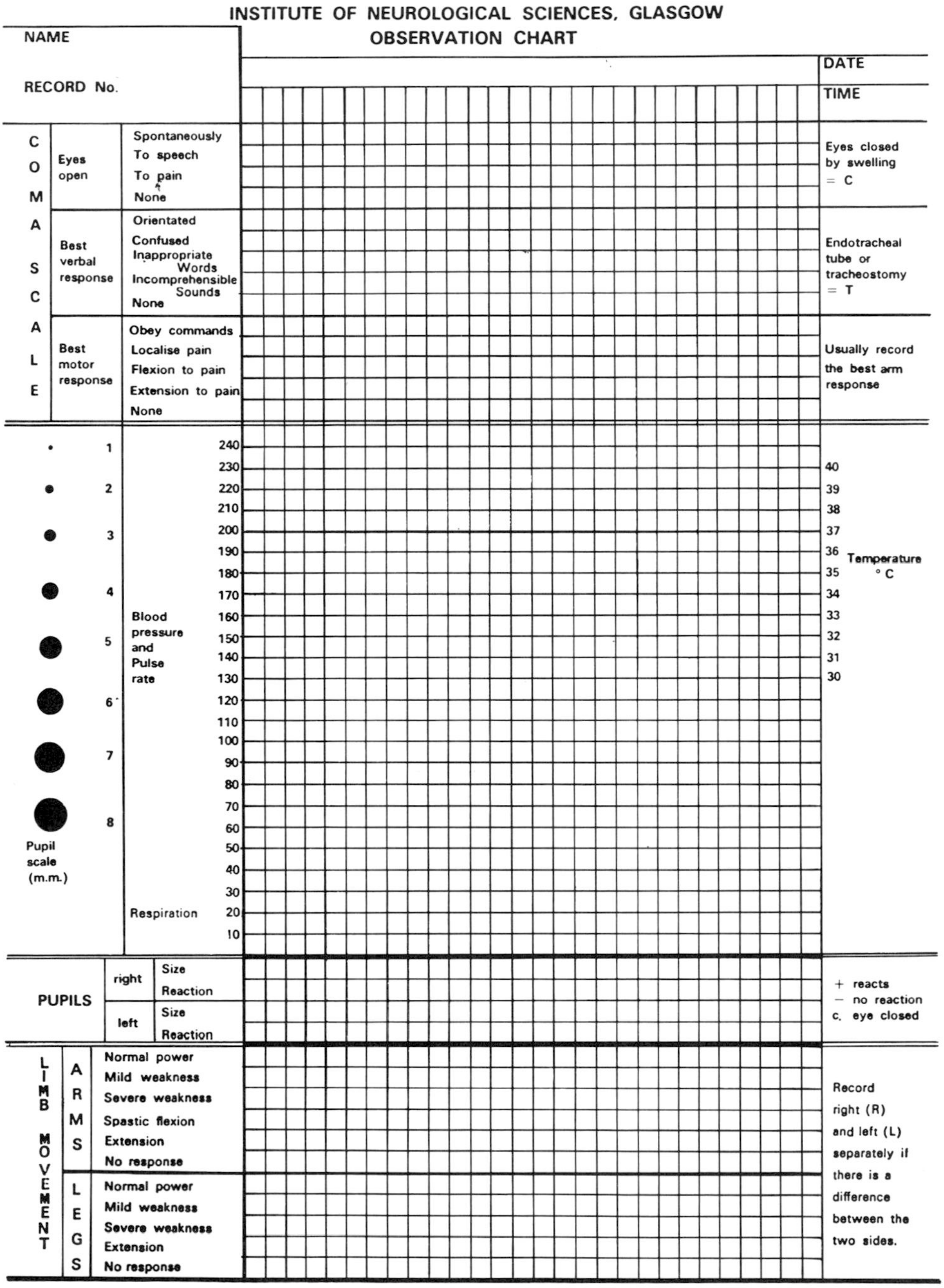

INSTITUTE OF NEUROLOGICAL SCIENCES, GLASGOW
OBSERVATION CHART

| NAME | | | | DATE |
| RECORD No. | | | | TIME |

C O M A	Eyes open	Spontaneously / To speech / To pain / None		Eyes closed by swelling = C
A S C A L E	Best verbal response	Orientated / Confused / Inappropriate Words / Incomprehensible Sounds / None		Endotracheal tube or tracheostomy = T
	Best motor response	Obey commands / Localise pain / Flexion to pain / Extension to pain / None		Usually record the best arm response

Pupil scale (m.m.): 1, 2, 3, 4, 5, 6, 7, 8

Blood pressure and Pulse rate: 240, 230, 220, 210, 200, 190, 180, 170, 160, 150, 140, 130, 120, 110, 100, 90, 80, 70, 60, 50, 40, 30

Respiration: 20, 10

Temperature °C: 40, 39, 38, 37, 36, 35, 34, 33, 32, 31, 30

| PUPILS | right | Size / Reaction | | + reacts |
| | left | Size / Reaction | | − no reaction / c. eye closed |

| LIMB MOVEMENT | ARMS | Normal power / Mild weakness / Severe weakness / Spastic flexion / Extension / No response | | Record right (R) and left (L) separately if there is a difference between the two sides. |
| | LEGS | Normal power / Mild weakness / Severe weakness / Extension / No response | | |

Figure 2. Full observation chart.

mistakenly interpreted as indicating severe brain stem dysfunction. Likewise some drugs, either locally instilled drops or systemically taken compounds, cause the pupils to be unreactive. Temporarily unreacting pupils can occur with an epileptic fit or with an episode of anoxia, owing to various combinations of systemic hypotension and hypoxemia with raised ICP. By contrast, metabolically induced coma does not affect pupil reactions. The clue to these spurious causes of nonreacting pupils is their occurrence either at a time when there is a relatively high level of responsiveness in other modalities, or when these other influences are known to be present. Before accepting pupils as unreacting, it is important also to be satisfied that an adequate light stimulus has been used; the feeble pen torch in a brightly lit intensive care unit is not enough.

Bilaterally unreacting pupils for a period of several hours usually indicate severe brain dysfunction, when all other influences have been reasonably excluded. However, too much reliance should not be placed on this sign alone. In the Data Bank study only two thirds of the observations of unreacting pupils in this series were associated with a low responsiveness score (3–5); by contrast, half of the cases with a coma score as low as this had reacting pupils, as did 10 percent of those who had no motor response.

Eye Movements

These may be abnormal as a result of depression of brain stem dysfunction as a whole or disconnection of the stem from rostral influences; focal damage in the brain stem; lesions in the pathways of the external ocular muscles; or damage to the vestibular apparatus and its nerve supply. They may therefore provide useful information about focal damage caused by impact or secondary developments, and they may also reflect the depth of coma. In uncooperative patients the eye movements can be elicited reflexly by head movements (oculocephalic) and by caloric stimulation (oculovestibular) (Table 2). Before eliciting oculocephalic reflexes, cervical spine fracture should be excluded. For the oculovestibular reflex, the head should be rotated 30 degrees to one side and flexed about 30 degrees; it should be established that the drum is intact, and that it is not obscured by wax.

For patients in coma a stronger stimulus is used than that employed in neuro-otological investigation. Ice-cold water is introduced in 20 ml amounts; before declaring the oculovestibular reflex to be absent, 100 ml should have been used. If the drum is recently perforated (by trauma), then cold water can be injected

Table 2. Eye movement scales

Spontaneous	1	Normal
	2	Conjugate roving
	3	Dysconjugate roving
	4	Lateral deviation
	5	Absent
Oculocephalic	1	Nil (normal)
	2	Full
	3	Minimal
	4	Absent
Oculovestibular	1	Nystagmus (normal)
	2	Conjugate tonic
	3	Dysconjugate tonic
	4	Absent

through a small catheter looped into the meatus, or into a needle guard introduced into the external canal.

For various reasons it is not always possible (or valid) to test all three kinds of movement; a method has therefore been devised to take account of limited data being available by constructing a composite eye score; these categories correlate well with outcome (Chapter 14). A high level of responsiveness (coma score >8) was almost always associated with intact eye movements. However, in patients with deeper coma, all grades of eye movement response were encountered (Table 3). Absent eye movements were associated with the lowest response on the coma scale in 75 percent of cases; high levels were very unusual. Some anomalous findings can be explained by the effects of depressant or anticonvulsant drugs. There are enough exceptions at the extremes to make it unwise to assume an absolute correlation between eye movements and other signs of responsiveness. On the other hand, eye movements graded as described above provide a good way of extending the assessment of degrees of severity that can be recognized in patients whose level of responsiveness is low.

Table 3. Eye signs associated with different coma scores in first 24 hours of coma

| | Coma Score (E + M + V) | | |
	3/4/5	6/7	>8
Composite eye movement scale	234	329	199
Absent	28%	7%	1%
Bad	24%	9%	2%
Impaired	22%	18%	12%
Good	26%	65%	85%

Respiration and Other Autonomic Features

Most of the clinical aspects of coma already described are reflections of brain stem dysfunction. This dysfunction may also give rise to disorders of respiration, heart rate, and blood pressure—as described in Cushing's classic triad of brain stem compression. Plum and Posner proposed that abnormalities of respiration were the most useful of these, and that they should be recorded as part of the assessment of the patient in coma.[24]

About 60 percent of 1000 patients in the Data Bank of severe injuries had one or more autonomic abnormalities during the first week, and more than half of these patients had more than one such autonomic abnormality. They were more commonly observed in patients whose response was low. However, only a minority of patients in the deepest coma at any one epoch showed such abnormalities. Moreover, they are liable to fluctuate considerably during any epoch and may be produced or aggravated by extracranial complications, such as hypoxia, hypovolemia, or pulmonary congestion and infection, as well as being sensitive to the effects of depressant drugs. When breathing patterns were mechanically monitored (p. 143), they were found to be very variable after recent structural brain damage such as head injury, and studies indicated that different patterns did not correlate closely with outcome.[15] It therefore seems unwise to consider respiratory abnormalities as a good index of the degree of coma, although they may be important diagnostically or as an indication for therapeutic intervention.

WAKEFUL REDUCED RESPONSIVENESS

When the eyes open spontaneously a patient may be said to be awake, and this will usually be associated with an aroused EEG pattern. However, some patients may remain in states of markedly reduced responsiveness and may be regarded by many doctors and nurses as still "in coma." It is important to distinguish a number of these states from coma—both in the early stages after injury, when the initial diagnosis is in question, and later when the duration of coma is a matter of consequence. In four of these states the patient is not only awake but is aware. None of these is at all frequent in association with head injury: the first three usually result from ischemic strokes; but patients who suffer a major stroke not infrequently fall and sustain a head injury, while patients who have had a primary head injury may suffer secondary cerebral vascular lesions. It is wise, therefore, to have these conditions in mind when there are doubts as to whether a patient is conforming to the usual pattern of a head injury.

Locked-In Syndrome

This syndrome, defined by Plum and Posner,[24] results from interruption of motor pathways in the ventral pons, usually by infarction. This state of de-efferentation leaves the patient tetraplegic and mute, but responsive and sentient; communication may be possible by code using blinking, or movements of the jaw or eyes, all of which are spared.

Akinetic Mutism

This was described by Cairns and associates[5] in a patient with a high brain stem lesion; it appears to resemble the *coma vigile* previously associated with typhoid. The state may fluctuate: occasional words may be uttered and some movement occur at times. Some patients who have recovered can recall events that occurred when they were mute.

Complete Aphasia

This may occasionally be mistaken for a state of reduced consciousness, but the preservation of normal motor function provides a clue to diagnosis.

Psychiatric States

These include schizophrenic catatonic stupor (now rarely encountered) and hysterical coma. In the latter state the EEG is normally aroused and eye movements (spontaneous, oculocephalic, and oculovestibular) are preserved to a degree incompatible with the apparent unresponsiveness of the patient.

Vegetative State

In contrast to the above conditions, which are associated with a functioning cerebral cortex and with awareness, the vegetative state implies that there is no cerebral cortical function, as judged behaviorally.[12] This can result from diffuse cerebral hypoxia (in patients with neocortical necrosis following "successful" resuscitation after cardiac arrest); the other common cause is severe shearing lesions in the white matter caused by the impact brain damage from head injury (p. 26). Patients in this state have quite a wide range of responses, including eye opening (with sleep and wake rhythms) and sometimes the ability to follow with the eyes; they usually make postural reflex adjustments with the limbs, and their hands may show a grasp reflex. These responses are often interpreted by relatives (and sometimes by nurses) as signs of returning consciousness and grounds for optimism regarding further recovery. But such responses can all occur at the subcortical level, and these patients never speak, nor do they make any response that is psychologically meaningful.

BRAIN DEATH

Like the vegetative state this is a product of modern intensive care, in that patients with such severe brain damage did not previously survive. But the problem of brain death is quite different, because the patient is dependent on a ventilator. However much is done, the heart always stops beating within a week or so, usually after a few days. Once brain death is established there is progressive dissolution of the organs, beginning with the brain, no matter how much artificial support is provided. If organ donation is a possibility, there is therefore need to discontinue ventilation while the organs (and in particular the kidneys) are still viable. But even when transplantation is not an issue (as indeed it relatively seldom is), it is still important to establish the diagnosis of brain death and to act appropriately by discontinuing ventilation. To continue artificial means of support once brain death has been declared deprives the patient of death with dignity and needlessly extends a harrowing experience for the relatives. Continuing to support brain dead patients may deny a chance of recovery to other patients, who cannot be admitted because the facilities are fully committed; it can also be bad for the morale of intensive care staff.

Although brain death and vegetative state are so distinct, public misunderstanding of the issues involved is inevitable, particularly when it appears, from reports by the press and the media, that doctors are not always clear in their minds about the difference. It was widely reported that Karen Quinlan's doctors believed that she would not survive without a ventilator, but she lived for years after the withdrawal of that support.[3] It is therefore essential to recognize the difference between the vegetative state and brain death (Fig. 3).

In the 20 years since Mollaret and Goulon[14] described *coma depassé* there has been extended debate about the medical, legal, and philosophical aspects of this artefact of nature. There is now widespread agreement that once brain death is confidently diagnosed, it is appropriate to discontinue mechanical ventilation, but there are differences between countries in the ways and means by which brain death is confirmed, and in the extent to which changes in legislation are regarded as necessary.[29] Many states in North America now have statutes that recognize that death can be declared prior to withdrawing ventilation, if it has been decided that the patient is brain dead. This protects those concerned from being held responsible for the patient's death, a defense that has been claimed (unsuccessfully) in a number of cases when the brain dead patient had suffered head injury from assault. The majority of these statutes do not specify the criteria by which brain death is to be determined, accepting that this is a technical matter for doctors and liable to change as more knowledge and experience is acquired. No

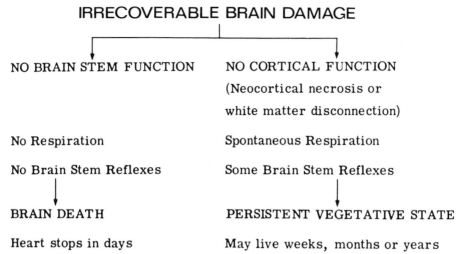

Figure 3. Differences between brain death and the vegetative state.

previous legislation had ever done more than rule that a person was dead when a doctor said so; these recent statutes simply indicate that brain death is one among several circumstances in which a doctor may declare a patient dead. These statutes dispose of any ambiguity about the doctor's action when he withdraws ventilation after brain death; he is then stopping doing something to a person who is already dead, not letting one of his patients die. It follows from this that the time of death is when brain death is declared, and not some later time when the heart stops.

The criteria used for diagnosing brain death reflect several underlying assumptions, or concepts. Differences in criteria between one country or institution and another, or between those in current use compared with those published 10 to 15 years ago, can mostly be traced to differing concepts of brain death. When the Ad Hoc Committee of the Harvard Medical School published its now famous report in 1968[1], the implicit assumption was that the whole nervous system had to be dead—cerebral cortex, brain stem and spinal cord. Its requirement that there be no motor activity in the limbs had to be modified when it became clear that spinal reflexes could not only persist after brain stem death, but often became more active the longer such a dead person continued to be ventilated. As experience with thousands of brain death cases each year has accumulated, there has also been a gradual realization that the EEG is not as relevant as was once believed. It has become apparent that once the brain stem is dead there is loss of activity not only downward to respiration but also upward to the cortex; even if residual activity persists for a time in parts of the isolated cortex, the outlook is the same—invariably there is cardiac asystole with 14 days, usually much sooner. This empirical observation of the consequences of brain stem death has now been made in many hundreds of cases in which ventilatory support has been maintained after brain death was clinically diagnosed.[11] The concepts underlying current criteria of brain death are that when the brain stem is dead, the brain is dead; and when the brain is dead, the person is dead.[8] It is acknowledged that death is a process and not an event, as was stated in the WMA Declaration of Sydney in 1968; what matters for the death of a person is not the point of death of different

87

organs or cells, but the certainty that the process has become irreversible by any technique of resuscitation; and a person cannot be considered alive because some organs or cells continue to function. This concept, and the shift of emphasis to the death of the brain stem, makes the EEG an irrelevant investigation, particularly in the view of some British neurologists and neurophysiologists.[16,21] The Harvard committee did not regard it as a mandatory examination, and this was emphasized by subsequent American commentators.[2,6,17,28] The statements of the American Neurological Association between 1973 and 1978 progressively relegate the role of the EEG in the diagnosis of brain death, although maintaining that it can be a valuable confirmatory test. Its main use, however, is to provide reassurance to physician and family rather than to make a clinical diagnosis more reliable—as Plum has observed.[22,23]

Criteria

With the above concepts in mind, it follows that the objective of diagnostic criteria is to determine that brain stem function has irreversibly ceased. The criteria published in 1976 by the UK Royal Colleges and their Faculties[7] reflect the changes to the Harvard recommendations that experience since 1968 has made necessary. They comprise two components, the pre-conditions and the tests. Only when the pre-conditions have been satisfied is it proper to proceed to the tests—and allegations of premature and mistaken suspicion of brain death usually prove to be the result of inadequate attention to the pre-conditions.

The pre-conditions are designed to establish that the depression of brain stem function (that the subsequent tests may show) cannot be due to reversible factors. There must be evidence of irremediable structural brain damage; in more than half the cases in Britain this is head injury, and in almost a third spontaneous intracranial hemorrhage. Other cases include those who have not responded to treatment for brain tumor or abscess, encephalitis, meningitis, or who have suffered an episode of cardiac arrest or profound hypotension. Factors that might be combining with structural damage to depress the brain stem must be excluded—depressant drugs (including alcohol), relaxant drugs (given to facilitate initial intubation or continued mechanical ventilation), hypothermia and gross metabolic imbalance. While some of these factors can be excluded by laboratory tests, the best safeguard against underestimating their influence is to allow enough time to elapse *before* undertaking confirmatory tests of the absence of brain stem function. It takes at least 6 hours in most instances to establish that irremediable structural brain damage has occurred; this gives time for initial resuscitation to be completed, and also allows alcohol levels to fall below a level that could account for complete unresponsiveness. If cerebral hypoxia has been the cause (or a main contributary cause) of brain damage, testing of brain stem function should be postponed for at least 6 hours. When the cause of the brain damage is in doubt, or when drugs are suspected but levels cannot be measured, it may be necessary to wait for 48 to 72 hours.

The tests consist of a series of brainstem reflexes—corneal, pupillary, gag, facial, and vestibulo-ocular (p. 83). If there is no response to any of these, the final and most crucial test is done. This is to confirm that there is no spontaneous respiratory movement when the patient is disconnected from the ventilator for a time sufficient to allow $PaCO_2$ to reach a level that will act as a strong stimulus to respiration, but not so high as to be depressant.

The duration of disconnection depends on the starting level of $PaCO_2$ (which is often low because of therapeutic hyperventilation) and the rate of CO_2 production (which is low in such patients). If 5 percent CO_2 and oxygen is administered until the $PaCO_2$ is about 45 mm Hg, then disconnection for 10 minutes will suffice. During this period 6 L per minute of oxygen should be administered through a tracheal catheter, to maintain oxygenation by diffusion. Patients with chronic respiratory insufficiency, accustomed to an abnormally high level of $PaCO_2$, require special consideration. Tests are customarily repeated, to exclude observer-error, after a period of approximately 30 minutes. The time interval that matters for diagnosis is that between the ictus producing apnea and the performance of tests on the first occasion.

DURATION OF ALTERED CONSCIOUSNESS

Using the Glasgow scale, duration of altered consciousness can now be defined in one of several different ways. One method would be determining when the patient is no longer "in coma" by the definition given; another would be to take progress on one component of the scale—such as when the patient speaks or first obeys commands. Many patients show a close correlation between the return of one function and another, but in a considerable number there is a discrepancy. In 700 patients emerging from coma during the first week after head injury, we observed about a quarter of these patients who could obey commands before they could speak, and a quarter who could speak before they could obey commands. Once patients are speaking it is obvious that the brain is functioning at a fairly high level—at this stage the distinction between expletive language (words), confused conversation, and normal orientation provides a useful means of grading brain dysfunction. However, there are several reasons other than coma why a patient does not speak. Children often remain mute with strangers, particularly given the frightening experience of recent injury; a patient may converse only in a foreign tongue; or he may be prevented from speaking by mechanical factors, such as endotracheal intubation or faciomaxillary injuries.

Post-traumatic Amnesia

Only 4 years after Symond's paper[30] it was proposed by Russell[25] that the recovery of *full* consciousness correlated with the quantum of brain damage that had occurred. He observed that the last readily recognizable function to return during the recovery from coma was on-going (anterograde) memory, and that the duration of altered consciousness could be assessed retrospectively from the patient's own account of when he regained his memory. The interval between the injury and this event was termed the post-traumatic amnesia (PTA). The end of PTA is when the patient begins to lay down continuous memory of on-going events—when he remembers today what happened yesterday and does not begin each day with a blank mind. He usually refers to this point in his recovery as the time when he first "woke up" or "came to." Some patients have occasional islands of memory prior to the return of continuous memory, but these can usually be identified by the patient as such. Sometimes the end of PTA can be precisely determined: the patient remembers the ward clock, or asking a visitor the date; or there is an event that acts as a marker, such as his transfer from one ward to another, or some family anniversary or national festival.

The patient's PTA does not end until some time after he has been judged by those around him to have "regained consciousness," usually because he has begun to speak. An approximate guide to the relationship between the return of speech and the end of PTA is that the interval from injury to the end of PTA is about four times longer than the interval until he first speaks (unless there has been a specific factor delaying the return of speech). However, relatives may remember when the patient first remembered their previous visit, or "became really sensible" or "was himself"; this usually correlates with the end of PTA. If tests of orientation are being given day by day, the end of PTA will be found to correspond closely with the end of spatial disorientation.

Even when PTA cannot be accurately estimated, it is almost always possible to judge whether it lasted for minutes, hours, days, or weeks. In fact it was a scale of this kind, approximately logarithmic, that Russell originally proposed and that he used to show the correlation between the PTA and the subsequent recovery of patients with head injury. This scale has now been used in many studies, and this is an expanded version:

> Less than 5 minutes—very mild
> 5 to 60 minutes—mild
> 1 to 24 hours—moderate
> 1 to 7 days—severe
> 1 to 4 weeks—very severe
> More than 4 weeks—extremely severe

The relationship between PTA and various other features of head injury was reviewed by Russell in 1946[27] and 1961.[26] Since then there have been further studies that have confirmed the close relationship between the duration of PTA and various sequelae of head injury.

It is often important to be able to assess the severity of injury long after the event, perhaps months or years later. The original notes are then seldom available, and even when they are they seldom contain as much information as is hoped. In such circumstances the PTA enables the severity of diffuse brain damage to be assessed without any data from witnesses, or the availability of any documents, because it depends on the patient's own account. In 1961 a Lancet editorial[14] agreed with the comment of an American author[4] that "PTA is the best yardstick for assessing severity of head injury." In spite of this, very few reports on head injury from North America or from continental Europe include PTA as a measure of severity. This may be because the degree of accuracy required in estimating the duration of PTA is misunderstood; or because of inappropriate use of data about PTA when they are used to define the severity in groups of patients (see below). The best way to describe a series of patients is either by the minimum duration of PTA or by the distribution of PTA durations. For example, the survivors among the 1000 patients in the Data Bank *all* had a PTA of more than 2 days; 94 percent more than a week; 80 percent more than 2 weeks; and 60 percent more than 4 weeks. A mean or average PTA with a standard deviation should never be quoted, because the distribution is not Gaussian. For example, a recent paper quoted a mean PTA of 37 days with a standard deviation of 43 days, which suggested that some patients had a negative PTA duration! Similarly, when comparing series of patients with "long" and "short" PTA, it is necessary to ensure that there is no overlap between the populations, i.e., that the shorter of the long, and the longer of the short durations are in fact distinguished. Failure to classify PTA in this way has led to some authors failing to find a correlation between PTA and various aspects of outcome.

PATHOLOGICAL SUBSTRATE OF ALTERED CONSCIOUSNESS
AFTER HEAD INJURY

Symonds has argued, from a clinical standpoint, that the difference between patients who remain unconscious for days or weeks rather than for minutes or hours could be in the *quantity* of brain damage, and not in the *kind* of lesion or its location.[31] He proposed that mild and severe concussion should be recognized; the most obvious pathological counterpart for this would be varying degrees of shearing damage of the white matter. There is some pathological evidence to support this view. Oppenheimer reported microglial stars in patients who had recovered from "concussion lasting only a few minutes," but who then died from an unrelated condition.[20] Moreover, Adams' group did not find (in human head injuries) any abnormality of nerve cell bodies (e.g., chromatolysis) in the brain stem of the kind previously described as a feature of concussion in animals, and which was an important part of the evidence adduced to support the view that primary brain stem damage is a consistent feature of blunt head injury. Indeed, attention is now shifting away from the brain stem as the site of the lesion responsible for the brief alteration of consciousness implied by the term concussion. An alternative explanation would be shearing lesions of a degree that tear only a few axons, but cause a stretch of many, with subsequent temporary failure of conduction in these nerve fibers. This would provide an explanation for the cumulative effect of repeated mild concussion[10] and would be compatible with the evidence that even mild concussion is associated with structural damage, albeit slight, which leaves its permanent mark in the brain.

However, the mechanisms underlying impaired consciousness after head injury are incompletely understood. There may be different explanations for brief concussion, for immediate deep and persisting coma, and for coma that develops secondarily after a lucid interval. It seems likely that the final common path for lesions that cause unconsciousness is inactivation of a sufficient proportion of the cerebral cortex. Cortical contusions by themselves are seldom of sufficient extent to bring about loss of consciousness. Certainly focal contusion and even laceration can be very marked (e.g., under a depressed fracture) without there being any *initial* impairment of conscious level. But severe contusions can lead to significant occupation of space once edema and local extravasation of blood develop around them; and *delayed or continued* coma may be due to this, even when there is not a discrete intracranial hematoma. With or without a hematoma the consequences are similar: raised intracranial pressure and internal herniations, which affect consciousness either by impairing perfusion of the cerebral cortex or by producing dysfunction in the ascending reticular system because of midbrain distortion, infarction, or hemorrhage.

Immediate coma that persists is probably due in most instances to widespread and severe impact damage to white matter, associated with disconnection of large areas of the cerebral cortex. Deep coma that persists is a consistent feature of those patients whose brains at autopsy show this lesion, and many of which have no marked cortical contusions or brain stem damage. Patients with head injury seldom show the phenomenon that is not infrequently seen after primary vascular lesions in the brain stem, namely, the very rapid development of either the vegetative state or the locked-in syndrome, without a preceding period of several days of sleep-like coma.

The traditional classification of *commotio cerebri* to describe patients with

91

brief unconsciousness and *contusio cerebri* for more prolonged and profound alteration of consciousness was based on a different, indeed almost an opposing, concept of clinicopathological correlation. According to that classification, clinicians were supposed to diagnose *commotio* when unconsciousness was brief, and *contusio* when it was prolonged (or there were focal signs). Most patients after head injury would now be considered to have a combination of *commotio* and *contusio,* if by these are meant (in modern pathological parlance) white matter shearing lesions and cortical contusions, respectively. Whether unconsciousness is initial or delayed, and transient or persisting, depends on the balance of the contribution of these two lesions, together with the degree of *compressio* (the third component of the traditional classification). If *compressio* is to include all patients with raised intracranial pressure and not to be confined to those with discrete intracranial hematoma, then it must be judged a factor in a high proportion of cases. But we would now have to consider also the contribution of other secondary events to continuing coma, in particular widespread hypoxic/ischemic brain damage. We now know that this may devastate the cerebral cortex (p. 35) and that such a lesion may develop within a few hours of the original injury, so that it may be very difficult clinically to distinguish between the effects of impact damage and of this secondary process.

SUMMARY

Discussions about head injury, whether at the bedside in the acute stage when decisions are being made about investigation or treatment, or later when reviewing the outcome of individual patients or of reported series in the literature, frequently focus on altered consciousness. Confusion about the definitions of concussion and coma, and about their supposed relation to pathology and prognosis, probably accounts for most of the controversy and uncertainty that is characteristic of spoken and written discussion about head injury. We have proposed a simple approach to these problems, with a clear distinction between what is observed at the bedside, and what is deduction and speculation about clinicopathological (or anatomical or physiological) correlations. The language that is used to describe the behavior of head injured patients shapes the way in which doctors come to think about them. That is why we have preferred to depend mostly on descriptive terminology and have tried to avoid using terms that imply interpretations that can seldom be verified. We propose that coma and clouded consciousness represent a continuum, but that there is considerable variation in the combinations of disordered function that are observed at various points along this continuum. For this reason it is unwise to seek to construct a series of levels that assume that certain degrees of abnormality in different functional modalities will always coincide. It is preferable to describe separately the degree of dysfunction in motor response, verbal behavior, eye opening, pupil reaction, and eye movement. Improvement or deterioration can then be recognized and described in an individual patient, and differences between single patients or series can be defined. That, in turn, will provide a reliable basis for diagnosis, prognosis, and management.

REFERENCES

1. AD HOC COMMITTEE OF THE HARVARD MEDICAL SCHOOL TO EXAMINE THE DEFINITION OF BRAIN DEATH: *A definition of irreversible coma.* J.A.M.A. 205:337–340, 1968.

2. BEECHER, H. K.: *After the "definition of irreversible coma."* N. Engl. J. Med. 281:1070–1071, 1969.

3. BERESFORD, H. R.: *The Quinlan decision: problems and legislative alternatives.* Ann. Neurol. 2:74–81, 1977.

4. BROCK, S.: *Injuries of the Brain and Spinal Cord.* Springer Publishing Co., New York, 1960.

5. CAIRNS, H., OLDFIELD, R. C., PENNYBACKER, J. B., et al.: *Akinetic mutism with an epidermoid cyst of the third ventricle.* Brain 64:273–290, 1941.

6. CHOU, S. N.: *Brain death.* Lancet i:282–283, 1981.

7. CONFERENCE OF MEDICAL ROYAL COLLEGES AND THEIR FACULTIES (U.K.): *Diagnosis of brain death.* Lancet ii:1069–1070, 1976.

8. CONFERENCE OF MEDICAL ROYAL COLLEGES AND THEIR FACULTIES (U.K.): *Diagnosis of death.* Br. Med. J. 1:322, 1979.

9. FROWEIN, R. A.: *Classification of coma.* Acta Neurochir. 34:5–10, 1976.

10. GRONWALL, D., AND WRIGHTSON, P.: *Cumulative effect of concussion.* Lancet ii:995–997, 1975.

11. JENNETT, B., GLEAVE, J., AND WILSON, P.: *Brain death in three neurosurgical units.* Br. Med. J. 281:533–539, 1981.

12. JENNETT, B., AND PLUM, F.: *Persistent vegetative state after brain damage.* Lancet i:734–737, 1972.

13. JENNETT, B., AND TEASDALE, G.: *Aspects of coma after severe head injury.* Lancet i:878–881, 1977.

14. LANCET: *The best yardstick we have.* ii:1445–1446, 1961.

15. LANCET: *Diagnosis of brain death.* ii:1064–1066, 1976.

16. LEGG, N. J. AND PRIOR, P. F.: *Brain death.* Lancet ii;1378, 1980.

17. MOHANDAS, A., AND CHOU, S. N.: *Brain death. A clinical and pathological study.* J. Neurosurg. 35:211–218, 1971.

18. MOLLARET, P., AND GOULON, M.: *Le coma depassé (memoire preliminaire)* Rev. Neurol. 101:3–15, 1959.

19. NORTH, J. B., AND JENNETT, S.: *Abnormal breathing patterns associated with acute brain damage.* Arch. Neurol. 31:338–344, 1974.

20. OPPENHEIMER, D. R.: *Microscopic lesions in the brain following head injury.* J. Neurol. Neurosurg. Psychiatry 31:299–306, 1968.

21. PALLIS, C.: *Prognostic value of brainstem lesions.* Lancet i:379, 1981.

22. PLUM, F.: *Brain death.* Lancet ii:379, 1980.

23. PLUM, F.: *Transplants—Are the donors really dead?* Br. Med. J. 282:565, 1981.

24. PLUM, F., AND POSNER, J. B.: *Diagnosis of Stupor and Coma.* ed. 3. F. A. Davis, Philadelphia, 1980.

25. RUSSELL, W. R.: *Cerebral involvement in head injury. A study based on the examination of 200 cases.* Brain 55:549–603, 1932.

26. RUSSELL, W. R.: *The Traumatic Amnesias.* Oxford University Press, Oxford, 1961.

27. RUSSELL, W. R., AND NATHAN, P. W.: *Traumatic amnesia.* Brain 69:280–300, 1946.

28. SHILLITO, J.: *The organ donor's doctor.* N. Engl. J. Med. 281:1071–1072, 1969.

29. SWEET, W.: *Brain death.* N. Engl. J. Med. 299:410–411, 1978.

30. SYMONDS, C. P.: *The differential diagnosis and treatment of cerebral states consequent upon head injuries.* Br. Med. J. 4:829–832, 1928.

31. SYMONDS, C. P.: *Concussion and its sequelae.* Lancet i:1–5, 1962.

32. TEASDALE, G., AND JENNETT, B.: *Assessment of coma and impaired consciousness.* Lancet ii:81–84, 1974.

33. TEASDALE, G., AND JENNETT, B.: *Assessment and prognosis of coma after head injury.* Acta Neurochir. 34:45–55, 1976.

34. TEASDALE, G., KNILL-JONES, R., AND VAN DER SANDE, J.: *Observer variability in assessing impaired consciousness and coma.* J. Neurol. Neurosurg. Psychiatry 41:603–610, 1978.

CHAPTER 5

Early Assessment
of the Head Injured Patient

How a head injured patient is regarded by those who see him in the early stages will determine his initial management. If this management is inappropriate the patient may suffer—from too much or too little care. If the risk of complications after mild injuries is overestimated, then unnecessary measures may be recommended (such as admission to hospital); but if real risks are overlooked then secondary events may already have done irreversible damage before they are recognized. Moreover it is difficult to judge the efficacy of alternative regimens if early assessment is inadequate, so that some patients selected are either too mildly injured to require such treatment or too badly affected to benefit. To some extent, therefore, early assessment implies classification of severity; but it also implies prognosis—of the likelihood of complications developing after milder injuries, and of the chances of recovery in the more severely affected. Early diagnosis also requires that head injuries be recognized as open or closed and that the extent of extracranial injuries be noted. In some cases the question of pretraumatic brain damage may arise, or of other kinds of cerebral disorders contributing to the present state (epilepsy, stroke, or drugs). This is the differential diagnosis of head injury—seeking answers to the question, is this patient's condition the result of head injury, and if it is, is head injury the only contributing factor?

It is *brain* damage, actual or potential, that requires assessment. Brain damage already sustained by the time of early examination may not be only that caused by impact, because secondary events can occur very rapidly. Whether or not it is judged that a reversible process is contributing to the present state of brain dysfunction will be crucial in deciding what to do. Investigations may be initiated with a view to possible surgical intervention, if a treatable lesion is suspected; but if the patient's state is considered to be static or improving, such active measures may not be required or justified.

Evidence of *actual* brain damage may relate to *diffuse* lesions, resulting from acceleration/deceleration, in the form of altered consciousness; or to *focal* damage, indicated either by neurological signs or by depressed fracture (including puncture wounds). Estimation of the risk of *potential* brain damage in effect means judging the likelihood of intracranial complications. In the absence of any direct evidence of brain damage (altered consciousness, focal neurological signs, or depressed fracture) the only clue to there having been violence to the head of a kind likely to lead to complications, such as intracranial hematoma or infection, may be the presence of a linear fracture of the vault or of the base of the skull.

95

EVIDENCE OF DIFFUSE BRAIN DAMAGE

Altered consciousness soon after injury is the clue to the brain damage already suffered. When first seen in the emergency department it is useful to record whether or not the patient is talking. If he is talking, is he orientated and rational? And if he is, can he remember everything about, and since, the accident? Amnesia for even a few minutes after a blow to the head is evidence of diffuse brain damage. The duration of this PTA normally exceeds by a considerable margin the length of time for which the patient was regarded as unconscious, because it includes the time during which he was awake but confused (p. 89). Football players are familiar with the phenomenon of the player who resumes the game after a brief concussion, who responds to situations appropriately and may even play confidently, but who subsequently has no memory at all of that part of the game. A period of PTA is not infrequently discovered on close questioning of patients whom reliable witnesses report never to have been unconscious at all after the injury.

In the patient already talking when first seen, it is vital to establish not only whether he has a period of PTA, but also to determine whether he is at present fully orientated. It is not enough to note that the patient can give his name and address, because overlearned material like this can be given as an almost automatic response; there are many instances of patients recorded by doctors as having been fully conscious, who have no subsequent memory of this encounter at all. This may apply likewise to interviews given by the patient to police officers or to others soon after an accident; subsequent denial of these statements by the patient, who cannot recall them, may take on a sinister significance unless doctors offer an explanation, based on the probability that the patient was still in the state of PTA when he made them.

In the patient who is not talking, it is essential to establish whether he has uttered any recognizable words since the injury. If he has uttered even a word or two it can be confidently concluded that he has not suffered severe impact damage of the white matter (p. 26); no patients in whom autopsy has disclosed this type of lesion have been reported as having talked at any time in the interval between injury and death. In the patient reported to have talked, and who will not now do so, some secondary intracranial event must be presumed to have occurred. In the Data Bank series of patients in coma[7] more than a quarter had talked at some stage after injury, prior to developing persisting unconsciousness; the proportion was similar for surviving and fatal cases, and it was similar in each of the three countries. This therefore confirmed an earlier report that patients who "talked and died" made up almost a third of deaths in one neurosurgical unit.[10] A subsequent study[11] showed that avoidable factors contributing to death were more often found in patients who had talked than in those who had been in continuing coma from the time of injury until death. Patients with an intracranial hematoma have more often talked (45%, compared with 10% of other patients); but about 20 percent of patients in coma who have previously talked have other secondary intracranial lesions (p. 170). Of patients in coma who are reported to have talked, 40 percent are said to have been completely lucid; this is much commoner in patients who have developed a hematoma.

Whatever the story of the conscious level prior to the present examination, what matters now is to assess the degree of impairment at the moment. This is best done by using the response scale previously described, together with other aspects of responsiveness, such as pupil size and reaction and the eye movements. Various local factors that may give rise to "false" signs in the eyes and pupils are discussed under focal signs (p. 98). It is necessary here to consider factors other than the degree of traumatic brain damage that may depress the level of responsiveness, and that may therefore lead to a mistaken assessment of the severity of the structural damage suffered. These factors may be *intracranial events,* such as a recent epileptic fit, so that the patient is still in the postictal state; or a stroke, hemorrhagic or ischemic, which preceded the head injury (and may indeed have been the cause of it).

Of more importance, however, are *extracranial factors* that influence the brain. The commonest are hypotension and/or hypoxia, associated with major extracranial injuries and the effect of drugs, in particular alcohol. Systemic disorders are a common feature in the early stages after head injury, especially when there are multiple injuries; in 100 patients arriving at an American neurosurgical unit, almost half had one or more serious disorders[9] (Table 1). Such patients may be unresponsive, perhaps with fixed pupils, and it is by no means uncommon for them to become much more responsive within minutes of restoring their blood pressure, or of correcting airway obstruction or inadequate ventilation. Assessment of the neurological status before and after resuscitation may indicate different degrees of "brain damage."

The effects of alcohol are less rapidly reversible, but an estimate of the contribution that is being made to the patient's state of coma by alcohol can be made from the blood alcohol level. In patients subsequently found to have suffered mild head injuries, it has been shown that no detectable confusion or disorientation occurs below a level of 200 mg/100 ml;[1] with a more severe traumatic lesion, the effect of alcohol might be greater. On the other hand, in habitual drinkers levels of over 300 mg/100 ml are compatible with the patient still talking and walking. It is of practical importance not to ascribe confusion (and certainly not coma) wholly or mainly to the effects of alcohol if the blood level is less than 200 mg; there is a case for having ready means of making an approximate estimate of alcohol in emergency rooms, preferably using breath analysis so as to avoid the need for blood samples.

The possibility that other drugs may be contributing to the patient's state may arise under certain circumstances, and toxicological tests may then be appropriate. Sometimes drugs have been given by previous medical attendants at the roadside, or at another hospital. In cases of multiple trauma there are still doctors unable to resist the reflex to give morphine, which not only affects the conscious

Table 1. Type and number of systemic insults noted in 100 patients with severe head injuries on arrival at a major trauma center

Type of Insult	Number	Associated with Multiple Injury
Hypotension	13	13
Anemia	12	11
Hypoxia	30	20
Hypercarbia	4	4
Total Insults	59	48
Total Patients	44	31

(From Miller, J. D., et al.,[9] with permission.)

level, especially when the brain is already damaged, but may constrict the pupils and limit their reactivity; it may also depress respiration. When there has been a fit the patient may have been given large doses of anticonvulsants, and these may combine with the postictal state to depress responsiveness. These various drugs may affect not only the responses of the coma scale but also the pupils and reflex eye movements. Occasionally hypothermia is a factor causing depression of consciousness and of other brain stem reflexes, when head injury has resulted in a patient lying exposed in winter at the roadside or perhaps in the mountains.

It should be part of the initial assessment of responsiveness to decide, if possible, whether the patient is static, improving, or deteriorating. The importance of establishing whether the patient has talked has already been stressed; it is less easy to determine whether the responsiveness of a patient who has been continuously unconscious has changed. But every effort should be made to glean information from those able to help—police, ambulance men, bystanders, relatives, and of course medical and nursing attendants from previous hospitals.

EVIDENCE OF FOCAL BRAIN DAMAGE

While any period of unconsciousness or of amnesia is evidence of brain damage, the absence of such features does not exclude the possibility of focal damage. Indeed many patients with compound depressed fracture, even those with brain oozing out of the wound, have never had any disorder of consciousness. When there has been a puncture wound, and the offending agent has been removed to leave only a tiny skin mark, there may be disbelief that the brain was actually penetrated—an error which can have costly repercussions (p. 198). Occasionally a blunt but focal blow, not occasioning either a scalp wound or a fracture, will produce focal signs without any alteration of consciousness. For example, dysphasia or weakness of an arm has been observed after a golf ball struck the side of the head, and hemianopia after a football struck the occiput. More often, evidence of focal brain damage is found in conjunction with either a skull fracture or altered consciousness, or both.

Focal signs are usefully classified into those indicative of brain damage (usually of the cerebral hemisphere, but occasionally of the brain stem and cerebellum) and those bespeaking cranial nerve dysfunction. In each case it is important to be aware of the possibility that the signs are due not to trauma, but to associated lesions. For example, hemiparesis or dysphasia may be due to a stroke, which precipitated the head injury, or they may be postictal, owing to a focal fit precipitated by the head injury. Occasionally a paralyzed arm proves to be due to brachial plexus injury, or a weak arm and leg to limited spinal cord injury. In the patient who is not fully conscious, and before complete assessment has been made, it is easy to jump to the conclusion that neurological signs must indicate traumatic brain damage.

Cranial nerve signs that may be evident at the stage of early assessment are facial weakness, trigeminal anesthesia, optic nerve lesions, and disorders of the external ocular nerves. The site of the lesions causing these may be intracranial, within the foramina of the skull base, or entirely extracranial; in the last case they may not be strictly regarded as evidence of brain injury. What matters most, however, is the confusion that each of these lesions can cause, by reason of the alternative interpretations that may be put upon them. For example, facial weakness that is due to involvement of the nerve in a petrous fracture may be regarded as evidence of contralateral cerebral hemisphere damage; dysconjugate eye movements that are due to peripheral lesions of the nerves to the ocular muscles may be interpreted as evidence of brain stem dysfunction; and pupillary abnormalities caused by lesions of the oculomotor or optic nerves in the orbit, or to mechanical damage to the globe, may be mistakenly regarded as evidence of tentorial herniation.

It may well be impossible to be certain where the site of the lesion is at this early stage after injury; however, it is important to consider the possibility that any of these signs may indicate lesions in a variety of different places and not to base management decisions on premature judgment.

SKULL FRACTURE

To the lay mind, and particularly to the legal mind, a fracture of the skull is an obvious mark of severity following a head injury. Thousands of heads are x-rayed in emergency rooms, but in only two or three cases in a hundred is there a fracture; consequently, radiologists write papers on the misuse of resources and demand that clinicians do better triage before x-rays are done. Neurosurgeons have long preached that assessment of the conscious level is more important than a skull x-ray, and this has been mistakenly taken to imply that they regard the detection of a fracture as unimportant, especially after milder injuries. In fact, it is in the patient whose consciousness is unimpaired, and who might otherwise be sent home as a trivial injury, that the finding of a fracture can be most significant, because it alerts the clinician to the risk of complications such as intracranial hematoma or infection.

Frequency of Skull Fractures

This varies according to the head injury populations studied: the more severe the injuries the more fractures are found (Table 2). Among accident/emergency room attenders fractures were more often found when there was evidence of brain damage on examination, or a history of unconsciousness after the injury; and among the brain damaged patients, fractures were more common in those who still had altered consciousness (Table 3).

In patients admitted to Scottish neurosurgical wards, a fracture was recorded in 65 percent, and in the severe injuries of the International Data Bank a radiological fracture was also found in 65 percent. The vault was involved three times as often as was the base, but sometimes there were fractures in both sites (Table 4).

Table 2. Frequency of skull fractures

	Number	Fracture	
A/E Attenders[12]	3558	3%*	
PSW Admissions[8]	1181	7%	
NSU Admissions[6]	424	65%	
Severe Injuries[7] (Data Bank)	974	65%	including clinical basal fractures
Deaths in NSU[5]	151	80%	at autopsy

*Of the 58 percent of attenders who were x-rayed.
A/E = Accident and emergency room; PSW = Primary surgical ward; NSU = Neurosurgical unit

Table 3. Skull x-rays and fracture in Scottish A/E attenders[12]

Evidence of Brain Damage	Percentage of 3558 Patients	Percentage X-rayed	Percentage with Skull Fracture (of X-rayed)
None	80	51	1.3
Any	20	84	5
Recovered from altered consciousness	15	88	2.6
Not fully conscious in A/E	5	76	15

Of those whose x-rays were reported to show neither a fracture of the vault nor of the base, a third had clinical signs of a fractured base: for the anterior fossa, orbital hematoma and CSF rhinorrhea; for the middle fossa, mastoid hematoma and CSF or bloody otorrhea. One or the other of these signs was recorded in 45 percent of the series of severe injuries, but they occurred almost twice as often in patients with radiological evidence of basal fracture (Table 5). A fractured base was much more often detected radiologically in patients with signs of a fractured base (Table 6).

Significance of Skull Fracture

A linear vault fracture in a conscious patient increases the risk of intracranial hematoma by about 400 times. In the Data Bank cases 77 percent of 437 patients with a hematoma had a skull fracture, but for children (under 15 years) the figure was only 63 percent. For extradural hematoma, which is liable to occur after mild injury, the fracture rate was 91 percent in adults and 75 percent in children. Although intracranial hematoma is a relatively rare complication, it can develop rapidly, and successful treatment depends on early detection (p. 180). For this reason it is generally accepted that a skull fracture calls for admission to hospital for observation, no matter how well the patient is. This in turn justifies the x-raying of many patients who are unlikely to have a fracture, because this may

Table 4. Skull fracture in 974 severe injuries

	Number	Percentage*
Vault only	435	45
Base only	35	4
Vault + base	167	17
All vault	602	62
All base	202	21
Any fracture	637	65
No radiological fracture	337	35
Clinical signs of base fracture; no radiological sign	102	10
No skull fracture, radiological or clinical	235	24

*11% of all patients had *depressed* fracture (18% of all vault fractures were depressed).
(Based on extended series from International Data Bank.[7])

Table 5. Incidence of clinical signs of basal fracture

In patients with		
Radiological basal fracture	175/202	87%
Vault fracture only	157/435	36%
No basal fracture on x-ray	259/772	34%
No radiological fracture	102/337	30%
All patients	453/1000	45%

(Based on extended series from International Data Bank.[7])

enable complications to be anticipated when there are no clinical clues. In patients in coma a fracture increases the likelihood of an intracranial hematoma by 20 times.

A fracture in association with a scalp laceration, or in communication with the paranasal air sinuses or the middle ear cavity, constitutes an open injury. This carries the risk of intracranial infection, which sometimes occurs when such fractures are overlooked initially (p. 198). It may be impractical to require an x-ray for every patient with a scalp laceration, but the clinician in the emergency room should always consider the circumstances of the injury and the nature of the wound in reaching a decision about the possibility of an underlying fracture. Detection of a basal fracture often requires special positioning and tomography, which may be impractical in the accident/emergency room, or in the early stages when patients are uncooperative or in coma. Even with good x-rays a proportion of basal fractures are not visualized and there is therefore a case for accepting a clinical diagnosis, at least in the first week; a decision as to whether or not there is a fracture can then be reached in the light of developments and further investigations.

Not all patients with a skull fracture are in a more serious state (*qua* brain damage already sustained) than those without a fracture. Many patients with a linear or depressed fracture are not initially unconscious, while serious brain damage can occur without fracture. Only 46 percent of 154 surviving head injuries with more than 24 hours PTA in one series had a skull fracture.[4] In the severe injuries of the Data Bank, a fracture was neither detected radiologically nor suspected clinically in 24 percent.[5,7] And no fracture was found even at autopsy in 20 percent of 151 consecutive fatalities coming to a neuropathological department from a neurosurgical ward. There is usually no skull fracture in association with the most severe kind of impact damage found in patients who reach hospital alive, namely, diffuse shearing lesions of white matter.

Table 6. Frequency of radiologically reported fracture of the base

Clinical Features		
No basal signs	27/540	5%
Any basal signs*	175/434	40%
Anterior fossa signs	88/192	46%
Middle fossa signs	129/302	43%

*Patients with both anterior and middle fossa signs counted only once.
(Based on extended series from International Data Bank.[7])

TECHNIQUE OF SKULL X-RAY

Those who claim that too many x-rays are taken and that they seldom affect the care of the patient often point to the poor quality of the films taken in emergency departments, or to the inadequacies of interpretation by untrained staff. In our view the practicalities of the situation will always demand that a sizable proportion of patients have skull x-rays in emergency departments, and that decisions about their management (in particular whether or not they are admitted) will depend on how these films are interpreted there and then—not a day or two later by trained senior radiological staff. It is therefore important to consider the main technical requirements for obtaining satisfactory films of the skull, and the rules for recognizing skull fractures. Much is made of the difficulties of securing reasonable radiographs from unreasonable patients, who are either unconscious or who are restless and unco-operative, often from a combination of recent injury and recent alcohol. In any event, patients in these states must be retained for observation until they are fully conscious, and x-rays can be deferred until then. Such difficult patients do not, however, account for all the unsatisfactory films taken in emergency departments. Indeed, one investigation some years ago showed that poor positioning and wrong exposure were more common causes of bad films than was patient movement, and that unsatisfactory films were common in patients recorded as having been fully co-operative.[5]

It is necessary to provide adequate equipment (with short exposure times) and to train radiographers properly; it is up to the clinician on the spot (if there is no radiologist) to request repeat films if those already taken are inadequate for diagnostic purposes. Films must be sharp; if there is blurring, because the patient moved, they should be repeated, if necessary after admission when the patient's condition has improved. Improper positioning of the patient or centering of the x-ray beam produces distortion, and normal features may be mistaken for fractures. It is important to include the whole skull, and lateral views should also include the upper cervical spine. Overpenetration is preferable to underpenetration, as it can be corrected by viewing the film in an especially bright light. Films taken in the ward, with portable equipment, are of limited value, but in patients with multiple injuries they should not be ignored.

Three views are taken routinely: posteroanterior (PA), Towne's or half axial PA view, and lateral (Fig. 1). To avoid disturbing the patient who is unconscious or has major facial injuries, films may be taken in the supine or "brow-up" position (Fig. 2); this is also useful for demonstrating fluid levels. In the lateral view, fractures are most clearly defined when the film is placed on the same side of the head as the suspected fracture. Although brain damage is often contre-coup, the skull fracture usually begins near the point of impact, so the site of any scalp injury is usually a reliable guide to its location. When the significance of a radiolucent line is uncertain or its location in doubt, a second x-ray with the film on the opposite side of the head can help.

Sometimes additional views are required; tangential views may confirm that a fracture is depressed and by how much, and a submentovertical view shows the base of the skull when a basal fracture is suspected. Stereoscopic views can be valuable in indicating the location of intracranial bone fragments after gunshot injury. In the investigation of a patient with a cerebrospinal fluid leak, special stereoscopic views and tomograms of the anterior fossa are employed to locate

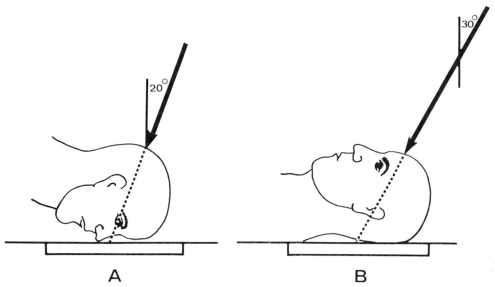

A   B

Figure 1. A, Posteroanterior (PA) view. Beam tilted 20 degrees down towards feet and centered on inion. **B,** Towne's view. Beam 30 degrees towards feet and centered on the junction of forehead and hair-line.

the fracture line and to detect angulated spicules, but these should be deferred until surgery is being planned a week or more after injury.

Interpretation

The *lateral view* may show fractures of the vault, but it will also have markings of normal structures, which should be identified (Figs. 3, 4, and 5). A calcified pineal gland may be visible in older patients, and the clinician is then alerted to look carefully for it on the axial views *(vide infra)*. After penetrating basal injuries, a brow-up view may show fluid levels in the sinuses, or air intracranially.

The *PA view* (Fig. 6) shows the orbits, the frontal bone, and, usually, the

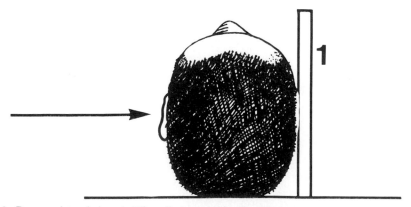

Figure 2. Brow-up lateral view. **1,** Film adjacent to side of scalp trauma.

103

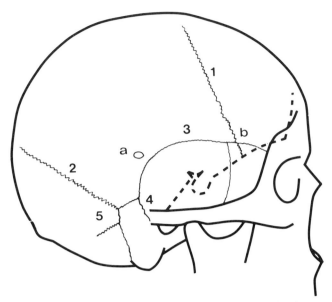

Figure 3. Position of normal sutures in the lateral view. **1,** Coronal; **2,** lambdoid; **3,** squamoparietal; **4,** mastoid; **5,** mendosal; **a,** pineal; **b,** pterion.

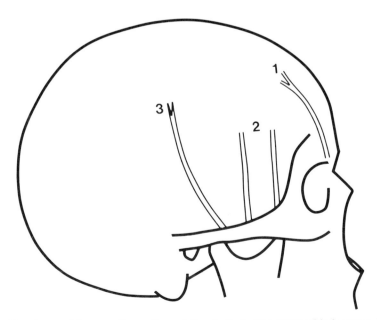

Figure 4. Vascular markings on the surface of the skull. **1,** The supraorbital artery; **2,** the deep temporal arteries; **3,** the middle temporal artery.

104

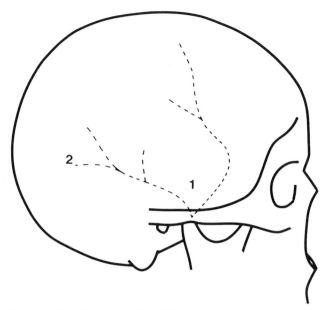

Figure 5. Lateral view of skull. Position of **1**, middle meningeal artery; and **2**, pineal gland.

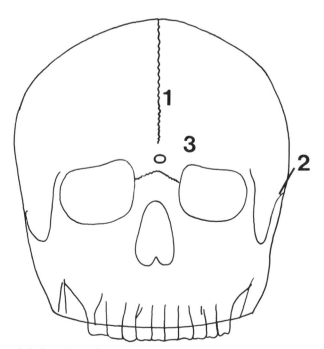

Figure 6. PA view of skull. **1**, Metopic suture; **2**, squamoparietal suture; **3**, position of pineal gland.

mastoid and petrous temporal bones. The occipital bone is shown best in the *Towne's view* (Fig. 7), and this projection distinguishes frontal from occipital fractures. In the latter the fracture line does not cross the shadow of the foramen magnum, whereas frontal fractures are frequently projected over it. The pineal gland should be sought in both PA and Towne's views, if it has been previously seen to be calcified in the lateral view, because displacement from its normal midline position may be a vital clue to a mass lesion on the surface of one cerebral hemisphere.

Fractures may be linear or comminuted; significant depression occurs only with comminution. Either linear or depressed vault fractures may be associated with a local scalp wound (externally compound), but dural tearing, entailing a risk of intracranial infection, is a complication only of depression. When a basal fracture line involves the paranasal sinuses or the middle ear cavity, it is sometimes said to be internally compound.

Distinct fracture lines rarely give rise to problems in interpretation; a more common difficulty is to decide that a particular line is *not* a fracture. Characteristically a fracture is straight, with parallel margins, and does not taper nor

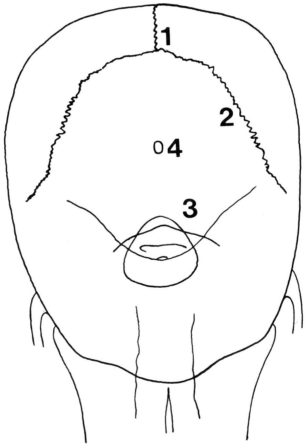

Figure 7. Towne's view of skull. **1,** Coronal suture; **2,** lambdoid suture; **3,** foramen magnum; **4,** position of pineal gland.

branch, but may have sudden angular changes in direction. Fractures tend to run across anatomical features, such as sutures or the grooves made by certain blood vessels. A fracture involves both tables of the skull and, if the x-ray is taken at right angles, produces a sharply defined line. The normal markings sometimes confused with fractures often involve only one table and have at least a faint margin of cortical bone. Moreover most of these markings are present on both sides of the skull and are symmetrical; fracture lines may go across the midline of the vault, but will seldom be symmetrical.

Age of Fracture

Some individuals sustain repeated head injuries and it may be difficult to determine whether the fracture that has been demonstrated is relevant to the present injury. As a fracture heals, its margins become less distinct, but the rate depends upon the patient's age, the width of the fracture, and its location. Fractures in children usually disappear within 6 months, but linear fractures in adults may remain sharp for several months and are rarely fully healed in less than 3 to 4 years.

Depressed Fractures

In the view at right angles to the fracture, depression may be missed and two views at right angles to each other are a minimal requirement. Depression can be suspected when there is an area of increased density close to the fracture line. The increased density may be due either to overlapping of the adjacent bone fragments or to a fragment being turned end-on to the x-ray beam. Tangential views are essential to confirm the diagnosis and to determine the extent of the depression.

Differential Diagnosis of Skull Fracture

Sutures

On the outer surface of the skull, suture lines are wavy, but on the inner surface they tend to be straighter and can sometimes be confused with a fracture. This is most likely to occur with the coronal and sagittal sutures. The normal positions of the various sutures should be known and determined in each skull view (Figs. 3, 6, and 7). The margins of the greater wing of sphenoid or squamous temporal bones are sometimes mistaken for fractures; more posteriorly, so too are the sutures around the mastoid bones and the lambdoid and Mendosal sutures. Rotated views are a particular cause of difficulty. The PA view shows a fissure laterally, produced by the junction of the squamous temporal and sphenoid bones with the frontal and parietal bones; this is distinguished from a fracture by its being present on both sides. In frontal views the metopic suture may be seen. It separates the two sides of the developing frontal bone and usually fuses at around 5 years old, but may persist into adult life. In the occipital bone there is sometimes failure of fusion between some of its six separate centers of ossification, but the persisting synchondroses run horizontally and are symmetrical on the two sides, whereas occipital fractures usually run vertically throughout the whole length of the bone.

107

Suture Diastasis

Separation of a suture by more than 2 mm is abnormal. Diastasis is likely to occur when a fracture runs into the lambdoid suture, but is sometimes falsely suspected when an obliquely taken film causes the normal sutures to appear of different widths.

Vascular Markings

Three sets of vessels may groove the outer surface of the skull, producing vertical lines in the lateral film: the supraorbital artery, two deep temporal arteries, and the middle temporal branch of the superficial temporal artery (Fig. 4). The lines produced by these vessels are usually straight, tapering, and bilateral.

Venous channels within the diploe cause wide, smooth translucencies with indistinct margins that usually run into venous lakes, but they can resemble large, stellate fractures.

The meningeal vessels on the inner surface of the skull produce branching, peripherally tapering lines, which are less sharp than fracture lines (Fig. 5) and are usually present bilaterally.

Scalp Wounds

Air may enter between the gaping margins of a large scalp laceration and can resemble a fracture on an x-ray, as can dressings applied to the scalp wound; neither of these artefacts will cause confusion if they are remembered by the clinician. Similarly dirt, glass, or stones in the patient's hair or in the wound can be mistaken for the double density of a depressed fracture or even for an intracranial foreign body.

Basal Skull Fractures

Fractures running into the basal air sinuses or the nasal cavity can sometimes be seen in "plain" films, but such an injury may be suspected by seeing fluid in an air sinus (maxillary antrum, the frontal or the sphenoid air sinuses), either as a result of bleeding from the fracture or because of escape of cerebrospinal fluid. In view "face-on" to the sinus its cavity appears opaque; in appropriately positioned lateral views a fluid level may be seen. In the sphenoid bone the degree of pneumatization varies, but partial pneumatization can be distinguished from a fluid level as the margin of the nonpneumatized part is covered by curving, cortical bone and the meniscus of a CSF collection forms a straight line that changes position with movement of the head.

Intracranial Air

Air can gain access to the inside of the skull through a fracture involving a paranasal sinus or the middle ear cavity, or, more rarely, in association with a compound depressed fracture of the vault. Intracranial air may be seen in the subarachnoid spaces of the basal cisterns, in the ventricles, or sometimes even within the brain itself. Superimposition of a mastoid air cell over the pituitary region, owing to improper positioning, can be confused with intracranial air.

108

When there is doubt, the shift of a translucent area with altered head position will confirm that it is indeed air.

Air in the head is certain evidence of a penetrating injury, which may be either small with a transitory communication, or large with a persisting fistula.

Conclusion

If there is a case for taking an x-ray at all, then skull x-rays can make an important contribution to the management of head injured patients. Every effort must be made to secure good quality films and to interpret them reliably. Inspection of a radiograph should always provide answers to the following questions:

1. Are the films satisfactory in respect to positioning, exposure, and lack of movement?
2. Can normal sutures and vascular markings be identified?
3. Is there a fracture of the vault, base, or both?
4. Is the vault fracture on the right or left, frontal or occipital, or elsewhere; is it depressed?
5. Is a basal fracture involving the air sinuses or middle ear?
6. Is there air in the intracranial cavity or fluid in a sinus cavity?
7. Is the pineal visible and if so is it displaced?
8. Are there any foreign bodies in the scalp or intracranially?

EXTRACRANIAL INJURIES

A third of head injuries admitted to hospital have another injury, elsewhere in the body. This is more common in road accidents, both to vehicle occupants and to pedestrians, because more than one impact is frequently sustained, whereas other injuries are uncommon with local injury to the head from assault or being struck by falling or swinging objects. As the acceleration/deceleration types of injury sustained in road accidents frequently result in continuous unconsciousness from the time of impact, it can be difficult to diagnose the other injuries since no complaint is made of pain elsewhere. If there is hypotension (without a massive scalp laceration) another injury should always be suspected, because head injury alone rarely produces shock.[3] Even without such a clue the initial assessment of a head injury should always include systematic search for evidence of another injury, especially in the trunk. Surgical emphysema, tire marks, or the impressed pattern of clothing may indicate that crushing has occurred; bowel sounds need to be listened for, and urine (obtained by catheter if necessary) inspected for blood. X-rays of chest and cervical spine should be a routine. Facial injuries are the commonest, and again adequate x-rays will enable a correct diagnosis to be made. Swelling or deformity of an extremity may point to a fracture or dislocation; peripheral pulses should always be checked at the wrist and ankle.

Pre-existing or coincident medical disease should not be forgotten. Is the patient diabetic, bronchitic, or hypertensive? Any of these may distort signs of systemic dysfunction after head injury and may need to be taken account of when planning management. Occasionally intracranial conditions are brought to light or precipitated by mild head injuries. For example, compensated hydrocephalus owing to aqueduct stenosis may begin to develop signs of intracranial pressure after head injury, perhaps because traumatic subarachnoid bleeding causes obstruction of venous pathways of CSF circulation and absorption. Sometimes normal pressure hydrocephalus may become symptomatic after mild head injury, as may benign intracranial hypertension (pseudotumor).

REFERENCES

1. GALBRAITH, S., MURRAY, W. R., PATEL, A. R., ET AL.: *The relationship between alcohol and head injury and its effect on the conscious level.* Br. J. Surg. 63:128–130, 1976.

2. GRAHAM, D. I., ADAMS, J. H., AND DOYLE, D.: *Ischaemic brain damage in fatal non-missile head injuries.* J. Neurol. Sci. 39:213–234, 1978.

3. ILLINGWORTH, G., AND JENNETT, B.: *The shocked head injury.* Lancet ii:511–514, 1965.

4. JENNETT, B.: *Epilepsy after Non-Missile Head Injuries.* ed. 2. Heinemann, London, 1975.

5. JENNETT, B.: *Significance of skull x-rays in the management of recent head injury.* Clin. Radiol. 31:463–469, 1980.

6. JENNETT, B., ET AL.: *Head injuries in neurosurgical units in Scottish hospitals.* Br. Med. J. 2:955–958, 1979.

7. JENNETT, B., TEASDALE, G., GALBRAITH, S., ET AL.: *Severe head injuries in three countries.* J. Neurol. Neurosurg. Psychiatry 40:291–298, 1977.

8. MACMILLAN, R., STRANG, I., AND JENNETT, B.: *Head injuries in primary surgical ward in Scottish hospitals.* Health Bull. 37:75–81, 1979.

9. MILLER, J. D., SWEET, R. C., NARAYAN, R., ET AL.: *Early insults to the injured brain.* J.A.M.A. 240:439–442, 1978.

10. REILLY, P. L., GRAHAM, D. I., ADAMS, J. H., ET AL.: *Patients with head injury who talk and die.* Lancet ii:375, 1975.

11. ROSE, J., VALTONEN, S., AND JENNETT, B.: *Avoidable factors contributing to death after head injury.* Br. Med. J. 2:615–618, 1977.

12. STRANG, I., MACMILLAN, R., AND JENNETT, B.: *Head injuries in accident and emergency departments at Scottish hospitals.* Injury 10:154–159, 1978.

13. VANCE, R. G.: *The healing of linear fractures of the skull.* Am. J. Roentgenol. 36:744–746, 1936.

CHAPTER 6

Special Investigations and Methods of Monitoring

Trauma is no respecter of geography and many head injuries have to be managed, for a time at least, outside of special centers. Clinical assessment and monitoring of responsiveness, and the place of skull x-ray, have already been discussed—these are methods available in all hospitals. This chapter is concerned with neuroradiological techniques for imaging the brain, and with the role of measurements of ICP and CBF, electrophysiological recordings, and biochemical abnormalities in blood, as means of monitoring brain dysfunction or damage (Fig. 1).

Imaging investigations are commonly done for diagnostic purposes, usually once only; they are repeated only infrequently. By contrast, monitoring implies continuous (or frequently repeated) acquisition of data, as a basis for observing

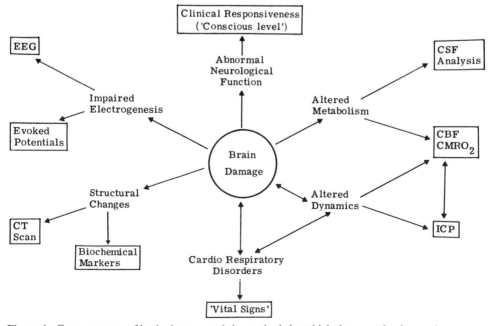

Figure 1. Consequences of brain damage and the methods by which these can be detected.

not only the state of the patient but also changes with time. Such changes may indicate a need for intervention by further investigation or by particular therapy and may be of prognostic significance.

Although relatively few patients require operative neurosurgery, many more need to go to a special unit in order to benefit from one or more of these technological developments. The emphasis in this chapter is therefore on the information yield of each, and the contribution of this to practical management, rather than on a detailed description of how the various procedures are carried out.

COMPUTER TOMOGRAPHY (CT Scanning)

Since computer tomography was developed in Britain by Hounsfield[45] and applied in a London neurosurgical unit by Ambrose,[3] the strategy of investigation for suspected intracranial conditions has been revolutionized. The availability of CT scanning alters the clinical approach not only to investigation but to management as a whole. Indeed it might be said there are now two kinds of head injury care: with and without CT scanning. However, availability is the key word—many thousands of head injuries are bound to be treated, for some years to come, in hospitals without CT scanners. For this reason there is need to define clearly the role of CT scanning in the management of head injuries, in particular the relative value of its wide use as a screening method for as many injuries as possible of a certain severity, as compared with its selective use only when specific complications or management decisions have to be considered.

This technique provides a densitometric map of a succession of brain slices, on a scale of 0 for water (black) to 500 + for bone (white); air is −500. Clotted blood is denser than normal brain, edema and infarcted brain less dense. Discrimination between normal and abnormal brain can sometimes be accentuated by the intravenous injection of iodine contrast compounds. This is of little value in the acute stage after head injury; later, when hematomas may be isodense with brain on the unenhanced scan, contrast injection may be helpful.

Securing Satisfactory Scans

Unless the patient keeps the head still for the duration of scanning for each slice, there will be movement artefacts. Some confused patients and young children may require sedation or anesthesia. Opinions will naturally differ as to the need and justification for this; these will depend in part on whether it is considered necessary to carry out a complete examination, with several slices. Some surgeons and radiologists believe that in the recently injured patient there is a place for a limited examination, restricted to one or two slices, which aims mainly to show whether there is a sizable hematoma or marked lateral shift, or both.

Abnormal Appearances

Much has still to be learned about the pathological correlation of various scan appearances after head injury. For this reason it is wiser to use primarily a descriptive classification for scan appearances, rather than to translate these directly into a particular pathological term.

Lateral displacement of the lateral ventricles, or the obliteration of the part of one ventricle, suggests local mass lesion, and this may be obvious on the same or on other slices (e.g., hematoma). The interventricular septum is often displaced to a greater extent than other midline structures.

Abnormally small ventricles, which are undisplaced, are frequently found after head injury in children. The ventricles are normally relatively small in children and it is not easy to know when this is a significant finding, except when the ventricles are so small as to be almost invisible and the subarachnoid cisterns around the brain stem are obliterated. It is believed that this appearance may reflect either diffuse edema or vascular engorgement; in the former case the density of the brain parenchyma would be expected to be reduced and in the latter increased. However, changes in the brain lipids after trauma may also affect tissue density, and the net effect of changes in these, in brain water and blood volume, may therefore be very variable.

Abnormally large ventricles may represent a pretraumatic state, particularly in older patients or in those who are chronic alcoholics (as a proportion of head injured patients are). In a younger patient, dilated ventricles in the acute state raise the possibility of an obstructive lesion, perhaps a posterior fossa hematoma. Dilatation of only one ventricle often occurs contralateral to a hematoma. If it is already some weeks since the injury, hydrocephalus may indicate an absorptive block from subarachnoid hemorrhage; more usually it reflects an atrophic process, owing to shrinkage of brain after a severe diffuse injury.

The pineal gland and choroid plexuses in the lateral ventricles are often calcified and will be seen on the scan as white (dense) areas. Lateral displacement of the pineal can be a useful clue to a mass lesion, especially if the ventricles are poorly visualized and their displacement not obvious; occasionally asymmetry of the choroid plexus calcifications will indicate a mass lesion.

Areas of Increased Density

In the first few days after injury, areas of markedly increased density (Hounsfield units > 50) usually indicate blood, if foreign bodies and calcification in normal structures are excluded. The size of these areas of hemorrhage may range from definite hematomas on the surface or in the substance of the brain, to smaller collections in the subarachnoid space; mottled areas in the brain substance, mixed with low density areas, are usually interpreted as "contusions," composed of a mixture of hemorrhage and edema. After a few days the density of extravasated blood is reduced, and by 2 to 3 weeks it may be isodense with brain. After 4 to 6 weeks the hemorrhagic area may show lower density than surrounding brain and this may persist. The place of scanning in the diagnosis of intracranial hematoma is discussed in more detail in Chapter 7.

Areas of Reduced Density

Areas of homogenous, reduced density, usually seen a day or more after injury, are believed to represent edema and are often associated with small ventricles. Areas of reduced density in the first 24 hours, associated with adjacent small areas of increased density, form a "salt and pepper" or mottled appearance, which is usually regarded as evidence of contusional damage. When such density is extensive but asymmetrical, it may be associated with shift.

Infarcted brain is also less dense than normal, and it may be that part of the mottling in "contusions" is due to small areas of infarction; much larger areas are sometimes seen and may take on the wedge shape that is typical of major vessel occlusion.

Intracranial air has extremely low density (very black) and will be recognized with appropriate window setting.

Hemorrhagic areas may, after 4 to 6 weeks, show a reduced density; such areas of "encephalomalacia" may persist permanently from hematoma or infarction.

Serial Scans

The development or the resolution of lesions may be observed by taking repeated scans. Contusions are often much more marked after 2 or 3 days than within 24 hours of injury; edema, infarction, and hemorrhagic extravasation probably account for this, and the combination may produce local swelling and shift of midline structures. It is uncommon, however, for a sizable intracranial hematoma to appear after an initially normal scan (or one showing only minor contusion); when it does, there is usually obvious clinical evidence of its presence. Late lesions, such as atrophy, hydrocephalus, and chronic subdural hematomas and hygromas, do of course take time to develop and occur in patients whose scan in the acute stage had been normal.

False Positives and Negatives

False positive scans appear to be rare after recent head injury and can usually be explained by movement artefacts or by the presence of foreign bodies (e.g., bone fragments), either in the brain or even in the scalp. Obliquely aligned slices may give a false appearance of shift. Rarely is a surgically significant intracranial hematoma found in the *acute* stage when the CT scan is normal; sometimes there is not a local area of increased density, but a lesion can be suspected from the ventricular shift or other mixed density abnormalities (p. 169). This was so in all three examples of false negative scans reported by Tans[104,105] among 60 hematomas; none of the three reported as negative had "normal" scans. An extradural hematoma at the vertex of the skull, however, may either be missed or its size underestimated in conventional horizontal slices.

Information Yield

CT scans make it possible to observe the presence, evolution, and resolution of lesions that could previously only be presumed on the basis of clinical features or deduced indirectly from angiographic or ventriculographic appearances. How often such abnormalities are found depends on the quality of the scans and on the skill with which they are interpreted. More information may be gleaned by the neuroradiologist who studies the scans at leisure next day than was evident to the hard-pressed junior neurosurgeon making a clinical decision during the night. In comparing reports about the frequency of occurrence of abnormalities in the recently injured, this fact of clinical life should be remembered.

In a consecutive series of 1000 head injuries managed in an American center where 24-hour scanning was available, only one third of newly arriving head injuries were scanned; half of these had a normal CT scan.[35] Moreover, more than 20 patients underwent surgery without prior scanning, usually for a depressed fracture or a rapidly developing intracranial hematoma. In patients scanned soon after injury, an abnormality was more often found when consciousness was impaired or there were focal signs; 85 percent of patients who had both these clinical features had an abnormal scan. However, almost half the patients who were in deep coma with abnormal motor activity had a normal scan.

In another American series of 300 patients, of which half were children, abnormalities were recorded in 58 percent of all cases; this ranged from 37 percent in the least serious to 91 percent of those in coma.[117] A study in Glasgow, confined to patients in coma for at least 6 hours, revealed abnormalities in over 80 percent. Half the cases had an intracranial hematoma; in the 60 severely injured patients without an intracranial hematoma the scan was normal in 35 percent of cases. Correlation with autopsy findings showed that a normal scan was compatible with severe hypoxic brain damage or with severe impact white matter damage.[97] Zimmerman and associates[116] reported that careful scanning, including thin slices in addition to routine cuts, will usually reveal indirect indicators of the latter lesion, in the form of small hemorrhagic lesions in the corpus callosum or the superior cerebellar peduncle, or blood in the lateral ventricles. Further circumstantial evidence is the absence of a skull fracture or contusions and the finding of normal or small and undisplaced lateral ventricles. However, it is important to recognize that a normal scan does not exclude severe brain damage, either primary or secondary.

While there is no doubt about the value of CT scanning in the diagnosis of intracranial hematoma, it is less certain what the contribution of CT scanning may be to the management of other problems. In prognosis it is of most value if taken in conjunction with the clinical data, when it may be useful in confirming what is already suspected from this. But when cases of similar clinical severity were compared in the Glasgow study, there was little difference between the outcome of patients with an abnormal as compared with a normal scan. In the patient who remains in coma after several days, however, the finding of evidence that is suggestive of diffuse white matter damage would make a poor outcome highly probable. A study of over 900 patients in Germany[61] has likewise emphasized that there may be discrepancies between clinical and CT findings and concluded that neither decisions about neurosurgical intervention nor prediction of outcome should be based on CT scanning alone.

As experience with CT scanning increases, the degree of its reliability will become clearer, in particular the significance that should be attached to a normal scan. More radiopathological correlations are required, but its value in the following contexts is already well established:

1. *Diagnosis of intracranial hematoma.* In replacing invasive investigations such as angiography and ventriculography in the investigation of patients in whom there is a suspicion of an intracranial hematoma, scanning finds its most important application. Because of its safety, it can be used also in cases in which suspicion is not high, and this may lead to the earlier detection of remediable lesions. Moreover, if the initial investigation is negative, it should be repeated without hesitation if the patient does not improve, although experience shows that most hematomas are present on the first scan.

2. *Diagnosis of "swollen brain" in children—distinction between edema and engorgement.* Some children in coma without a hematoma may have vascular engorgement and so might respond to decongestive therapy, as distinct from those with edema.[14,86,114]

3. *Diagnosis of diffuse white matter impact injury.* The characteristic features

of this lesion may be recognized;[116] taken together with the patient's condition this may make it possible to make a prediction about outcome more confidently and at an earlier stage than could be done on clinical grounds alone.

4. Increased understanding of the mechanism of injury. Knowing where contusions are in the brain is of limited value to the clinician concerned with planning therapy or making a prognosis. However, it is likely that the correlation disclosed between fracture sites and contusions, both in scans and in brains at autopsy, will improve understanding of the mechanisms of injury. Zimmerman and associates[115] suggest that a distinction can be made between multiple contusions on the inferior surface of the frontal and temporal lobes, which are due to acceleration/deceleration injury (frequently without fracture) and localized contusion in the frontal and parietal lobes, which appears more often to be due to local impact.

5. Detection of late complications. The demonstration of increasing ventricular enlargement in a patient with either persisting or increasing disability may lead to the diagnosis of hydrocephalus responsive to shunting.

CT Scan and Skull X-rays

It has been argued that if a scan can be done there is no need for a skull x-ray. However, a linear fracture or a depressed fracture may not be seen on the scan and yet may be of importance. A linear fracture of the vault increases the risk of an intracranial hematoma. Although this lesion will usually be evident on CT scan, it may develop after the first scan has failed to show its presence; if a fracture has been demonstrated, this would indicate an increased need to consider a repeat scan because it increases the likelihood that a hematoma will develop (p. 163).

In most places, and for most injuries, plain x-ray will likely remain the usual preliminary investigation for recently head injured patients. The finding of a fracture may then be useful in selecting which of the less severely affected patients should have a CT scan, which may involve transfer of the patient to a special center.

CEREBRAL ANGIOGRAPHY

Angiography is still used because the facilities for CT scanning are not universally available, nor are they likely to be in the foreseeable future. Moreover, even when a CT scan can be performed it may fail to show surface collections that are less than 1 cm thick or are isodense with the brain tissues. Angiography may therefore be required to clarify the result of a scan; it is also the only way of making a precise diagnosis of a vascular complication of head injury.

Only those who have received practical training should carry out cerebral angiography—even in expert hands the method has a small risk of grave complications.

Catheterization of the cerebral arteries following puncture of a distant artery is being increasingly used as a means of reducing the sequelae of direct puncture in the neck; it also usually makes a more complete examination possible. In particular, the carotid tree can readily be shown on both sides—a wise maneuver in view of the frequency of bilateral lesions after trauma. Both carotid trees may be visualized by direct puncture of one carotid artery if compression of the opposite artery is carried out, but this is not a reliable technique. It is important to have a series of films (usually five during the 7 seconds after injection) in order to compare the arterial and venous phases, which provide different information. The arterial and the late venous phases are of most value in indicating space-occupying complications after head injury, but extracerebral collections in frontal or occipital regions may be overlooked unless appropriate oblique views are taken in addition to the usual anteroposterior and lateral films.

Abnormalities

Vascular Displacement

SUPRATENTORIAL MASS. Lateral shift of the anterior cerebral and pericallosal arteries and of the internal cerebral vein indicates a mass lesion in one hemi-sphere, but not whether it is due to hematoma or to swelling. Rotation of the film may give a false impression of arterial shift; the vein is nearer the center of the skull and is less prone to this artefact. The likely site of the displacing lesion can often be deduced from the nature of the vascular displacement. Thus, frontal lesions bow the anterior cerebral artery laterally (Fig. 2I) and shift the vein less than do more posterior lesions, which cause a more "square" arterial shift (Fig. 2II). Temporal lesions produce characteristic displacement of the middle cerebral artery in the axial views (Fig. 2III); upward bowing of the middle cerebral is less

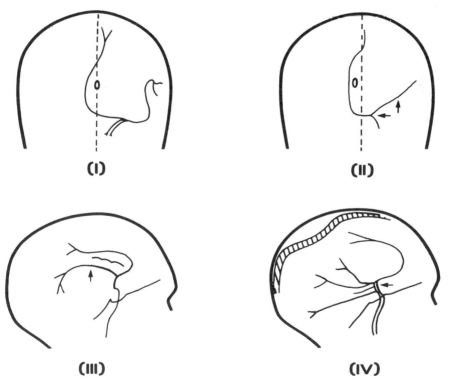

Figure 2. Angiographic features of intracranial hematomas. **(I)** frontal; **(II)** temporal; **(III)** temporal (lateral view); **(IV)** subfrontal (arterial phase) and sagittal extradural (venous phase).

117

reliably detected in the lateral view, because even mild rotation of the head can produce apparent upward displacement.

The lack of lateral shift does not exclude a mass lesion above the tentorium. Lesions in the parieto-occipital region can be angiographically silent, while bilateral lesions may "balance" each other.

TRANSTENTORIAL HERNIATION. A shift from the supratentorial to the infratentorial space can be detected by displacement of either of the branches of the proximal intracranial portion of the internal carotid artery—the posterior communicating and anterior choroidal arteries—or of the posterior cerebral artery, or of the basal veins. Downward displacement can be seen in the lateral view. On the anteroposterior view the same vessels may be seen to be displaced medially.

INFRATENTORIAL MASS. This lesion may be suspected if there is evidence on carotid angiography of hydrocephalus (upward sweep of the anterior cerebral and pericallosal arteries on the lateral view, and lateral bowing of the striothalamic vein in the axial view). Detection of hematomas from the displacement of the vessels in the posterior fossa is not easy, and diagnosis seldom depends upon vertebral angiography.

Avascular Areas

Most often an avascular area in the recently head injured patient will indicate a hematoma, but distinction from infarction may not be easy, if the mass is clearly intracerebral. It is not always obvious that the avascular lesion is on the surface and not in the brain. In the venous phase of the angiogram, there may be a clear gap between the skull and the small vessels on the surface of the brain; oblique views may be needed to show this appearance when the clot is not in the common lateral site. Clots at the vertex are difficult to detect, but they may displace the venous sinuses away from the bone (Fig. 2IV). Also elusive are clots situated subfrontally; upward and backward displacement of the proximal anterior cerebral artery may be the clue (Fig. 2IV).

When the angiogram shows a meningeal vessel displaced away from the skull, or leaking contrast, there is no doubt that the lesion is an extradural hematoma. This diagnosis is also favored if the avascular area is related to a skull fracture crossing the meningeal groove. A well-localized, lentiform-shaped collection also suggests an extradural clot, unless the suspicion is of a chronic subdural hematoma. With an acute subdural hematoma the lesion is usually widespread and crescentic.

Abnormalities of Transit Time

Contrast usually appears in the venous channels on angiograms 5 to 7 seconds after carotid injection. Marked slowing *may* indicate a reduced blood flow caused by raised ICP, but it can also occur with systemic hypotension. Pseudo-occlusion of the carotid artery (little or no flow above the siphon) is indicative of arrested circulation and is clearly a very grave sign.

Unduly rapid transit is sometimes observed. It may indicate luxury perfusion and correlates with rapid clearing of tissue peaks on cerebral flood flow studies (p. 133). Capillary blush or early venous filling may be very localized or can affect the whole temporal lobe. However, the clinical significance of this appearance after recent head injury remains uncertain.

Vascular Spasm

Irregular narrowing of segments of the cerebral arteries, characteristic of "spasm," are seen in the angiograms of a proportion of head injured patients. Most of these patients prove to have subarachnoid bleeding, and there is a correlation between the extent of spasm in the vertebrobasilar system after experimental head injury and the degree of hemorrhage into the basal cisterns.[75] Estimates of the incidence of spasm after head injury have varied. Suwanwela and Suwanwela[101] found it in almost 20 percent of their own series of 350 patients, but noted that previous reports ranged from 3 to 71 percent. Spasm may be local, in association with cortical contusions, but the vessels of the circle of Willis and the proximal parts of the major cerebral arteries are more commonly affected. Spasm may be seen within the first day or two of injury and can last for 2 or 3 weeks.

Some observers have considered that patients showing vascular spasm cannot be distinguished in clinical state or subsequent course from other head injured patients. On the other hand, it is clear that spasm sometimes can produce neurological dysfunction and ischemic damage. Marshall and associates[73] have described a series of patients who showed signs of posterior fossa dysfunction after head injury and in whom this could be attributed to spasm in the vertebrobasilar territory. Macpherson and Graham[72] have found correlations between the presence of spasm, intracranial hematoma, and ischemic damage after head injury.

Vascular Injury after Head Trauma

Frieckman and colleagues[36] reviewed 345 patients who had angiography after head injury—in almost all cases a closed injury—and showed that 62 (18%) had lesions of the extracranial and intracranial arteries. More than one vessel was involved in one third of cases. Abnormalities of the external carotid system were present in 24 patients; in 15 of these there was a rupture or AV fistula of the meningeal vessels. Intracranial vessels were affected in 38 patients. The abnormalities seen included stenosis, occlusion, aneurysm, AV fistulae, and rupture of a vessel and tearing of the intima. The internal carotid was involved in 27 cases, the meningohypophyseal trunk in 16 cases, and cortical vessels in 19 cases. In many of these patients a basal skull fracture was present, giving a clue to the likelihood of damage to vessels at the base of the brain.

Injury to the major neck vessels may also occur in the head injured patient as a consequence of trauma to the neck, as from whiplash. Spasm or thrombosis of the extracranial portion of the internal carotid is reported and in some cases can lead to hemiplegia developing at an interval after injury. The vertebral arteries can be damaged if a hyperextension injury of the neck occurs at the same time as a head injury.

Repeat Angiography

In the majority of patients it is necessary to perform only one study. However, a second investigation is indicated if the patient develops new features or fails to improve, and a second study can be strikingly different from one taken within the first few hours of injury. Cronqvist and Tylen[25] repeated angiography in 14 patients out of a total of 36 cases in whom the original angiograms showed a temporal contusion and found that in 8 of the 14 patients the lesion had increased in size.

VENTRICULOGRAPHY

After the introduction of angiography, the use of ventriculography in head injury declined. Ventriculography can only indicate that there is displacement of the ventricular system; it gives less information than either angiography or computer tomography about the nature of a lesion responsible for the shift. The introduction of air or other contrast material into the ventricles of a patient with a space-occupying lesion can produce a rise in intracranial pressure, even if precautions are taken against this by preliminary aspiration of CSF; this was one of the reasons that ventriculography fell out of favor. In the head injured patient the ventricles are often compressed and distorted. This might be expected to give rise to problems in performing ventriculography, but in one recent series this was said to be surprisingly rare.[7] Today the use of ventriculography with water-soluble contrast media lies mainly in clarifying the nature or size of a posterior fossa expanding lesion when inadequate information has been given by either angiography or computer tomography.

RADIOISOTOPE IMAGING

Two kinds of study can be performed with the use of suitable isotope labelled molecules: in a conventional brain scan the isotope is injected intravenously and its distribution within the cerebral vessels and brain tissues is followed; in isotope cisternography the isotope is introduced into the CSF in order to detect abnormal patterns of flow. Both techniques find their greatest application after head injury at a stage when late complications, such as a chronic subdural hematoma or hydrocephalus, are suspected.

Isotope Encephalography

Brain scanning may be performed as a *dynamic study* in which pictures are taken in rapid sequence within the first few seconds after an intravenous bolus of tracer. This method gives information about the distribution of tracer, and hence blood flow, through the two hemispheres and will sometimes indicate the presence of an avascular lesion such as a subdural hematoma.

In *static scanning* imaging is carried out after a finite interval—usually between 30 minutes and 3 hours after intravenous injection. The most commonly used agent is sodium pertechnetate ($Na^{99m}TcO_4$), but a wide variety of compounds have been used. What they all have in common is that they do not cross the normal blood-brain barrier but, in damaged brain or when vascular permeability is increased, they enter the brain and produce an area of heightened activity on the scan. Isotope scanning is seldom used in the acute phase of head injury because any associated skull or scalp lesion will also show as enhanced uptake at this stage, and this may be difficult to distinguish from an intracranial lesion. The greatest use made of isotope scanning has been in the detection of subacute and chronic subdural hematomas.

The most characteristic sign of a chronic subdural hematoma is a crescent-shaped area of increased uptake seen in the anterior or posterior view. In other patients there is an increased uptake over the whole of the hemisphere, either uniformly or in a patchy distribution. These appearances are not specific to subdural hematoma and are also seen in empyema, meningitis, and certain tumors.

120

The so-called "doughnut sign"[44] denotes an area of high uptake surrounding a central area in which there is no uptake.

It is the capsule of the hematoma that is probably responsible for the enhancement of the scan: when this is positive the surgeon usually finds a well-formed membrane at operation. False negative scans are thus common only in patients studied within the first few days after injury. Cowan and associates[23] found only 50 percent positive scans in patients studied within 10 days of injury, at a stage when the capsule is often minimal, but in patients who were scanned 10 days or more after injury, 91 percent of scans were positive.

Although computer tomography is superior in detecting an acute intracranial hematoma, when the suspicion is of a chronic subdural hematoma the two techniques of scanning may be equally useful. Cornell and colleagues[21] found that in 90 percent of patients with a chronic subdural hematoma the results of the two investigations corresponded; indeed, when there was disagreement, the more common finding was of a positive radioisotope scan when the CT scan was negative. This observation reflects the failure of CT scanning to demonstrate chronic hematomas that are isodense with the brain, particularly when these are bilateral and there is no midline shift.

Radioisotope Cisternography

In radioisotope cisternography the tracer is injected into the CSF, either by lumbar or ventricular puncture. The circulation of the CSF is then followed by serial static scanning. Cisternography after head injury is used either in order to confirm the presence of, or to localize the site of a cerebrospinal fluid leak in patients with a basal fracture (Chapter 8). Alternatively, in the later stages after injury, it can be used in the investigation of patients suspected of having hydrocephalus (Chapter 11), but is a less reliable method of investigating such patients than is a period of continuous monitoring of intracranial pressure.[89]

ULTRASOUND ENCEPHALOGRAPHY

Shift of the midline structures above the tentorium can be detected by ultrasound, using one-dimensional A mode techniques. Exactly what structures are responsible for the echo from the midline is uncertain; echoes may also be obtained from the walls of the lateral ventricle and from the surface of hematomas. It was at one time hoped that this cheap and portable technique might prove useful in detecting complications, particularly in patients who are in general hospitals at a distance from centers equipped for neuroradiology. Although a high reliability has been reported by committed experts,[27,50] the variability in the hands of the average user has led many surgeons[103] and radiologists to regard this as an unreliable method.

Automated methods have been used in an effort to increase the accuracy of the detection of the cerebral midline. Brisman and associates[10] compared standard scanning and automated scanning using the "Midliner" and angiography. The Midliner did not detect 19 percent of shifts, but was better than standard scanning in this respect. Klinger and colleagues,[56] on the basis of a large collaborative study of three neurosurgical clinics in Germany, also found a low false negative rate, but they noted that as many as 18 percent of their scans were unsatisfactory. They came to the conclusion that even computerized methods of detecting the midline were not sufficiently reliable for routine use in the management of head injury.

In the hands of those who have acquired both enthusiasm and expertise (and who do not have access to CT scanning), echoencephalography may have some value in the management of head injured patients, as it is a rapid method that can be carried out on a restless patient. We do not recommend it in other circumstances.

MONITORING INTRACRANIAL PRESSURE AFTER HEAD INJURY

The frequency with which ischemic brain damage and pathological evidence of raised ICP has been found at autopsy after head injury in recent reports (Chapter 2) reflects what clinicians have long recognized, namely, that many of the processes that affect the brain after head injury are eventually space-occupying. The observation that brain was often squeezed out of surgical openings in the dura after recent head injury indicated a rise in ICP, and this generated an interest in measuring intracranial pressure in head injured patients as early as 1922.[46] Continuous measurements of intracranial pressure were pioneered by Guillaume and Janny[41] and were applied systematically to head injury patients by Lundberg.[67,69] Since then much has been learned by the measurement of intracranial pressure, both in patients with brain injury and in experimental animals. However, there is still no general agreement either about the value of intracranial pressure measurements in routine practice or, if pressure is to be monitored, about which method is most appropriate.

Methods of Measuring Intracranial Pressure

Intracranial pressure can be measured most simply by connecting the CSF through a catheter to an open, fluid-filled manometer; the height of the fluid then indicates the level of pressure inside the head. In practice this is not a useful method because the likelihood of infection is too great, and because it does not provide a continual record. Intracranial pressure can vary widely, even over minutes, and all methods currently employed rely on transducing the pressure into continuous electrical signals. They can then be displayed on an oscilloscope or written out on a chart recorder. Data may also be stored and analyzed by computer.

Variations in method are mainly in the site where intracranial pressure is sensed. Clinically intracranial pressure is measured from the ventricles or from the subarachnoid, subdural, or extradural spaces. Brain tissue pressure measurements are largely confined to experimental studies.[81]

Measurement of Ventricular Fluid Pressure

This is the original method of measuring ICP and it is still widely regarded as the most reliable for routine use. A burr hole or twist drill hole is made in the right frontal region, anterior to the coronal suture and in the line of the pupil. A plastic catheter is then passed into the ventricle, entry being signalled by a slight increase and then a reduction in resistance. It might be expected that the shift and compression of the ventricles that is so common after head injury would make catheterization difficult, yet this seldom seems to be the case.[7]

In some methods the transducer is located on the tip of the ventricular catheter, but most workers have found it convenient to lead the catheter to a transducer either mounted on a bedside stand or placed externally on the patient's head. In both of the latter cases, the transducer is available for recalibration and adjustment of zero drift (Fig. 3).

Another method is to connect the ventricular catheter to a subcutaneous reservoir; after the skin is closed access to the CSF spaces is gained by inserting a fine needle through the skin into the reservoir. This method makes for easier repetition of studies, but infection is common and the reservoir may have to be removed at a second operation.

In all methods the system is calibrated against a zero reference level; this may be the level of the right atrium in a recumbent patient,[11] but Lundberg employed the approximate level of the uppermost part of the CSF system.[68] Certainly, when a patient's head is displaced above or below the level of the heart, the reference point should be related to the position of the head and should approximate to the level of either the tip of the ventricular catheter in the frontal horn, or the foramen of Munro.

Because intraventricular pressure measurements are made from naturally fluid-filled spaces, the quality of recording is high, and rapid changes in pressure can be seen. Moreover, access to the ventricle provides the possibility of measuring the "tightness" of the brain by determining the effects of induced perturbations of CSF volume upon the level of pressure. Miller and colleagues[76,80] have performed extensive studies, in patients and animals, of the effect of withdrawing from or adding to the ventricles small aliquots of fluid (1 ml); the immediate change in ICP is a measure of compliance (or tightness). They have described the effects of various pathological processes and of therapeutic maneuvers upon this.[63,79] The height of the intracranial pulse produced by the arterial pulsation has also been employed as a measure of tightness[4] as has the variation in intracra-

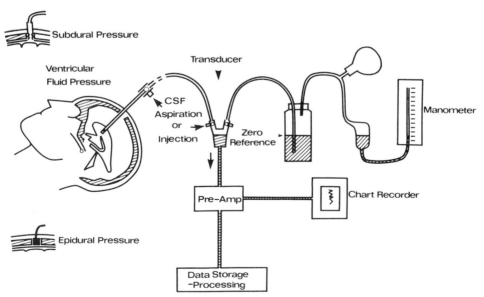

Figure 3. Techniques for continuous measurement of intracranial pressure.

nial pressure over time.[102] Another advantage of intraventricular records lies in the possibility of withdrawing fluid from the ventricle as a means of controlling intracranial pressure, at least temporarily.

The most serious disadvantages of this method are the risks of producing hemorrhage along the catheter track and of introducing infection. Intracranial hematoma as a complication of ventricular catheterization has been recorded in only isolated cases. Estimates of the risk of infection vary: it has been reported to occur in only 1 percent of large series;[100] but most experienced users admit to a rate of 3 to 5 percent[48,49,93] and some as high as 10 percent.[34] The chances of infection seem to increase with the number of times the system is manipulated, and with the duration of monitoring; they may also be increased by concurrent administration of steroids. It seems that it is only when monitoring is continued beyond 3 days that the risk of infection becomes appreciable; within this period, provided that the procedure is carried out with the full respect that it deserves, the risk is minimal.

Measurement of Subdural or Subarachnoid Pressure

A number of workers have sensed pressure from the supratentorial, subdural, or subarachnoid spaces. Some have implanted pressure transducers into this space, but the more customary method has been to incise the dura and connect the fluid in the subdural or subarachnoid space to an externally mounted transducer. Vries, Becker, and Young[113] described a method that has been adopted in a number of centers. The hole in the skull is made with a specially manufactured drill so that, once the dura has been opened, a hollow metal bolt is screwed into the opening and an exact fit obtained. The bolt is connected to the transducer by means of hollow plastic tubing and the system is irrigated occasionally to ensure patency of the bolt. It is not necessary to employ specifically manufactured bolts. Kindt and colleagues[55] have obtained satisfactory recordings merely by inserting a standard plastic three-way stopcock into the twist drill hole in the skull. It is also possible to record from a plastic catheter in the subdural space, a useful technique in a patient whose ventricles prove difficult to catheterize, as often occurs after a bone flap has been lifted.

The advantage of subdural pressure recordings lies in the simplicity with which the space can be entered, as compared to tapping the ventricle in a head injured patient. The risk of intracerebral hemorrhage is avoided, but the infection rate does not appear to be substantially less than with intraventricular measurements[93] (although the consequences may be less serious). One disadvantage of measurements from the supratentorial space is that, when the brain is swollen, the space may become obliterated and pressure readings then lost. This can often be overcome by irrigating the system, but if this has to be done frequently it may increase the risk of infection; it also occasionally produces a loculated collection of fluid, and pressure in this may not accurately reflect the overall intracranial pressure. This may explain the occasional observation of an apparently rising intracranial pressure, some days after injury, in a patient who is making an apparently satisfactory recovery.

Measurement of Extradural Pressure

Extradural pressure measurements are usually made by inserting a transducer into the skull so that the diaphragm is applied to the dura. Measurements made this way have been shown to approximate to intradural pressure, but there may be a time lag before this is achieved. Even within the normal intracranial pressure range the level of pressure measurements in the extradural space can be 1 to 2 mm Hg higher than the intradural pressure; when intracranial pressure is elevated the discrepancy may be considerable.[22]

The main disadvantage of extradural measurements lies in the rigorous technical requirements that must be satisfied. Thus it is important that the transducer lies absolutely flat on the dura,[28] otherwise stresses and strains in the dura can distort the measurements. Another major problem with extradural pressure measurements, as with all implanted pressure-sensitive devices, is electronic: the possibility of a drift from the baseline. Unless this can be checked and recalibration carried out, erroneous readings may be obtained.

Telemetry

There are a variety of implantable devices that will transmit a signal through the skin to an external receiver. This method may reduce the risks of infection and may also permit measurement of intracranial pressure in very restless patients. As yet, technical difficulties have prevented these devices from becoming simple and cheap enough to pass into routine clinical use. The need for a second operation in order to remove the device is another drawback.

Recording and Display of Pressure Records

Much useful information can be rapidly and simply obtained by visual review of the tracing, noting the basal level of pressure and whether various waves are present. Some workers record the data electronically and process them to produce frequency distributions showing the proportion of time during which intracranial pressure has been in particular ranges.[12,57] Such histograms are usually skewed, and both the degree of "skewness" and the range of variation in different epochs can be used to indicate worsening of the intracranial state or improvement in response to therapy.[112]

Definition of Raised Intracranial Pressure

The normal intracranial pressure is about 10 mm Hg. A continuous record shows pulsatile components, reflecting heart beat and respiration, and may show transient increases to extremely high levels, as when intrathoracic pressure changes in coughing and in straining. There is general agreement that a sustained level above 15 mm Hg is abnormal,[78] but the levels quoted have varied between series, and different levels may have changing significance for diagnosis and treatment (Table 1).

Lundberg[69] and Johnston, Johnston, and Jennett[51,52] suggested that, when ICP is reported, levels above 20 mm Hg should be regarded as moderately elevated and sustained levels above 40 mm Hg as severely elevated. This simple system should be generally acceptable and its use would facilitate comparisons; these are difficult to make because of the inconsistencies in many previous reports.[59]

A high level of ICP may be sustained over several hours, but transient, wave-like elevations are also common. Lundberg drew attention to three different types:

Table 1. Significance of different levels of intracranial pressure after head injury[78]

	ICP mm Hg
Normal	<10
Abnormal	>10
Further investigation	>15
Unequivocally raised	>20
Threshold for therapy	>30
Likelihood of mass	>40

A Waves or plateau waves rise suddenly and persist for at least 5 minutes above a level of 50 mm Hg before falling precipitously, even to below the original level. These waves usually emerge at variable intervals from a background of elevated pressure and can be precipitated by activity, by changes in $PaCO_2$, and by injection of air or saline into the ventricles. They may be accompanied by neurological deterioration, but are less common after head injury as compared with patients with posterior fossa tumors. They are rapidly aborted by withdrawal of CSF.

B Waves are rhythmic oscillations at ½- to 2-minute intervals and are of lesser amplitude than a plateau wave—10 to 50 mm Hg. Although they have been related to periodic breathing of the Cheyne-Stokes type, their origin is still debated. Nevertheless, they are an important sign that intracranial compensation is failing.

C Waves are more frequent, 4 to 8 per minute, and are of even smaller amplitude. They correspond to variations in blood pressure of the Traube-Herring-Meyer type.

It is common to observe an episodic change in ICP that cannot be easily recognized as one of the classic wave forms, and some workers describe "preplateau" waves, which start and stop in the same abrupt way as plateau waves, but fail to reach 50 mm Hg. It may be that no clearly distinct subdivisions exist, and patients may show a spectrum of events (Fig. 4).

Incidence

So numerous are the factors that can raise intracranial pressure after head injury that it is not surprising that the level is often abnormal when severely injured patients are monitored. Langfitt analyzed 280 patients from six previous reports (Table 2).[59] Just over one third of patients had either moderate or severe intracranial hypertension, but the varying circumstances under which ICP had been recorded and the variable definitions made interpretation difficult.

The most detailed report of ICP after head injury is that of Miller and colleagues (Table 3).[78] More than 80 percent of head injured patients who were in coma when admitted to hospital had raised intracranial pressure (defined as over 11 mm Hg), and the pressure was almost invariably high in patients with space-occupying intracranial complications (the only exceptions were patients with a cerebrospinal fluid leak through a basal skull fracture). After a hematoma was evacuated, raised intracranial pressure continued to be a problem in half of the patients. In the absence of an intracranial hematoma, raised intracranial pressure is less common; even among such patients who are in coma, only a third have abnormal ICP and the level is rarely more than moderately elevated.[34,78]

126

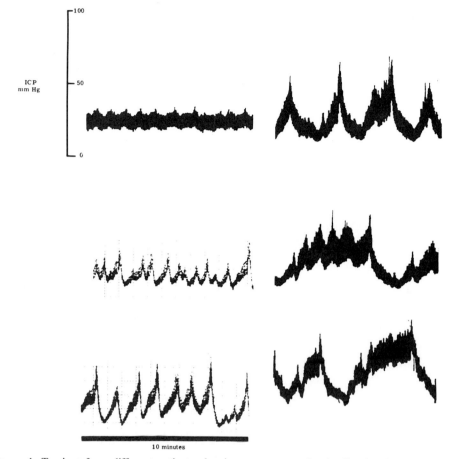

Figure 4. Tracings from different patients showing a spectrum of episodic elevations in intracranial pressure.

Significance

Despite its frequency, the meaning of raised intracranial pressure after head injury is much debated: Does brain damage cause raised intracranial pressure or does raised intracranial pressure cause brain damage? A recent review[77] acknowledges that the answer to both questions is "yes." Sometimes raised intracranial pressure merely reflects swelling of a brain already irretrievably damaged. At

Table 2. Levels* of intracranial pressure in 280 head injured patients derived from six reports summarized by Langfitt[59]

	Normal	Raised		
		Mild	Moderate	Severe
No. of patients	70	108	53	49
Percentage	25	39	19	17

*Normal <10 mm Hg; Mild >10, 11–29, or <30 mm Hg; Moderate >30, 31–50, or <60 mm Hg; Severe >50 or >60 mm Hg

Table 3. Intracranial pressure in severely head injured patients on admission to a neurosurgical unit, after hyperventilation and evacuation of mass lesions, and after further treatment by CSF drainage and mannitol with persisting raised ICP[77]

| | | On Admission | | | | In ITU | |
| | | | | | | Postoperative + Hyperventilation | After Further Therapy |
Diagnosis	No.	0–11 mm Hg	11–20 mm Hg	21–40 mm Hg	>40 mm Hg	>20 mm Hg	>20 mm Hg
Diffuse Injury	98	26	44	26	2	32 (33%)	8
Mass Lesion	62	2	17	29	14	32 (52%)	15
All patients	160	28	61	55	16	64 (40%)	23

other times raised intracranial pressure certainly can impair or even halt cerebral blood flow, so that ischemic brain damage results. Yet most investigators believe that the rate of cerebral blood flow in a head injured patient does *not* correlate closely with the level of intracranial pressure (p. 134).

In head injured patients who have only diffuse brain damage (i.e., no intracranial mass or hematoma), raised intracranial pressure may be largely a reflection of the degree of brain damage, with both the incidence and the level of raised intracranial pressure correlating with a patient's clinical state.[34,78] Thus an elevated pressure is associated in the early stages with clinical evidence of more profound damage to the brain and with a worse eventual outcome. Yet very severe degrees of diffuse white matter damage can be sustained without any evidence of raised intracranial pressure, during either clinical monitoring[51,52] or postmortem examination.[2] Sometimes it is undeniable that a rise in intracranial pressure is associated with, or even precedes, clinical deterioration and intracranial herniation.[20] But it must be questioned again whether the change in intracranial pressure is any more than another sign, although an early one, of a worsening intracranial situation.

There is least doubt that raised intracranial pressure can be a mechanism resulting in brain damage in patients with intracranial hematomas. Bruce and colleagues[13] found a correlation between perfusion pressure and cerebral blood flow only in patients with mass lesions. On the other hand, Enevoldsen[30] found that ICP levels below 45 mm Hg did not affect blood flow. When systemic arterial pressure is in the normal range, an increase in intracranial pressure above 40 mm Hg can be associated with a decline in blood flow, even in a previously normal brain, and an intracranial pressure above this threshold was associated with an increasingly severe clinical state in a series of patients with intracranial mass lesions.[78] Yet, even among patients with an intracranial hematoma there is no consistent point at which intracranial pressure will always cause a reduction in cerebral blood flow or will indicate a particular extent of brain shift.

Perhaps a fall in cerebral blood flow results from raised ICP only when cerebral compression is well advanced, while before this occurs, distortion and shift of the brain are more important. Indeed, in the early stages the various compensatory mechanisms may prevent anything more than a minimal rise in intracranial pressure, and it is here that measurements of intracranial elastance are claimed to be helpful. When this is tested by adding 1 ml of fluid to the ventricles, or alternatively, withdrawing the same volume, a change in intracranial pressure of less

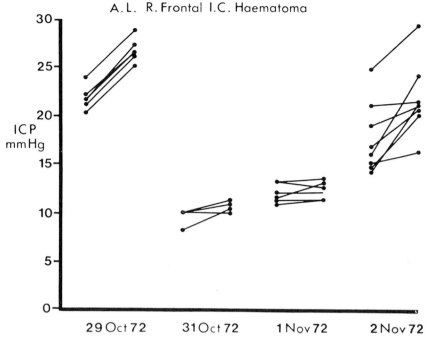

Figure 5. Intracranial pressure responses to 1 ml change in CSF volume in a patient with a post-traumatic frontal intracerebral hematoma. After the first observations, partial aspiration of hematoma was carried out, resulting in reduction of mean pressure and sensitivity in 31 October, 1972; thereafter, both mean pressure and sensitivity increased, requiring formal craniotomy and evacuation of further hematoma. (From Miller and Pickard,[80] with permission.)

than 2 mm Hg indicates adequate compensatory reserve; a rise of 5 mm Hg or more can indicate the need for treatment[80] (Fig. 5).

Value of Measuring Intracranial Pressure

Three uses for continuing intracranial pressure measurements have been suggested: in diagnosis, in prognosis, and in determining both the need for treatment and its effectiveness.[48]

Diagnosis

Intracranial pressure is usually, although not invariably, elevated when measurements are made in a patient who has a significant acute intracranial hematoma. Yet when CT scanning is freely available, ICP measurements have little part in the diagnosis of this complication because the indications for investigation by CT scanning can be based upon simple clinical criteria. In the patient whose initial scan is negative, the subsequent development of a space-occupying lesion is uncommon, and when it does occur it is usually accompanied by clinical signs. However, in a patient who has been rendered inaccessible to clinical assessment by sedative or paralyzing drugs, a rise in intracranial pressure may be the only indication of the need for repeated scanning; this may be especially useful in the postoperative period.

Prognosis

Many authors have sought to relate levels of intracranial pressure to outcome after head injury. Langfitt[59] reviewed several previous studies[8,13,52,54,111] and concluded that elevated intracranial pressure had little effect upon prognosis unless the pressure had increased to an extremely high level. The surprisingly high rate of bad results among the group of patients with normal pressure reflects case selection in the original series, which included an unrepresentatively high proportion of deeply unconscious patients with diffuse white matter injury—in whom intracranial pressure is typically normal. Langfitt commented that "severe intracranial hypertension carries with it a poor prognosis; nevertheless, approximately one third of the mortality and severe morbidity is in patients with little or no intracranial hypertension."

Several recent studies have emphasized the relationship between intracranial pressure levels and outcome, although the stage at which intracranial pressure was measured, and the methods of reporting elevated levels, varied between the different reports (Table 4). Some of these reports mention the need to take a patient's age and clinical state into account. Thus, Collice and associates[20] found, in children under 15 years of age, that there was not a significant relationship between intracranial pressure level and outcome, and that children under 8 years of age would recover after even severely raised intracranial pressure. These and other workers acknowledged the need also to take account of a patient's neurological state when considering prognosis because "ICP levels are of less significance than clinical signs of severe cerebral and brainstem dysfunction."[78]

In an adult patient an extremely high and sustained level of intracranial pressure that is resistant to therapy can reliably indicate irretrievable brain damage. Yet these levels are found in relatively few patients, and in them there is almost always clear clinical evidence of poor prognosis. Intracranial pressure measurements probably add only marginally to the accuracy of prognosis derived from a statistical analysis based on assessment of neurological dysfunction combined with age.

Table 4. Numbers of patients and bad outcomes* in different ICP ranges

Author	ICP Reported	ICP mm Hg	No. of Pts.	Bad Outcome	ICP mm Hg	No. of Pts.	Bad Outcome	ICP mm Hg	No. of Pts.	Bad Outcome
Collice et al.[20]	Highest value of baseline	0–15	41	20%	16–45	17	47%	>45	15	87%
Papo & Caruselli[88]	After admission	0–20	24	83%	20–50	49	82%	>50	9	100%
Miller et al.[78]	Admission	0–20	89	36%	20–40	71	45%	>40	16	75%
Miller et al.[77]	During monitoring in ITU	0–20	96	22%	>20	64	64%	—	—	—
Fleischer et al.†[34]	Sustained elevation	0–20	26	54%	>20	14	71%	—	—	—

*Bad outcome = Dead (Collice); or Dead/Vegetative/Severe (Papo & Caruselli, Miller et al., and Fleischer et al.).
†All patients had negative angiograms.

Treatment

The value of intracranial pressure monitoring should be judged by the difference it makes to management and to an improved outcome for the monitored patient. Unfortunately, it is here that evidence is least conclusive and opinions are most conflicting.

It is necessary to separate the undoubted contribution of intracranial pressure measurements to our understanding of intracranial events after head injury from the application of these concepts to the management of an individual patient. Once a particular measure has been shown in a careful study to raise, or conversely, to reduce raised intracranial pressure, it may not be necessary to continue demonstrating this effect in every patient before taking appropriate action. An intracranial hematoma can be evacuated, an abscess can be drained, and hypoxia, hypercarbia, hypotension, and other causes of cerebral swelling can be prevented or corrected without demonstrating that there is raised intracranial pressure in a particular patient. Thus part of the debate about the contribution of pressure *measurements* to management centers upon the value of various forms of treatment that are aimed at relieving raised intracranial pressure without regard to its specific cause. Many of these therapeutic techniques are now part of routine care for the patient in coma, and monitoring of pressure is not required in order to justify their use. However, certain other methods carry a substantial hazard, and their effect on outcome remains controversial. These include extreme hyperventilation, osmotics, high-dose steroids, and barbiturate-induced cerebral depression. It would seem justifiable to use such regimens only when ICP measurements have shown that in this individual patient the ICP was in fact high in spite of more conventional measures. Moreover, continued monitoring during treatment may help to evaluate the actual contribution of these methods to the control of ICP, which is of course only one benefit that they might confer.

Intensive systems of management that are aimed at controlling intracranial pressure have been reported to result in improved outcome both in adults[7,74] and in children.[14] The criteria for inclusion in each study, whether data were recorded prospectively or retrospectively, and the basis for making comparisons need careful scrutiny. Measurement of intracranial pressure on a routine basis has been only one component of the so-called intensive regimens, and there is no conclusive evidence that, by itself, intracranial pressure measurement can substantially affect the outcome of a head injured patient. Nor would it be realistic to expect it to do so.

Indications for Monitoring Intracranial Pressure

The risk of a hematoma or other surgically remediable intracranial complication is small among patients who do not have impairment of consciousness. Even those who are enthusiastic about intracranial pressure measurement monitor, as a routine, only patients who are not obeying commands, and some monitor only those with abnormal motor responses to painful stimulation. By contrast, the frequency of raised intracranial pressure after evacuation of an intradural hematoma makes it a circumstance in which measurements can be of great value. They may also be helpful in determining the need for surgery in patients with a "silent" intradural hematoma in whom it is decided to adopt a conservative, expectant policy (see p. 172).[106] Management of raised pressure that has been caused by cerebral engorgement provides another indication. In a patient who has been shown not to have a hematoma, the value of pressure measurements is debatable, and Fleischer and colleagues[34] considered that there might be no reason to monitor pressure in a head injured patient once the presence of an intracranial mass has been excluded by CT scanning.

In deciding whether to recommend that a particular hospital should undertake the monitoring of intracranial pressure, local circumstances, such as the personnel available and the sort of patient population encountered, will usually indicate what is appropriate. The degree of expertise needed to manage intracranial pressure monitoring, and in particular, to interpret and then act upon its results, should not be underestimated. Experienced users share their reservations about recommending that intracranial pressure measurements be instituted for no purpose other than monitoring head injured patients, particularly in a unit in which the necessary neurosurgical and neuroanesthetic expertise are not immediately available throughout the day and night. Many believe in restricting its use to neurosurgical centers where other reasons for monitoring and treating intracranial pressure will also apply.

MEASUREMENT OF CEREBRAL BLOOD FLOW AND METABOLISM

Most secondary brain damage after head injury is ultimately the result of focal or generalized reduction in cerebral blood flow (CBF). When this is sufficiently severe and persistent it produces structural changes; the frequency of ischemic brain damage at autopsy after head injury has already been noted (Chapter 2). It was therefore natural to apply the methods evolved over the last 15 years for measuring CBF in man to head injured patients, to seek both a practical guide to treatment and in the hope of finding correlations between abnormal CBF and either initial severity or ultimate outcome. That the results have been disappointing, and that no clear picture has emerged reflect both the complexity of the problem and the inherent limitations of the techniques that have so far been developed.

Measurement of Regional Cerebral Blood Flow in Man

The most commonly employed method depends upon measuring the rate of clearance from the brain of a radioactive tracer—usually the inert gas ^{133}xenon— which is soluble and readily diffusible between blood and brain tissue. The tracer is administered either by the intracarotid or intravenous injection of a solution or by the inhalation of the gas. After administration is discontinued the rate of clearance from the cerebral tissues depends upon two factors: the rate of cerebral blood flow and the diffusibility of xenon between brain and blood.

Until recently it was possible to produce only a two-dimensional map of blood flow, usually of the lateral aspect of the cerebral hemisphere. This picture is dominated by the blood flow in the cerebral cortex but there are contributions from deeper structures and there is also considerable overlap between adjacent regions of the brain. When there is localized disease this may produce a large area of underperfusion, yet this may be under-represented on the two-dimensional map, because it is overshadowed by surrounding areas of better perfusion. Recently introduced methods of measuring blood flow in the brain in three dimensions may overcome this problem but share some of the other limitations of cerebral blood flow measurements.

Accurate measurements of blood flow with any isotope clearance technique depend upon the tracer achieving a uniform partial pressure throughout the tissue being studied. When there is an area of inhomogeneously damaged brain, xenon may diffuse between areas of relatively low and high perfusion; this will again have the effect of causing an underestimation of the extent of any area of low perfusion. An important contribution to the calculation of values of cerebral blood flow is a knowledge of the partition coefficient of xenon. This expresses the relative solubility of xenon in brain and blood and has been determined for normal brain but apparently not for injured brain. This limits the value of any comparisons, whether between different regions in the same brain, between serial studies in the same patient, or between different groups of patients. Also, although it is normally possible to separate the fast clearance of isotope from the gray matter from the slow clearance from the white matter, the differences between these two components of the cerebral circulation become much less distinct in the presence of brain damage or low blood flow.

Cerebral Blood Flow after Head Injury

Several studies have shown that in individual head injured patients the overall level of cerebral blood flow may be normal (usually 50 to 55 ml/100 g/min), extremely low, or extremely high.[5,13,15,30,33,86,87] The usual findings in the first few days after injury, when consciousness is impaired, is that cerebral blood flow is subnormal; subsequently, in patients who recover, the level returns to normal, but in those who either deteriorate or stay in coma there is usually a further reduction in blood flow. An alternate finding has been of an abnormally high (hyperemic) level of cerebral blood flow in the early stage, particularly in certain young patients who have severe diffuse brain damage. Studies of cerebral blood flow in patients with an intracranial hematoma have usually been limited to only the affected side. Before operation the usual finding is of lower blood flow than in a comparable patient with a diffuse injury.[5,13] Obrist and colleagues,[86] using an inhalation technique, found that a hematoma was usually associated with an asymmetrical flow, lower levels being recorded on the side of the clot. After evacuation of a hematoma blood flow may remain depressed or may increase, and changes usually correlate with the patient's clinical course.

The most commonly observed focal abnormality of blood flow within the cerebral hemisphere has been one or more areas of high blood flow.[31,53,87] Indeed several workers have detected regions that appeared to contain a third, extra-fast component that dominates the first few minutes of clearance, the so-called "tissue peak." This component may be equivalent to an area with a blood flow between 170 and 300 ml/100 g/min and can account for up to 40 percent of the perfusion of an affected region. Such tissue peaks have been correlated with the angiographic appearance of arteriovenous shunting and a capillary blush; both findings have been most commonly disclosed in patients observed to have cerebral contusions at operation. Areas of focally reduced blood flow have been seen only rarely, but this is certainly merely a reflection of the technical factors referred to above.

Dynamic Aspects

AUTOREGULATION. The ability of the brain to maintain a constant blood flow when perfusion pressure changes has usually been tested by infusion of angiotensin in order to raise the blood pressure. Within the first week of injury, some impairment of autoregulation is common, although it rarely affects the whole of the cerebral hemisphere; indeed in one study[17] 83 percent of patients had focally disturbed autoregulation.

Increases of blood pressure have been found to increase the size of a hyperemic area and to disclose further areas of focal hyperemia. These areas have been correlated with regions that were seen to be damaged at the time of operation; on the other hand, Bruce[13] could not define a pattern of relationship between autoregulatory impairment and cortical lesions and, indeed, found little difference in autoregulatory function in different regions of the same hemisphere.

In some head injured patients who have clinical (and often eventually pathological) evidence of severely damaged brain, an increase in perfusion pressure does not affect CBF. This stability does not indicate a responsive vasculature, but possibly one that is compressed by edema;[31] it has been termed "false autoregulation." However, the assumption that the angiotensin used to increase blood pressure has itself no effect on cerebral vessels is probably incorrect. Pickard and colleagues[1] have shown that angiotensin, when applied locally around the pial vessels, produces vasoconstriction and also has this effect when administered into the carotid artery, in a dose that does not affect systemic blood pressure. The possibility that systemically administered agents may have additional, direct effects upon CBF when the blood-brain barrier is defective[71] limits their use in investigating the diseased brain's circulation.

RESPONSE OF THE CEREBRAL CIRCULATION TO CARBON DIOXIDE. A sudden change of $PaCO_2$ will normally alter blood flow by 4 to 6 percent for every millimeter of change in CO_2. Clinical studies indicate that some CO_2 responsiveness is preserved, but in the early stages after head injury it is reduced to half of normal.[15,37,87] However, in one study[33] the absence of reactivity was noted in 44 percent of a series of patients tested within 4 days of injury; patients showing the lowest CO_2 reactivity have usually been the most severely injured and have an extremely poor prognosis.[18,87]

It is known from many experimental studies that the responses of the cerebral circulation to changes in CO_2 and to changes in blood pressure may be dissociated. CO_2 responsiveness is often retained when autoregulation is lost and this is probably customary after head injury, although the number of observations is limited. On the other hand, experimental brain stem injury has been reported to produce an impaired CO_2 responsiveness while autoregulation is preserved.[32,96]

Intracranial Pressure and Cerebral Blood Flow

Studies of cerebral blood flow have usually been carried out in patients with either normal or, at the most, mildly raised intracranial pressure, and a consistent relationship has not emerged.[17,30,33,59,87] The report of Bruce and colleagues[13] is distinctive because a high proportion of patients had raised intracranial pressure. In that study it was only in patients who had an intracranial space-occupying lesion that there was any correlation between the level of cerebral blood flow and intracranial pressure (or perfusion pressure) (Fig. 6). Moreover, even in this group the evidence for the relationship depended upon a small number of patients with an extremely high intracranial pressure; there was no obvious relationship when intracranial pressure was less than 60 mm Hg. The absence of an obvious relationship between blood flow and perfusion pressure may seem at odds with the observation that autoregulation is often disturbed after head injury, but may reflect the dominant role of cerebral function and metabolism as determinants of the level of blood flow.

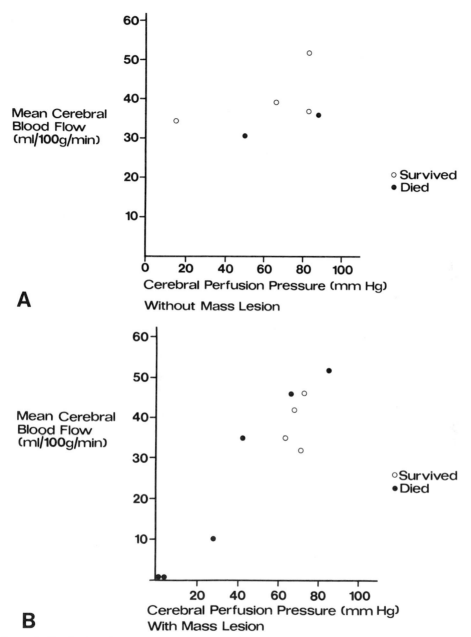

Figure 6. Cerebral perfusion pressure and cerebral blood flow in head injured patients. **A,** Without mass lesion; **B,** with mass lesion. (Data derived from Bruce and associates.[13])

Cerebral Metabolic Rate

From a knowledge of the rate of cerebral blood flow and the difference in content of oxygen of cerebral arterial and venous blood, it is possible to calculate the cerebral metabolic rate for oxygen (p. 46). In clinical studies blood has

135

usually been obtained from the internal jugular vein but this may be contaminated by extracranial blood and so not truly represent cerebral venous findings. Another problem is that blood flow has usually been measured in only one hemisphere at a time, whereas jugular venous blood is derived variably from both hemispheres. The normal brain consumes oxygen at a rate slightly above 3 ml/100 g/min, but the $CMRO_2$ has been found to be reduced to one third or one half of normal among severely head injured patients.[13,15,37] In such patients, however, there are wide individual variations. Although extremely high levels of intracranial pressure, and indeed coma, tend to be associated with a lower level of metabolism, measurement of cerebral metabolic rate has been a disappointing index of prognosis. Cold commented that he could not identify a critical low level of $CMRO_2$ and that values as low as 0.4 ml/100 g/min could be followed by survival.[15]

Some workers have studied changes in $CMRO_2$ as a means of identifying the benefits of various treatments. Thus the administration of mannitol or elevation of perfusion pressure or hyperventilation can increase $CMRO_2$.[6,13,37] However, the clinical implications of measurements of $CMRO_2$ are unclear and they do not provide information of value in routine clinical practice.

Blood Flow and Outcome

In patients who die or who fail to recover, the level of cerebral blood flow has usually been found to be lower than in those who survive to make good recoveries (Table 5).[60] The correlation between low blood flow and bad outcome has often depended upon a minority of patients with very low blood flows whose poor prognosis was evident on clinical grounds. On the other hand, very high levels of blood flow have also been found to relate to bad outcomes,[87] and in some patients evoked electrocortical activity may be absent even though cerebral blood flow is high.[40] These observations indicate an uncoupling of the link between cerebral metabolism and blood flow (p. 52) and may be an illustration of the so-called "luxury perfusion syndrome." Although it has been suggested that blood flow may be used as a guide to prognosis, the measurements probably add little to what can be gained from clinical examination.

Table 5. Intracranial pressure, cerebral blood flow, and outcome

Authors	Outcome	n	ICP mm Hg	Range	CBF ml/100g/min	Range
Bruce et al.[13]	Survive	9	36	10–77	41.0	32–52
	Dead/vegetative	5	61.4	22–112	24.4	0–46
Fieschi et al.[33]	Recover or extra-cerebral death	7	5	—	32.0	—
	Cerebral death	3	17	—	46.6	—
Cold & Jensen[17]	Survive ± dementia	14	19	3–30	37	20–71
	Dead/vegetative	4	17	10–25	33	27–40

ELECTROPHYSIOLOGICAL ASSESSMENT OF BRAIN FUNCTION

The changes in the electrical activity of the brain that accompany neural activity have been studied in the hope that the findings might provide a measure of brain damage that would be more direct, more sensitive, and more objective than clinical examination. Two methods have been employed: recording of the sponta-

136

neous electroencephalogram, and the analysis of the electrocerebral responses that can be evoked by defined, specific, sensory stimuli.

The Electroencephalogram

More than a quarter of a century ago, Dawson carried out serial electroencephalograms of head injured patients,[26] and several subsequent workers have reported on the value of the investigation in the monitoring of progress, in the diagnosis of complications such as a hematoma, and as an index of prognosis.[99] The most common finding is of slowing on the EEG, to an extent that correlates with severity of head injury. Changes in frequency accompany clinical improvement or deterioration; individual patterns, however, vary considerably and the nonspecific changes that accompany impairment of consciousness often mask those resulting from complications. With a hematoma the EEG may show an increase in slow activity or suppression of amplitude on one side, or there may be a decrease in activity on both sides of the brain. Such slow wave activity may be rhythmic or arrhythmic, but it is not clear whether the EEG changes are due directly to the effect of the hematoma on the underlying brain or whether they reflect brain stem compression, in which generalized rhythmic slow wave activity is common. With an intracerebral hematoma there may be few specific EEG changes.

The interpretation of the EEG after head injury requires considerable experience, not least because it is difficult to obtain reliable records in restless patients. Artefactual abnormalities may result from swelling of the scalp, which reduces the voltage, and from arterial pulsation in the scalp, resulting in slow waves. If there are lacerations or operative incisions that make it necessary to place electrodes in unusual positions, the result may be an apparent asymmetry.

More quantitative information about the level of electrocerebral activity than is obtained by the usual "eyeball" analysis of the EEG can be derived by computer analysis of the spectrum of frequencies or by integration of the voltage within a particular record. However, frequency and voltage may change in different directions, so there may be times when a single index of overall cerebral electrical activity will obscure important events. Sophisticated methods of analysis may therefore offer little advantage over standard EEG recordings, and, because these have found little place in clinical practice, interest has centered recently upon the electrocerebral events that occur in response to specific stimuli.

Evoked Cerebral Potentials

The changes in electrocerebral potential that ensue when a single brief stimulus is applied to a sensory nerve reflect the passage of the stimulus through subcortical structures, or the events consequent on its arrival in the cortex. The amplitude of the change resulting from a single stimulus is so small that, when recorded via a scalp electrode, it is lost against the background EEG. Clinical studies of evoked responses have been made feasible by the development of methods for storing electronically the response to a single stimulus, so that the results of a train of successive stimuli can be averaged. This process multiplies the changes specific to the sensory stimulus and largely eliminates EEG and other background activity. The resulting wave forms consist normally of a number of peaks with characteristic amplitude and latency, according to the response being studied and the technique of recording. In the near-field technique the potentials recorded are those occurring between a pair of closely spaced electrodes; a small alteration of position of one electrode on the scalp causes changes in what potential is recorded. In far-field techniques the electrodes are widely spaced—usually one is on the skull and the other is on the mastoid process. Precise placement of electrodes is not critical, yet a wide range of events can be detected.

The evoked responses currently studied after head injury include visual, somatosensory, and auditory near-field and far-field responses. In the somatosensory evoked responses a peripheral nerve is stimulated electrically—usually the median nerve at the wrist. Just before each peripheral stimulus, a synchronizing pulse is sent to trigger the computer averaging. Similarly, with visual and auditory responses, averaging is triggered along with the generation of the light or sound stimulus. When a patient shows an abnormal response it is important to consider whether the peripheral sensory organs and pathways are functioning and whether the pathways conducting the response at spinal, brain stem, and subcortical levels are intact before inferring that there is damage within the appropriate area of the cerebral cortex. The auditory far-field response consists of a complex series of potentials, which reflect various components in the auditory pathway, the early events being correlated with potentials in the auditory nerve and subsequent potentials relating to successive parts of the pathways within the brain stem and hemispheres. The ability to identify events within the brain stem has led to this response being referred to sometimes as the "brain stem evoked response."

Following Larson's demonstration of the feasibility of studying somatosensory evoked responses after head injury,[62] the use of a comprehensive range of evoked responses was described by Greenberg and colleagues.[38] The latter authors reported on 51 severely head injured patients,[39] all of whom were unresponsive to verbal commands for at least 4 days. In 89 percent of cases the patient was first studied within the first 9 days of injury (mean time was the third day); a comprehensive range of potentials was studied and abnormalities were frequent (Fig. 7). There was a correlation between abnormalities in evoked responses and outcome, and between individual responses and clinical findings in the acute stage. When visual responses were normal but somatosensory and auditory responses abnormal, this was held to reflect damage predominantly in the brain stem, and this finding correlated with the presence of abnormal eye movements or pupil responses. Abnormal cortical potentials correlated with the presence of abnormal motor responses (decortication and decerebration) and with the subsequent duration of coma. This finding supports the concept that the cerebral hemispheres may be more vulnerable to damage from diffuse impact forces than the brain stem (p. 22).

The most appropriate method for analyzing evoked potential recordings is unresolved. Both changes in amplitude and alterations in the latency of different peaks can occur and make it difficult to interpret abnormal records in an exact manner. The most profitable approach may be to study simply how many waves can be detected and so judge overall complexity of response.

There are practical limitations to the use of evoked potentials. To perform the comprehensive study of visual, somatosensory, and auditory responses with present techniques takes 2 or more hours, during which time skilled operators must be constantly present. Technical developments may improve upon this and also reduce the very considerable capital cost of equipment. Meanwhile, it is important to clarify whether evoked potential studies can discover more than can be found by routine clinical methods, and also whether there may be selected

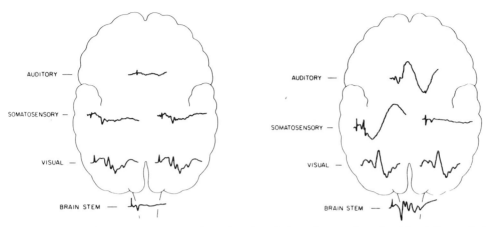

Figure 7. Brain images with the approximate location of sites of generation of multimodality evoked potentials. *Left:* The visual evoked potential is practically normal, while the somatosensory and auditory near- and far-field evoked potentials are absent in this comatose patient, suggesting brain stem dysfunction. *Right:* The right parietal lobe response to left median nerve depolarization is absent in a patient with dense left hemiparesis. All other multimodality evoked potentials were almost normal in this patient. (From Greenberg, Becker, Miller, et al.[39] Reprinted with permission of the American Association of Neurological Surgeons, Publishers of the Journal of Neurosurgery.)

clinical circumstances in which they can offer advantages. One of these may be when the patient has received muscle relaxants or central nervous system depressants, either of which render him inaccessible to clinical examination. The value of evoked responses as a means of continuous monitoring of head injured patients is currently under study. Even if the technical problems are overcome, sensory evoked responses may provide only a very limited warning of a deteriorating intracranial situation. Experimentally, after middle cerebral artery occlusion, the somatosensory evoked response is usually maintained despite considerable reductions in cerebral blood flow, until the latter falls to a critical threshold level of about 15 to 17 ml/100 g/min, when the response disappears abruptly.[9] Although this event appears to precede the establishment of permanent brain damage, the value of the response as an indication of the adequacy of cerebral perfusion is limited by the absence of premonitory changes. On the other hand, although the level of CBF at which activity disappears appears to be similar with any electro-cortical event, other evoked responses may show progressive changes before this occurs.[29,107]

BIOCHEMICAL MARKERS OF BRAIN DAMAGE

The discovery of emboli consisting of brain tissue in the lungs of the severely head injured patient was an extreme illustration of the way that substances may leak from damaged brain and enter the bloodstream or the cerebrospinal fluid.[70] Lesser degrees of leakage are probably a common occurrence and the identification of substances that are derived from the brain may be useful in first confirming the presence of brain damage and then perhaps in indicating its severity, and so a patient's prognosis. Interest was first directed to identifying enzymes in the blood that were specific to the brain, as distinct from those that might be released from injuries to other organs in the patient with multiple injuries. Lindblom showed that isoenzymes of lactic dehydrogenase were present in abnormally high levels in the blood in a series of patients with brain contusions.[65,66] The maximum level of activity of this enzyme could be related to prognosis.[90,91,110] However, the identification of brain-specific isoenzymes of lactic dehydrogenase is technically difficult, and creatine kinase may be a more useful index because its isoenzyme CK_{BB} is almost brain-specific.[43] The time course of the rise in enzyme activity in the blood varies with the nature of brain damage; high levels within the first 24 hours reflect primary damage, whereas activity caused by secondary complications appears later.

The detection of nervous system-specific proteins may be an even more specific indication of brain damage than studies of isoenzymes. Radioimmunoassay techniques have been employed to determine the level of myelin-basic protein (MBP) in the blood and CSF of head injured patients.[108] Levels were significantly raised on admission in patients with severe intracerebral damage and rose at 4 to 6 days after injury in patients with extracerebral hematomas, this time course paralleling that observed for brain isoenzymes. The mean level between 2 to 6 days after injury was higher in those patients who had poor outcomes (Fig. 8).

A preliminary study has shown that the maximum levels of serum myelin basic protein correlate with the patient's responsiveness as assessed by the Glasgow Coma Scale.[109] How much biochemical markers of brain damage add to what can be detected clinically has still to be discovered.

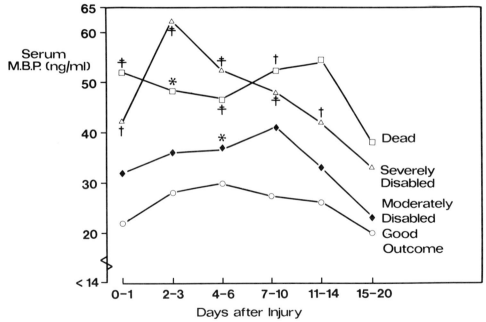

Figure 8. Mean serum myelin-basic protein (M.B.P.) in head injured patients by outcome. The numbers are good outcome 51, moderate disability 40, severe disability 28, and death 38. Results significantly greater than control: *p 0.05, †p0.01, ‡p 0.001. Comparison of results between outcome groups indicates that serum M.B.P. in severely disabled patients was greater than in those with good outcome between days 2 and 6 (p 0.01), and levels in patients who died were greater than in those with good outcome between days 4 and 6 (p 0.05). (From Thomas, Palfreyman, and Ratcliffe,[108] with permission.)

The demonstration that complex brain-specific molecules gain access to the blood stream after head injury has raised the possibility that they may initiate immunological response, which can then in turn be directed against the brain itself. Such mechanisms may contribute to the pathophysiological processes responsible for either early or late complications of injury. Although the clinical value and theoretical significance of these measurements are at present unclear, they seem likely to be a topic of increasing interest. Not the least of the attractions is that all that is required of the clinician is the withdrawal of a blood sample at the appropriate time, which may then be stored for later analysis.

CSF Biochemistry

In cerebral ischemia the ratio of lactate to pyruvate increases (p. 47), and Enevoldsen and colleagues[30] observed that a rising CSF lactate and a falling pH preceded increases in intracranial pressure and changes in cerebral blood flow in severely head injured patients. However, many factors other than brain damage can affect the CSF acid-base status, and these include such common components of head injury as respiratory changes and subarachnoid hemorrhage. Prognostically, a high level of CSF lactate correlates with a bad outcome,[24,58] but only at extreme levels is the relationship reliable. The major limitation of measurements made in the CSF is that they are an extremely imperfect way of reflecting events within the cells of the brain itself.

CARDIORESPIRATORY MONITORING

Cardiorespiratory dysfunction is common after severe head injury and it is important to recognize and to analyze. It may reflect brain damage and therefore be of diagnostic or prognostic significance. The dysfunction itself, whatever its cause, may threaten cerebral oxygenation, which makes it vital to treat the condition appropriately. When there are pulmonary complications (or associated chest injury) it is often difficult to judge the relative contribution to cardiorespiratory abnormalities of pulmonary and cerebral factors.

We are concerned here largely with the measurement of cardiorespiratory function, not with indications for therapy, which are discussed elsewhere. There is, however, a tendency to confuse observations or measurements with the action to which they may properly lead. For example, "inadequate respiratory function" may be taken to mean "requiring assisted ventilation"; however, there is considerable controversy about indications for ventilation, and these should be clearly distinguished from observations about respiratory function.

Respiratory function is reflected in PaO_2 and $PaCO_2$. These are the end results of several factors, particularly ventilation and metabolic rate (of O_2 consumption and CO_2 production); but they are also influenced by the oxygen content of the inspired air and by any factors that adversely affect gas exchange in the lungs. It is surprising how often the level of the PaO_2 is quoted without reference to whether the patient is breathing air or an oxygen-enriched mixture. Metabolic rate can vary markedly after head injury, being increased when there is excessive muscle activity and reduced by muscle relaxants or hypothermia. The consequences of change in respiratory function will be different in patients who are breathing spontaneously, whose chemoreflex activity is preserved, than in those whose ventilation is controlled or assisted. Failure to acknowledge this simple

141

physiological fact may account for some of the differences between the statements of anesthesiologists on the one hand and of surgeons on the other.

A *raised PaCO$_2$* can only result from alveolar ventilation that is inadequate relative to CO$_2$ production (hypoventilation). No matter how severe the venous admixture (owing to shunting or ventilation/perfusion abnormality), the PaCO$_2$ cannot rise to even the mixed venous level (normal value 46 mm Hg). When venous admixture occurs in a spontaneously breathing patient, PaCO$_2$ will not rise and indeed will usually fall, because of chemoreflex stimulation of ventilation resulting from the associated hypoxemia.

Hypoxemia in the recently head injured patient is common, but is not usually due to hypoventilation (i.e., PaCO$_2$ is commonly normal or low). The cause is more often venous admixture, caused by areas of lung having a low ventilation/perfusion ratio, such that blood leaves the lungs inadequately oxygenated. This may be the result of structural changes in alveoli (from aspiration or pulmonary edema), or of pulmonary hemodynamic changes, possibly owing to neurogenic influences from brain damage. The PaO$_2$ can usually be restored to at least 100 mm Hg by breathing oxygen-enriched gas. With 100 percent inspired oxygen, if the lungs are normal, the PaO$_2$ should rise to above 600 mm Hg; the extent to which it falls short of that level is a measure of the severity of the effective pulmonary arteriovenous shunting.

The PaO$_2$ and the PaCO$_2$ represent, therefore, the end result of a series of interacting physiological processes. The effect of respiratory dysfunction of blood gases can be summarized as follows:

1. If there is *hypoventilation,* whether the patient is spontaneously breathing or is on assisted ventilation, then the PaCO$_2$ will rise, and PaO$_2$ will fall.
2. If there is *venous admixture* (effective shunting) the effect will differ.
   a) *Spontaneous breathing* —PaO$_2$ down; PaCO$_2$ normal or down.
   b) *Assisted ventilation* —PaO$_2$ down (unless breathing oxygen-enriched air); PaCO$_2$ up.

What effect hypoxemia has on oxygen availability in the brain depends on the effect that PaO$_2$ has on the saturation of the hemoglobin (in accordance with the oxyhemoglobin dissociation curve), on the hematocrit, and on cerebral blood flow. Hypercapnia will affect the pH environment of the neurons; its effect on the intracranial hemodynamics will depend on various local variables, in particular the elastance of the brain and the cerebrovascular reactivity[85] (p. 53).

The level of PaO$_2$ that will definitely threaten cerebral oxygenation depends on many factors. For example, if cardiac output, oxyhemoglobin saturation, and hemoglobin content are all reduced by modest amounts (each of which alone would not be significant), there may be an important affect on the brain. But if PaO$_2$ falls to 70 mm Hg, there is very little decrease in saturation, because this is the flat part of the oxygen dissociation curve. As an example, if the hematocrit is 30 and the PaO$_2$ is 60 to 70 mm Hg, correcting the hemoglobin is about five times more effective in raising the oxygen content of the blood than is restoring the PaO$_2$ to 100 mm Hg, and at least four times as effective as raising the PaO$_2$ to 400 mm Hg.

Because important therapeutic decisions may depend on laboratory reports on blood gas levels, it is important to be aware of the errors that can arise owing to faults in technique. Whenever possible *arterial* samples should be taken, but if this is difficult, arterialized capillary blood can be used (from a well-warmed finger or a baby's heel); venous blood from a warm hand approximates to this.

Care is needed to avoid any air bubbles and to close the end of the syringe with a cap, having used a standardized amount of heparin. Time of sampling and of analysis should always be noted; if this interval is expected to exceed 10 minutes, the sample should be kept in crushed ice. If oxygen analysis will be delayed, a glass rather than a plastic syringe should be used. Blood-gas analysis requires disciplined and well-trained technicians, who are aware of the need to check the membranes of the electrodes frequently, and who will repeat analysis on duplicate samples whenever possible, and always when a result is abnormal. Similarly, the clinician should not act on the basis of a single abnormal result, if this is unexpected; he should have the estimation repeated on another sample.

End-expired CO_2 ($P_{EI}CO_2$) can be measured using a rapid infrared analyzer, but this may not be valid if tidal volume is inadequate, as when breathing is shallow and rapid. The best check of the validity of the measurements is to write out the recording, in order to confirm that a $PaCO_2$ plateau is reached in most breaths; it is also important to calibrate the equipment regularly with accurate gas mixtures. End-tidal CO_2 (reflecting alveolar CO_2) will approximate to arterial CO_2, provided alveolar dead space is not significantly increased.

Respiratory frequency is traditionally recorded by nurses at the bedside. Because the pattern of breathing is often irregular it is essential that such "eye-ball" records made by nurses be based on sufficiently long periods of observation—at least a minute. Respiratory frequency may be increased owing to pyrexia, hypoxia, metabolic acidemia, afferent influences from the lungs when there are pulmonary complications, or, in conscious patients, owing to anxiety, pain, or even hysteria. All these should be considered before ascribing tachypnea to neurogenic mechanisms that are supposedly related to brain damage.

Increased frequency on its own is an unreliable measure of hyperventilation; indeed it has been shown to correlate poorly with $PaCO_2$ in brain damaged patients.[84] Change to a slower rate may be significant, but it is often not recognized that a number of normal individuals have respiratory rates of 8 to 10 per minute. Frequency above 30 per minute in adults must be regarded as abnormal; most patients breathing at this rate have pulmonary complications or are hypoxic, or both. Central neurogenic ventilation is a rare occurrence.[84]

Minute ventilation can be recorded using a simple respirometer and clearly gives more information than does a simple measure of frequency. However, North and Jennett[84] also showed that in brain damaged patients even minute ventilation was poorly correlated with $PaCO_2$; it must be regarded, therefore, as an inaccurate reflection of ventilatory sufficiency.

Respiratory pattern is traditionally considered a useful diagnostic and prognostic guide; in particular, periodic (including Cheyne-Stokes) breathing is usually regarded as of serious significance. Except when abnormal patterns are very marked, they are readily overlooked on routine clinical monitoring, as was revealed when a series of brain damaged patients had respiratory movements continuously recorded by impedance pneumography (Fig. 9). This method is readily set up, using stick-on sensors on the skin of the chest, connected to a direct-writing recorder.[83] In a large series of recently brain damaged patients, three patterns were recognized: normal, periodic, and irregular.[84] These occurred with about equal frequency in a series of 227 patients with acute brain damage of various etiologies in a neurosurgical unit (90 had recent head injury). Patients frequently had mixed patterns, particularly if observed over several hours (Fig. 10), but sometimes there would be more than one type of breathing within a few

143

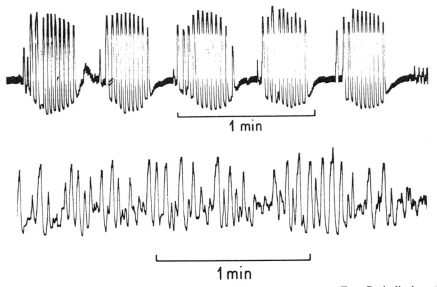

Figure 9. Abnormal patterns of respiration on impedance pneumogram. *Top:* Periodic breathing. *Bottom:* Ataxic breathing.

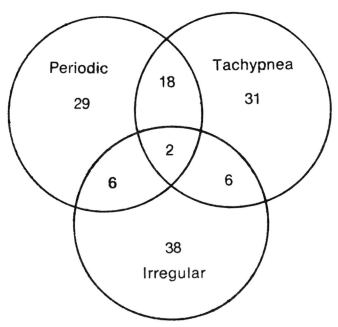

Figure 10. Frequency of different breathing patterns in acutely brain damaged patients. Note that some patients had two or three different abnormalities. (From North and Jennett,[84] with permission.)

144

minutes (Fig. 11). Only when grossly irregular (ataxic) breathing was observed could the lesion be localized reliably—this indicated medullary damage.

As ventilation increases (from the normal value of 6–7 liters/min) it has to reach 70 liters/min before the oxygen consumption of breathing itself contributes even 10 percent of the total resting body consumption; this would be equivalent to very gentle walking. The minute ventilation of brain damaged patients with respiratory frequency more than 30/min might be about 30 liters/min. If the lungs were normal this would represent no more of a work load from breathing than would walking at 2 km/hr. The work of breathing would be greater if there were decreased lung compliance, but even with the most severe emphysema the work of breathing is only equivalent to that occasioned by normal walking. Patients who are breathing rapidly may also have general body spasticity and perhaps tonic spasms, and the oxygen consumption attributable to these may be considerable. It is important not to put undue emphasis on the notion that the breathing itself is in some way diverting oxygen from the brain, because there is no physiological basis for such an assertion.

Cardiovascular function, which attracts so much attention in general intensive care units, is of rather less significance after head injury. Systemic *hypotension* is, however, important—both in the diagnosis of extracranial injury (p. 228) and because of the threat to cerebral oxygenation that it poses (p. 54). *Heart rate* can vary from many causes after recent head injury, and the bradycardia classically associated with cerebral compression is relatively seldom encountered. As emphasized when we discuss acute intracranial hematoma, it is a late sign of midbrain compression and should not be relied upon or waited for; in young, athletic subjects, the normal heart rate is often <60/min, and this may cause unjustified anxiety after head injury.

EKG abnormalities, in particular ST depression, are frequently observed in the first few hours (sometimes days) after acute brain damage. These have most often been reported after spontaneous (nontraumatic) subarachnoid hemorrhage, probably because such patients are frequently observed in medical as distinct from surgical wards. These observations are associated with structural changes in cardiac muscle[82] and are believed to result from release of catecholamines owing to cerebral damage.

The frequency with which various autonomic abnormalities were recorded in

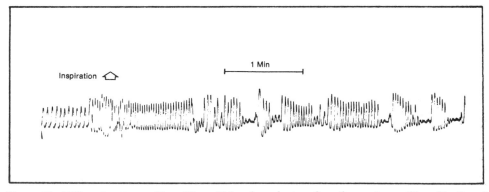

Figure 11. Different patterns of breathing within a few minutes of continuous trace. (From North and Jennett,[84] with permission.)

145

Table 6. Frequency of autonomic abnormalities after recent severe head injury

	2–3 Days		Any time in first week	
Periodic respiration	88/802	11%	181/857	28%
Respiration>30/min	172/121	24%	298/916	33%
Pulse>120/min	201/777	26%	334/974	34%
BP>160 mm Hg	126/754	17%	213/968	22%
Temperature>39°C	129/779	17%	222/961	23%

the Data Bank severe injuries is shown in Table 6. The incidence was similar in the three countries. Although these are associated with a less good outcome (p. 323), these abnormalities occur in patients whose brain damage is already obviously more severe, as indicated by other features. Autonomic abnormalities are also readily influenced by extracranial factors. For these reasons they are not reliable indicators of severity, nor are they powerful predictors.

CONCLUSION

Computer tomography has rapidly established its importance. On the other hand, it may seem that we have taken an unduly cautious attitude towards the use of various other tests that have been developed in the last decade. We believe that, in the present state of knowledge and of medical practice, this is justified. Reports on the use of intracranial pressure are certainly now numerous, although they still come from a small proportion of the centers treating severe injuries. Reports on CBF and on evoked potentials have come from only a handful of centers. It is therefore too soon to judge the role of these techniques as useful clinical tests, as distinct from research tools. At present most head injuries in most countries are managed without such investigative techniques, and for this reason alone it is unwise to base methods of management on their availability.

REFERENCES

1. ACAR, U., AND PICKARD, J. D.: *Effects of angiotensin II on pial arterioles.* Proc. Physiol. Soc. 14–15 July. J. Physiol. 284:58–59, 1978.

2. ADAMS, J. H., MITCHELL, D., GRAHAM, D. I., ET AL.: *Diffuse brain damage of immediate impact type—its relationship to "primary brainstem damage" in head injury.* Brain 89:235–268, 1977.

3. AMBROSE, J.: *Computerised transverse axial scanning. II. Clinical application.* Br. J. Radiol. 46:1023–1047, 1973.

4. AVEZAAT, C., VAN EIJNDHOVEN, J., DE JONG, D., ET AL.: "A new method of monitoring intracranial volume/pressure relationships." In Beks, J. W. F., Bosch, D. A., and Brock, M. (eds.): *Intracranial Pressure, III.* Springer-Verlag, Berlin, 1976, pp. 308–313.

5. BALDY-MOULINIER, M., AND FREREBEAU, PH.: "Cerebral blood flow in cases of coma following severe head injury." In Brock, M., Fieschi, C., Ingvar, D., et al. (eds.): *Cerebral Blood Flow.* Springer-Verlag, Berlin, 1969, pp. 216–218.

6. BALDY-MOULINIER, M., ROQUEFEUIL, B., ESCURET, E., ET AL.: "Hemodynamic and metabolic modifications into the brain following short lasting or prolonged changes of arterial pressure and PaCO₂ in comatose patients." In Harper, M., Jennett, W. B., Miller, J. D., et al. (eds.): *Blood Flow and Metabolism in the Brain.* Churchill Livingstone, Edinburgh, 1975, pp. 13.34–13.37.

7. BECKER, D. P., MILLER, J. D., WARD, J. D., ET AL.: *The outcome from severe head injury with early diagnosis and intensive management.* J. Neurosurg. 47:491–502, 1977.

8. BECKER, D. P., VRIES, J. K., YOUNG, H. F., ET AL.: "Controlled cerebral perfusion pressure and

ventilation in human mechanical brain injury: prevention of progressive brain swelling." In Lundberg, N., Ponten, V., and Brock, M. (eds.): *Intracranial Pressure, II.* Springer-Verlag, Berlin, 1975, pp. 480–484.

9. BRANSTON, N. M., SYMON, L., CROCKARD, H. A., ET AL.: *Relationship between the cortical evoked potential and focal cortical blood flow following acute middle cerebral artery occlusion in the baboon.* Exp. Neurol. 45:195–208, 1974.

10. BRISMAN, R., BUCHANAN, D. S., AND ROSEGAY, H.: *Reliability of technicians in computerised and standard A-mode midline echoencephalography.* J. Neurosurg. 41:736–739, 1974.

11. BROCK, M., AND HARTUNG, C.: "Glossary of definitions, standards and abbreviations." In Brock, M., and Dietz, H. (eds.): *Intracranial Pressure, I.* Springer-Verlag, Berlin, 1972, pp. 372–375.

12. BROCK, M., ZYWIETZ, C., MOCK, P., ET AL.: "Reliability and reproducibility of ICP frequency analysis." In Beks, J. W. F., Bosch, D. A., and Brock, M. (eds.): *Intracranial Pressure, III.* Springer-Verlag, Berlin, 1976, pp. 288–294.

13. BRUCE, D. A., LANGFITT, T. W., MILLER, J. D., ET AL.: *Regional cerebral blood flow, intracranial pressure and brain metabolism in comatose patients.* J. Neurosurg. 38:131–144, 1973.

14. BRUCE, D. A., SCHUT, L., BRUNO, L. A., ET AL.: *Outcome following severe head injuries in children.* J. Neurosurg. 48: 679–688, 1978.

15. COLD, G. E.: *Cerebral metabolic rate of oxygen (CMRO$_2$) in the acute phase of brain injury.* Acta Anaesth. Scand. 22:249–256, 1978.

16. COLD, G., ENEVOLDSEN, E., AND MALMROS, R.: "The prognostic value of continuous intraventricular pressure recording in unconscious brain injury patients under controlled ventilation." In Lundberg, N., Ponten, V., and Brock, M. (eds.): *Intracranial Pressure, II.* Springer-Verlag, Berlin, 1975, pp. 517–521.

17. COLD, G. E., AND JENSEN, F. T.: *Cerebral autoregulation in unconscious patients with brain injury.* Acta Anaesth. Scand. 22:270–280, 1978.

18. COLD, G. E., JENSEN, F. T., AND MALMROS, R.: *The cerebrovascular CO$_2$ reactivity during the acute phase of head injury.* Acta Anaesth. Scand. 21:222–231, 1977.

19. COLD, G. E., JENSEN, F. T., AND MALMROS, R.: *The effects of PaCO$_2$ reduction on regional cerebral blood flow in the acute phase of brain injury.* Acta Anaesth. Scand. 21:359–367, 1977.

20. COLLICE, M., ROSSANDA, M., BEDUSCHI, A., ET AL.: "Management of head injury by means of ventricular fluid pressure monitoring." In Beks, J. W. F., Bosch, D. A., and Brock, M. (eds.): *Intracranial Pressure, III.* Springer-Verlag, Berlin, 1975, pp. 101–109.

21. CORNELL, S. H., CHIU, L. L., AND CHRISTIE, J. H.: *Diagnosis of extracerebral fluid collections by computed tomography.* Am. J. Roentgenol. 131:107–110, 1978.

22. CORONEOS, N. J., McDOWALL, D. G., GIBSON, R. M., ET AL.: *Measurement of extradural pressure and its relationship to other intracranial pressures.* J. Neurol. Neurosurg. Psychiatry 36:514–522, 1973.

23. COWAN, R. J., MAYNARD, C. D., AND LASSITER, K. R.: *Technetium-99m pertechnetate brain scans in the detection of subdural haematomas: a study of the age of the lesion as related to the development of a positive scan.* J. Neurosurg. 32:30–34, 1970.

24. CROCKARD, H. A., AND TAYLOR, A. R.: *Serial CSF lactate/pyruvate values as a guide to prognosis in head injury coma.* Eur. Neurol. 8:151,1972.

25. CRONQVIST, A., AND TYLEN, U.: *Repeat angiography in temporal contusions.* Acta Radiol. (Diagn.) 18:161–166, 1977.

26. DAWSON, R. E., WEBSTER, J. E., AND GURDJIAN, E. S.: *Serial electro-encephalography in acute head injuries.* J. Neurosurg. 8:613–630, 1951.

27. DE VLEIGER, M., AND DE RIDDER, J. H.: *Use of echoencephalography.* Neurology (Minneap.) 9:216–223, 1959.

28. DORSCH, N. W. C., AND SYMON, L.: "The validity of extradural measurements of the intracranial pressure. In Lundberg, N., Ponten, V., and Brock, M. (eds.): *Intracranial Pressure, II.* Springer-Verlag, Berlin, 1975, pp. 403–408.

29. EISENBERG, H. M., TURNER, J. W., TEASDALE, G., ET AL.: *Monitoring of cortical excitability during induced hypotension in aneurysm operations.* J. Neurosurg. 50:595–602, 1979.

30. ENEVOLDSEN, E. M., COLD, G., JENSEN, F. T., ET AL.: *Dynamic changes in regional CBF, intraventricular pressure, CSF pH and lactate levels during the acute phase of head injury.* J. Neurosurg. 44:191–214, 1976.

31. ENEVOLDSEN, E. M., AND JENSEN, F. T.: *Autoregulation and CO_2 responses of cerebral blood flow in patients with acute severe head injury.* J. Neurosurg. 48:689–703, 1978.

32. FENSKE, A., HEY, D., THEISS, R., ET AL.: "Regional cortical blood flow in the early stage of brainstem oedema." In Harper, Jennett, Miller, et al. (eds.): *Blood Flow and Metabolism in the Brain.* Churchill Livingstone, Edinburgh, 1975, pp. 1.12–1.15.

33. FIESCHI, C., BATTISTINI, N., BEDUSCHI, A., ET AL.: *Regional cerebral blood flow and intraventricular pressure in acute head injuries.* J. Neurol. Neurosurg. Psychiatry 37:1378–1388, 1974.

34. FLEISCHER, A. S., NETTLETON, S. P., AND TINDALL, G. T.: *Continuous monitoring of intracranial pressure in severe closed head injury without mass lesions.* Surg. Neurol. 6:31–34, 1976.

35. FRENCH, B. N., AND DUBLIN, A. B.: *The value of computerised tomography in 1000 consecutive head injuries.* Surg. Neurol. 7:171–183, 1977.

36. FRIECKMAN, N., SARTOR, K., AND MATSUMOTO, K.: "Angiographic demonstration of vascular injuries following head injury and its significance." In Frowein, Wilcke, Karimi, et al. (eds.): *Advances in Neurosurgery 5.* Springer-Verlag, Berlin, 1978, pp. 116–123.

37. GENNARELLI, T. A., OBRIST, W. D., LANGFITT, T. W., ET AL.: *Vascular and metabolic reactivity to changes in PCO_2 in head injured patients.* In Popp, Bourke, Nelson, et al. (eds.): *Seminars in Neurological Surgery: Neural Trauma.* Raven Press, New York, 1979, pp. 1–8.

38. GREENBERG, R. P., MAYER, D. J., BECKER, D. P., ET AL.: *Evaluation of brain function in severe human head injury with multimodality evoked potentials. Part I. Evoked brain injury potentials, methods and analyses.* J. Neurosurg. 47:150–162, 1977.

39. GREENBERG, R. P., BECKER, D. P., MILLER, J. D., ET AL.: *Evaluation of brain function in severe human head trauma with multi-modality evoked potentials. Part II. Localisation of brain dysfunction and correlation with post-traumatic neurological conditions.* J. Neurosurg. 47:163–177, 1977.

40. GREENBERG, R. P., SAKALAS, R., MILLER, J. D., ET AL.: "Multimodality evoked potentials and CBF in patients with severe head injury." In Ingvar and Lassen (eds.): *Cerebral Function, Metabolism and Circulation.* Munksgaard, Copenhagen, 1977, pp. 498–499.

41. GUILLAUME, J., AND JANNY, P.: *Manometrie intracranienne continue. Interet de la methode et premiers resultats.* Rev. Neurol. 84:131–142, 1951.

42. HASS, W. K., KOBAYASHI, M., HOCHWALD, G. M., ET AL.: "Relationship of cerebral metabolic rate to brain stem injury." In Harper, M., Jennett, W. B., Miller, J. D. et al. (eds.): *Blood Flow and Metabolism of the Brain.* Churchill Livingstone, Edinburgh, 1975, pp. 13.39–13.40.

43. HEDMAN, G., AND RABOW, L.: *CK_{BB}-isoenzymstegring som tecekn pa hjarnparenkyn-skada.* Svenska Lakarsallskapets Riksstamma, Stockholm, 1978.

44. HOLLOWAY, W., EL GAMMAL, T., AND POOL, W. H., JR.: *Doughnut sign in subdural haematoma.* J. Nucl. Med. 13:630–632, 1972.

45. HOUNSFIELD, G. N.: *Computerised transverse axial scanning. I. Description of the system.* Br. J. Radiol. 46:1016–1023, 1973.

46. JACKSON, H.: *The management of acute cranial injuries by the early exact determination of intracranial pressure and its relief by lumbar drainage.* Surg. Gynecol. Obstet. 34:494–508, 1922.

47. JANNY, P., JOVAN, J. P., HANNY, L., ET AL.: "A statistical approach to long term monitoring of intracranial pressure." In Brock, M., and Dietz, H. (eds.): *Intracranial Pressure, I.* Springer-Verlag, Berlin, 1972, pp. 59–64.

48. JENNETT, B.: "Closing comments." In Beks, J. W. F., Bosch, D. A., and Brock, M. (eds.): *Intracranial Pressure, III.* Springer-Verlag, Berlin, 1976, pp. 343–346.

49. JENNETT, B., AND JOHNSTON, I.: "The uses of intracranial pressure measurements in clinical management." In Brock, M., and Dietz, H. (eds.): *Intracranial Pressure, I.* Springer-Verlag, 1972, Berlin, pp. 353–356.

50. JEPSON, S. T.: *Echo-encephalography. IV. The midline echo; an evaluation of its usefulness for diagnosing intracranial expansions and an investigation into its sources.* Acta Chir. Scand. 121:1–151, 1961.

51. JOHNSTON, I. H.: "Intracranial pressure changes after head injury." In Vinken and Bruyn (eds.): *Handbook of Clinical Neurology 23.* North-Holland Publishing Co., Amsterdam, 1975, pp. 199–222.

52. JOHNSTON, I. H., JOHNSTON, J. A., AND JENNETT, B.: *Intracranial pressure changes following head injury.* Lancet ii:433–436, 1970.

53. KASOFF, S. S., ZINGESSER, L. H., AND SHULMAN, K.: *Compartmental abnormalities of regional cerebral blood flow in children with head trauma.* J. Neurosurg. 36:463–470, 1972.

54. KELLY, P. J., IWATA, R., MCGRAW, C.P., ET AL.: "Intracranial pressure, cerebral blood flow and prognosis in patients with severe head injuries." In Langfitt, McHenry, Reivich, et al. (eds.): *Cerebral Circulation and Metabolism.* Springer-Verlag, Berlin, 1975.

55. KINDT, G.W.: "Simplification of intracranial pressure monitoring." In Lundberg, N., Ponten, V., and Brock, M. (eds.): *Intracranial Pressure, II.* Springer-Verlag, Berlin, 1977, pp. 381–383.

56. KLINGER, M. KAZNER, E., GRUMME, T.H., ET AL.: *Clinical experience with automatic midline echo-encephalography: co-operation study of three neurosurgical clinics.* J. Neurol. Neurosurgical Psychiatry 38:272, 1975.

57. KULLBERG, G.: "A method for statistical analysis of intracranial pressure recordings." In Brock, M., and Dietz, H. (eds.): *Intracranial Pressure.* Springer-Verlag, Berlin, 1972, pp. 65–69.

58. KURZE, T., TRANQUALA, R., AND BENEDICT, I. C.: *Spinal fluid lactic acid levels in acute cerebral injury.* In Caveness and Walker (eds.): *Head Injury.* J. B. Lippincott, Philadelphia, 1966, pp. 254–259.

59. LANGFITT, T.W.: "Incidence and importance of intracranial hypertension in head injured patients." In Beks, J. W. F., Bosch, D. A., and Brock, M. (eds.): *Intracranial Pressure, III.* Springer-Verlag, Berlin, 1976, pp. 67–72.

60. LANGFITT, T. W., OBRIST, W. D., GENNARELLI, T. A., ET AL.: *Correlation of cerebral blood flow with outcome in head injured patients.* Ann. Surg. 186:411–414, 1977.

61. LANKSCH, W., GRUMME, TH., AND KAZNER, E.: "Correlations between clinical symptoms and computer tomography findings in closed head injuries." In Frowein, Wilcke, Karimi-Nejad, et al. (eds.): *Advances in Neurosurgery 5.* Springer-Verlag, Berlin, 1978, pp. 27–30.

62. LARSON, S. J., SANCES, A., ACKMANN, J. J., ET AL.: *Non-invasive evaluation of head trauma patients.* Surgery 74:34–40, 1973.

63. LEECH, P., AND MILLER, J. D.: *The Intracranial volume-pressure relationships in primates. 3. The effect of mannitol and hyperventilation.* J. Neurol. Neurosurg. Psychiatry 37:1105–1111, 1974.

64. LEGIER, J., AND RINALDI, I.: *Gross pulmonary embolisation with cerebral tissue following head trauma.* J. Neurosurg. 39:109–113, 1973.

65. LINDBLOM, A.: *The pattern of serum LDH isoenzymes and S-GOT after traumatic brain injury.* Scand. J. Rehab. Med. 4:61–72, 1971.

66. LINDBLOM, U., VRETHAMMAR, T., AND ABERG, B.: *Isoenzymerav mjolksyredehydrogenas vid hjarnskada.* Nord. Med. 77:337–340, 1967.

67. LUNDBERG, N.: *Continuous recording and control of ventricular fluid pressure in neurosurgical practice.* Acta. Psychiatry Neurol. Scand. (Suppl.) 149, 1960.

68. LUNDBERG, N.: "Monitoring of the intracranial pressure. In Critchley, M., O'Leary, J. L., and Jennett, B. (eds.): *Scientific Foundations of Neurology.* Heinemann, London, 1972, pp. 356–371.

69. LUNDBERG, N., TROUPP, H., AND LORIN, H.: *Continuous recording of the ventricular fluid pressure in patients with severe acute traumatic brain damage. A preliminary report.* J. Neurosurg. 22:581–590, 1965.

70. MAAS, A. I. R.: *Cerebrospinal fluid enzymes in acute brain injury. II. Dynamics of changes in CSF enzyme activity after experimental brain injury.* J. Neurol. Neurosurg. Psychiatry 40:655–665, 1977.

71. MACKENZIE, E. T., MCCULLOCH, J., O'KEANE, M., ET AL.: *Cerebral circulation and norepinephrine: relevance of the blood brain barrier.* Am. J. Physiol. 231:483–488, 1970.

72. MACPHERSON, P., AND GRAHAM, D. I.: *Correlation between angiographic findings and the ischaemia of head injury.* J. Neurol. Neurosurg. Psychiatry 41:122–127, 1978.

73. MARSHALL, L. F., BRUCE, D. A., BRUNO, L., ET AL.: *Vertebrobasilar spasm: a significant cause of neurological defect in head injury.* J. Neurosurg. 47:560–564, 1978.

74. MARSHALL, L. F., SMITH, R. W., AND SHAPIRO, H. M.: *The outcome with aggressive treatment in severe head injuries. I. The significance of intracranial pressure monitoring.* J. Neurosurg. 50:20–25, 1979.

75. MCCULLOCH, D., NELSON, K. M., AND OMMAYA, A. K.: *The acute effects of experimental head injury on the vertebro-vascular circuit: angiographic observations.* J. Trauma II:442–478, 1971.

76. MILLER, J. D.: *Volume and pressure in the craniospinal axis.* Clin. Neurosurg. 22:76–105, 1975.

77. MILLER, J. D.: *Intracranial pressure monitoring.* Br. J. Hosp. Med. 19:497–503, 1978.
78. MILLER, J. D., BECKER, D. P., WARD, J. D., ET AL.: *Significance of intracranial hypertension in severe head injury.* J. Neurosurg. 47:501–516, 1977.
79. MILLER, J. D., AND LEECH, P. J.: *Effects of mannitol and steroid therapy on intracranial volume-pressure relationships in patients.* J. Neurosurg. 42:274–281, 1975.
80. MILLER, J. D., AND PICKARD, J. D.: *Intracranial volume-pressure studies in patients with head injury.* Injury 5:265–268, 1974.
81. NAKATANI, S., KOSHINO, K., MOGAMI, H., ET AL.: "Brain interstitial fluid pressure measurement in head injury patients." In Shulman, K., Marmarou, A., Miller, J. D., et al. (eds.): *Intracranial Pressure, IV.* Springer-Verlag, Berlin, 1980, pp. 39–44.
82. NEIL-DWYER, G., WALTER, P., CRUICKSHANK, J. M., ET AL.: *Effect of propranolol and phentolamine on myocardial necrosis after subarachnoid haemorrhage.* Br. Med. J. 4:990–992, 1978.
83. NORTH, J. B., AND JENNETT, S.: *Impedance pneumography for the detection of abnormal breathing patterns associated with brain damage.* Lancet ii:212–213, 1972.
84. NORTH, J. B., AND JENNETT, S.: *Abnormal breathing patterns associated with acute brain damage.* Arch. Neurol. 31:338–344, 1974.
85. NORTH, J. B., AND JENNETT, S.: *Response of ventilation and of intracranial pressure during rebreathing of carbon dioxide in patients with acute brain damage.* Brain 99:169–182, 1976.
86. OBRIST, W. D., DOLINSKAS, C. A., GENNARELLI, T. A., ET AL.: *Relation of blood flow to CT scan in acute head injury.* In Popp, Bourke, Nelson, et al. (eds.): *Seminars in Neurological Surgery: Neural Trauma.* Raven Press, New York, 1979, pp. 41–50.
87. OVERGAARD, J., AND TWEED, W. A.: *Cerebral circulation after head injury. I. Cerebral blood flow and its regulation after closed head injury with emphasis on clinical correlation.* J. Neurosurg. 41:531–541, 1974.
88. PAPO, J., AND CARUSELLI, G.: *Long-term ICP monitoring in comatose patients suffering from head injuries. A critical survey.* Acta Neurochir. 39:187–200, 1977.
89. PICKARD, J. D., TEASDALE, G. M., MATHESON, M., ET AL.: "Intraventricular pressure waves— the best predictive test for shunting in normal pressure hydrocephalus." In Shulman, K., Marmarou, A., Miller, J. D., et al. (eds.): *Intracranial Pressure, IV.* Springer-Verlag, Berlin, 1980.
90. RABOW, L.: *Isoenzymes of lactic dehydrogenase as a prognostication in patients with contusio cerebri.* Scand. J. Rehab. Med. 4:90–92, 1972.
91. RABOW, L., HEBBE, B., AND LIEDEN, G.: *Enzyme analysis for evaluating acute head injury.* Acta Chir. Scand. 137:1240–1244, 1971.
92. RABOW, L., AND HEDMAN, G.: *CK_{BB}-isoenzymes as a sign of cerebral injury.* Proceedings of the VIth European Congress of Neurosurgery. Acta Neurochir. 28:108–112, 1979.
93. ROSNER, M. J., AND BECKER, D. P.: *Intracranial pressure monitoring: complications and associated factors.* Clin. Neurosurg. 23:494–519, 1976.
94. ROSSANDA, M., BOSELLI, A., CASTELLI, C., ET AL.: *Effects of changes in $PaCO_2$ on CBF cerebral oxygenation and EEG in severe brain injuries.* Eur. Neurol. 8:169–173, 1972.
95. ROSSANDA, M., COLLICE, M., PORTA, M., ET AL.: "Intracranial hypertension in head injury. Clinical significance and relation to respiration." In Lundberg, N., Ponten, V., and Brock, M. (eds.): *Intracranial Pressure, II.* Springer-Verlag, Berlin, 1975, pp. 475–499.
96. SHALIT, M. N., REINMUTH, O. M., SHIMOJYO, S., ET AL.: *Carbon dioxide and cerebral circulatory control. III. The effects of brainstem lesions.* Arch. Neurol. 17:342–353, 1967.
97. SNOEK, J., JENNETT, B., ADAMS, H., ET AL.: *Computer tomography for recent severe head injury in patients without acute intracranial haematoma.* J. Neurol. Neurosurg. Psychiatry (in press).
98. SOMER, H., KASTE, M., TROUPP, H., ET AL.: *Brain creatine kinase in the blood after acute brain injury.* J. Neurol. Neurosurg. Psychiatry 38:572–576, 1975.
99. STOCKARD, J. J., BICKFORD, R. G., AND AUNG, M.: "The electro-encephalogram in traumatic brain injury." In Vinken and Bruyn (eds.): *Handbook of Clinical Neurology 23.* North-Holland Publishing Co., Amsterdam, 1975, pp. 317–367.
100. SUNDBARG, G., KJALLQUIST, A., LUNDBERG, N., ET AL.: "Complications due to prolonged ventricular fluid pressure monitoring in clinical practice." In Beks, J. W. F., Bosch, D. A., and Brock, M. (eds.): *Intracranial Pressure, III.* Springer-Verlag, Berlin, 1976, pp. 348–352.
101. SUWANWELA, C., AND SUWANWELA, N.: *Intracranial arterial narrowing and spasm in acute head injury.* J. Neurosurg. 36:314–323, 1972.

150

102. SZEWCZYKOWSKI, J., DYTKO, P., KUNICK, A., ET AL.: "Determination of critical ICP levels in neurosurgical patients; a statistical approach. In Lundberg, N., Ponten, V., and Brock, M. (eds.): *Intracranial Pressure, II.* Springer-Verlag, Berlin, 1975, pp. 392–393.

103. TALLALA, A., AND MORIN, M. A.: *Acute traumatic subdural haematoma: a review of 100 consecutive cases.* J. Trauma 11:771–776, 1971.

104. TANS, J. TH. J.: *Computed tomography of intracerebral haematoma.* Clin. Neurol. Neurosurg. 79:285–295, 1976.

105. TANS, J. TH. J.: *Computed tomography of extracerebral haematoma.* Clin. Neurol. Neurosurg. 79:296–306, 1976.

106. TEASDALE, G., GALBRAITH, S. AND JENNETT, B.: "Operate or observe? ICP and the management of the 'silent' traumatic intracranial haematoma." In Shulman, K., Marmarou, A., Miller, J. D. et al. (eds.): *Intracranial Pressure, IV.* Springer-Verlag, Berlin, 1980, pp. 36–38.

107. TEASDALE, G., ROWAN, J. O., TURNER, J. W., ET AL.: "Cerebral perfusion failure and cortical electrical activity." In Ingvar and Lassen (eds.): *Cerebral Function, Metabolism and Circulation.* Munksgaard, Copenhagen, 1977, pp. 23.14–23.15.

108. THOMAS, D. G. T., PALFREYMAN, J.W., AND RATCLIFFE, J. G.: *Serum basic protein assay in diagnosis and prognosis of patients with head injury.* Lancet i:113–115, 1978.

109. THOMAS, D. G. T., RABOW, L., AND TEASDALE, G.: *Serum myelin basic protein, clinical responsiveness, and outcome of severe head injury.* Proceedings of the VIth European Congress of Neurosurgery. Acta Neurochir. (Suppl.) 28:93–95, 1979.

110. THOMAS, D. G. T., AND ROWAN, T. D.: *Lactate dehydrogenase in head injury.* Injury 7:258–261, 1976.

111. TROUPP, H., KUURNE, T., KASTE, M., ET AL.: "Intraventricular pressure after severe brain injuries. Prognostic value and correlations with blood pressure and jugular venous oxygen tension." In Brock, M., and Dietz, H. (eds.): *Intracranial Pressure, I.* Springer-Verlag, Berlin, 1972, pp. 222–226.

112. TURNER, J. M., MCDOWALL, D. G., GIBSON, R. M., ET AL.: "Computer analysis of intracranial pressure measurements: clinical value and nursing response." In Beks, J. W. F., Bosch, D. A., and Brock, M. (eds.): *Intracranial Pressure, III.* Springer-Verlag, Berlin, 1976, pp. 283–285.

113. VRIES, J. K., BECKER, D. P., AND YOUNG, H. F.: *A subarachnoid screw for monitoring intracranial pressure.* J. Neurosurg. 39:416–419, 1973.

114. ZIMMERMAN, R. A., BILANIUK, L. T., BRUCE, D., ET AL.: *Computed tomography of paediatric head trauma: acute general cerebral swelling.* Radiology 126:403–408, 1978.

115. ZIMMERMAN, R. A., BILANIUK, L. T., DOLINSKAS, C., ET AL.: *Computed tomography of acute intracerebral haemorrhagic contusion.* Comput. Axia. Tomogr. 1:271–280, 1977.

116. ZIMMERMAN, R. A., BILANIUK, L. T., AND GENNARELLI, T.: *Computed tomography of shearing injuries of the cerebral white matter.* Radiology 127:393–396, 1978.

117. ZIMMERMAN, R. A., BILANIUK, L. T., GENNARELLI, T., ET AL.: *Cranial computed tomography in diagnosis and management of acute head trauma.* Am. J. Roentgenol. 131:27–34, 1978.

CHAPTER 7

Intracranial Hematoma

This complication can transform a seemingly mild head injury into a life-threatening situation within hours. Although only a minority of patients admitted to hospital after head injury develop an intracranial hematoma, this lesion accounted for 75 percent of a series of patients who "talked and died,"[87] and two thirds of fatal injuries in which death was judged to have been potentially avoidable.[54] Many disabled survivors after head injury have had a hematoma evacuated in time to save their lives, but too late to restore brain function fully. The interest of neurosurgeons in this surgical complication is indicated by the considerable number of reports of operated cases.[16,47,48,66,85,105] However, it is difficult to make direct comparisons between different series because of the various ways of classifying hematomas: by interval since injury (acute, subacute, and chronic), or by site (extradural, subdural, and intracerebral). Hitherto most series were of surgical patients, but with occasional reference to clots discovered at autospy. CT scanning has now introduced another clinical group—those diagnosed radiologically but not going to surgery. CT scanning is also making it possible to recognize much more reliably than was usually possible from operation or from angiography the presence of multiple lesions. Thus, an appreciable number of extradural hematomas are associated with underlying contusion or intradural hematoma, while a second lesion on the other side of the brain is not uncommon. For these two reasons, recent series of patients, whose diagnosis has depended on CT scanning, may differ in some respects from those previously classified by angiography and operative findings.

PATHOLOGY AND CLASSIFICATION

Site

Extradural hematomas are mostly temporal or temporoparietal, resulting from damage to the anterior or posterior branches of the middle meningeal vessels (Fig. 1). Hooper[43] considered the hemorrhage to be arterial in origin in two thirds of cases, but Wood-Jones[112] pointed out that the vein was more closely related to bone, and Paul[82] stated that bleeding was always venous in origin. At operation the separated dura often seems to be diffusely hemorrhagic, which is compatible with experimental evidence that dural separation may occur at impact, with subsequent rapid bleeding from the dura into this space.[5,22] Frontal hematomas are

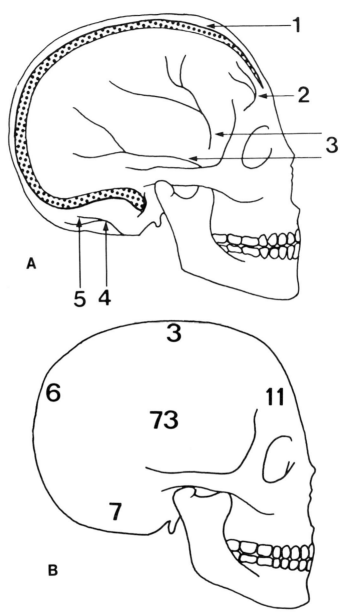

Figure 1. A, Distribution of vessels from which epidural hematomas may arise: (1) sagittal sinus, (2) anterior meningeal artery, (3) middle meningeal artery, (4) posterior meningeal artery, (5) transverse sinus. **B,** Percentage distribution of site of epidural hematoma in the series of Jamieson and Yelland.[49] (Redrawn from Jamieson.[47])

either at the pole or along the base of the anterior fossa. A torn venous sinus accounts for a minority of extradural clots. These may be in either the occipital region or the posterior fossa (and sometimes in both sites) or under the vertex, sites in which they may be missed unless appropriate radiological techniques are used.

154

Intradural hematomas (Fig. 2) include those which are confined to the subdural or intracerebral sites, and the more common "burst lobe." This consists of a mixture of *subdural and intracerebral* clot, with cortical lacerations. In 80 percent of cases this lesion affects the temporal pole and in most of the rest the frontal pole (Fig. 3) (hence the alternative term "compound polar injury"). The relative contribution of the subdural and intracerebral component varies, but there is a sizable subdural hematoma in most cases. Indeed, this was probably the lesion in most patients hitherto reported as having "acute subdural hematoma."

Pure subdural hematomas, without underlying cortical laceration, do sometimes occur soon after injury—usually caused by rupture of veins bridging the cortex to the sinuses (sphenoparietal[63] or transverse and petrosal[12]). Occasionally arterial bleeding is responsible,[17,40,79] and this can even follow mild injury.

Pure intracerebral hematomas, distinct from surface contusions or lacerations,

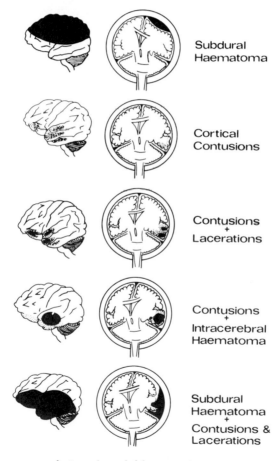

Intradural Haematomas

Figure 2. Spectrum of intradural hematomas. (Modified from Hooper, R., "Indications for surgical treatment." In Vinken, and Bruyn (eds.): *Handbook of Clinical Neurology 24.* North Holland Publishing Co., Amsterdam, 1976, pp. 637–667.)

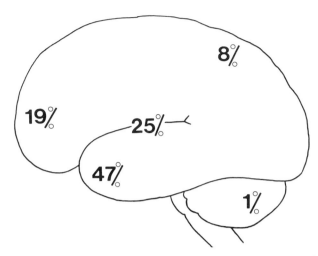

Figure 3. Distribution of cortical damage in 222 patients with "complicated" subdural hematomas. (From Jamieson, K. G., and Yelland, J. D. N.: *Surgically treated traumatic subdural haematomas.* J. Neurosurg. 37:137–149, 1972, with permission.)

are rather more common in the frontal than the temporal lobe, but their mechanism of production is unclear.

It is suggested that hematomas are best classified as extradural only, intradural only, and mixed extradural and intradural; intradural clots are futher designated as subdural, intracerebral, or both. More than one site may harbor intradural collections and both sides of the head are affected in a third of cases.

Time after Injury

Authors have usually distinguished between three types: acute hematomas, commonly defined as those presenting in the first three days after injury; subacute hematomas; and chronic collections (more than 2 to 3 weeks). There is, however, no uniformity of nomenclature (Table 1).

In the first 2 weeks after injury most clots are solid and cannot be satisfactorily evacuated through burr holes alone. Half of these acute hematomas are diagnosed (and evacuated) within 24 hours of injury, and 20 percent in the next 2 days. Chronic subdural hematomas are liquid, and when the preceding incident of trauma can be identified it is usually 3 or 4 weeks prior to diagnosis and operation, sometimes longer; this applies both to adults and children. These chronic lesions present quite a different clinical and therapeutic problem from the acute hematoma (first 2 weeks after injury). We see no need to identify a subacute category, although this is used by some clinicians for cases presenting (or diagnosed, or treated) between 3 days and 2 to 3 weeks after injury.

Previous reports in the literature reveal that more than half of extradural hematomas, irrespective of whether they were associated with an intradural hematoma, were operated upon within 24 hours of injury. This lesion thereafter became increasingly uncommon, although chronic collections, which presented weeks or months after injury, were recorded.[45,94] In the case of intradural lesions, even when only acute and subacute hematomas are considered, rather less than half presented in the first day.

156

Table 1. Variations in temporal classifications of hematomas in different series

Authors	Interval between Injury and Diagnosis or Operation	
	Acute	Chronic
Voris 1941[111]	24 hrs	
Thomas & Gurdjian 1973[107]	"	>10 days
Richards & Hoff 1974[88]	"	
Ransohoff et al. 1971[86]	<2 days	
Laudig et al. 1941[63]	<3 days	
Browder 1943[10]	"	
Harris 1971[36]	"	
Tallala & Morin 1971[101]	"	
Fell et al. 1975[21]	"	
Gurdjian & Thomas 1974[34]	<3 days	>2 weeks
Lewin 1966[65]	"	"
Jamieson (extradural) 1968[49]	"	"
Loew & Kivelitz (subdural) 1976[66]	"	"
Gurdjian & Webster 1958[34]	<3 days	>3 weeks
McKissock et al. 1960[69]	"	"
McLaurin & Tutor 1961[72]	"	"
Jamieson (intradural) 1972[50,51]	"	"
Ramamurthi 1976[85]	"	"
Rosenørn & Gjerris 1978[90]	"	"
Echlin et al. 1956[18]	7 days	
Philips & Azariah 1965[83]	"	

(From Teasdale and Galbraith[105])

Sometimes an intracerebral hemorrhage is considered to relate to an injury weeks or even years before it is discovered. Bolinger[8] names this "spat-apoplexie" (or delayed traumatic hematoma), and he postulated that arterial necrosis caused by trauma led to this hemorrhage. Conclusive evidence for the association is lacking.[3] The diagnosis is sometimes the subject of medicolegal claims,[2,32] but probably can be supported only when the antecedent injury was of some severity and when the interval is no more than a few weeks, during which there have been persisting symptoms.

Frequency of Hematomas

Estimates of the overall incidence of hematomas based on clinical reports vary greatly, as would be expected from the different admission policies that determine the population of general hospitals or of neurosurgical units (Table 2). In general hospitals 1 to 6 percent is the range, while two large European neurosurgical series recorded 26 percent and 30 percent of head injured patients with hematomas. Epidemiological studies in Scotland indicate that 1.2 percent of patients admitted to hospital after head injury develop a surgical hematoma; the annual occurrence rate is 4.5 per 100,000 population.[55]

The proportional distribution of different types of hematoma varies, again through local, organizational influences (Table 3). City hospitals admitting many unselected severe road traffic injuries soon after the accident will have more

Table 2. Incidence of intracranial hematoma among head injured patients admitted to hospital

Source of Data		Period Covered	Total Admissions	Intracranial Hematomas
Galbraith et al.[26]	General hospital	1 yr	918	0.8%
Steadman & Graham[95]	General hospital	1 yr	484	2.3%
Kalyanaraman et al.[59]	Head injury unit	2¾ yr	2000	3.5%
Gillingham[30]	Head injury unit —general hospital	1 yr	1132	5.7%
Jamieson & Yelland[49–51]	General hospitals	11 yr	11,000	6.3%
Klonoff & Thompson[61]	Neurosurgical ward—general hospital	1 yr	279	11.5%
Pia et al.[84]	General surgical wards	11 yr	1790	10%
	Neurosurgical clinic	22 yr	3793	26%
Scottish Head Injury Management Study[55]	3 Neurosurgical units	2 yr	785	30%

(From Teasdale and Galbraith[105])

intradural hematomas.[92] Regional units will have more patients referred somewhat later, often after definite deterioration, and there will be more extradural and "pure" subdural and intracerebral hematomas in such a population. About 25 percent of patients have an extradural hematoma, but more than a third of these have an intradural clot also; less than a fifth of patients, therefore, have a "pure" extradural hematoma. At all stages after injury, an intradural hematoma is the commoner finding (Table 4), and about a third of all patients have a mixed intradural lesion (burst lobe.)

Table 3. Incidence of different types of traumatic hematoma

Source of Data	Total Cases	Extradural only (%)	Extradural + Intradural (%)	Subdural only (%)	Subdural + Intracerebral (%)	Intracerebral (discrete) (%)
London McKissock et al.[69,70]	298	42			58	
Cincinnati McLaurin et al.[71]	137	11	9	3	10	
Brisbane Jamieson & Yelland[49–51]	763	13	11	34	36	6
Richmond Becker et al.[4]	62	19		42	39	
International Collaborative Study[57] Glasgow, Rotterdam, Groningen, Los Angeles	487	16	7	22	34	20
Glasgow Teasdale & Galbraith[105]	180	24	9	31	23	13
Giessen Pia et al.[84]	980	20		70		10

(From Teasdale and Galbraith[105])

Table 4. Types of hematoma at different times after injury

Time between Injury and Operation	n	Extradural Alone	Extradural + Intradural	Intradural Alone
1st day	87	22%	11%	67%
2–3 days	42	18%	8%	74%
3 days–2 weeks	51	17%	2%	81%

(From Teasdale and Galbraith[105])

Only 2 to 3 percent of traumatic hematomas are in the posterior fossa, where extradural hematomas are as common as intradural. The former arise either from the meningeal branch of the occipital artery or from the transverse sinus; intradural hematomas are almost always a mixture of cerebellar and subdural blood, usually involving bridging veins from the sinus, and there may also be an occipital surface clot above the tentorium.

DIAGNOSIS

Delayed diagnosis or inappropriate surgery for intracranial hematoma are the most frequent causes of avoidable mortality and morbidity after head injury. Successful surgery depends on operating soon enough and on using the right approach; that depends on maintaining a high index of suspicion in high risk cases and proceeding to investigation in time to provide accurate enough localization for adequate exposure of the clot.

It is not possible to distinguish reliably on clinical grounds between extradural and intradural hematomas, nor between clots in different regions of the skull. Yet surgery must sometimes be undertaken without the benefit of CT scanning or angiography. For this reason, as well as to indicate the circumstances in which a hematoma should be suspected, it is important to consider which clinical features are associated with different kinds of hematoma. There are, however, no classical features that are reliable in this respect—indeed one reason why diagnosis is so often delayed appears to be an undue expectation that the syndrome described in textbooks will always happen. Our investigations indicate that these clinical presentations occur only in a minority of patients with intracranial hematoma. This observation depends partly on our own experience in Glasgow, and partly on reviewing some of the larger reported series that include enough information for useful analysis.

Age Incidence

Hematomas tend to affect older head injured patients, and this is so whether the incidence is analyzed for all hospital admissions for head injury, for admissions to a neurosurgical ward, or for patients who are in coma. This is because the intradural hematomas, which account for two thirds of all cases, are more common in the older age groups. The peak incidence of extradural hematoma is in the second and third decades, and of intradural hematoma in the fifth and sixth decades. Forty percent of extradural hematomas and only 10 percent of intradural hematomas are under 20 years of age; of the hematomas occurring in patients under the age of 20 years, 40 percent are extradural, compared with less than 10 percent of patients over 40 years (Fig. 4).

159

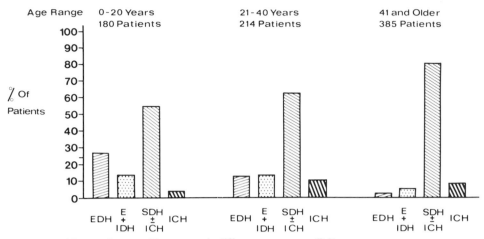

Figure 4. Incidence of types of hematoma in different age ranges.[49-51]

Impaired Consciousness

Deteriorating level of consciousness is the most consistent clinical feature of a significant intracranial hematoma in the acute stage after injury. When coma follows recovery from immediate post-traumatic unconsciousness, there is said to have been a lucid interval. However, this classic sequence was recorded in only 12 percent of extradural and 13 percent of intradural hematomas in the large series from Brisbane.[49-51] Others claim a higher incidence with extradural hematoma: 26 percent[70] and 42 percent.[43]

About 40 to 50 percent of patients with hematoma have not been unconscious immediately after injury, but this is seldom the case when a burst lobe is subsequently found. If these cases are added to those with a lucid interval, the proportion of patients who talked at some stage prior to surgery proves to be over 80 percent for pure extradural, subdural, or intracerebral hematomas in Jamieson's series;[49-51] this occurred in only 50 percent of patients with a burst lobe. Other patterns of change in conscious level occur: patients may remain unconscious or be conscious continuously between injury and operation; or they may regain consciousness and retain it until operation.

From these considerations, and from the relative frequency of different types of hematoma, it is possible to conclude what kind of hematoma a given patient is most likely to have—but this can never be an accurate prediction. Almost half the patients with the classical sequence have a burst lobe, and half the patients not initially unconscious have a pure subdural hematoma (Table 5).

Neurological Symptoms and Signs

In patients who are conscious, *headache* is an early indication of developing compression but, by itself, is rarely sufficient grounds for making a presumptive diagnosis. *Vomiting,* irritability, and restlessness are also often quoted as features of intracranial hematoma; none of these on its own is a reliable indicator, but their development in a patient previously unaffected should arouse suspicion. *Neck stiffness* can be due to a hematoma, and this should always be considered before a lumbar puncture is performed.

160

Table 5. Types of hematoma in patients with different patterns of consciousness in series of Jamieson and Yelland[49-51]

Pattern of Consciousness	All Sites n	All Sites %	Extradural Alone %	Extradural + Intradural %	Intradural %
Always conscious	192	27	15	7	78
Conscious becoming unconscious	124	17	15	14	71
Unconscious becoming conscious	106	15	19	12	69
Unconscious, then conscious, then unconscious*	96	13	5	16	79
Always unconscious	197	28	9	11	80

*Classical sequence

Weakness and Abnormal Posture

Deteriorating consciousness is often associated with weakness of the opposite limbs, particularly when the clot is situated laterally. As compression progresses, abnormal motor responses may appear, and extension or abnormal stereotyped flexion predominate; eventually there may be no response from the limbs. The development of abnormal motor patterns in a patient previously known to have had a better level of response probably reflects midbrain compression or ischemia and is an indication for urgent decompression. However, Feldman has emphasized that extensor motor responses can result from a disorder at any level of the motor pathway.[19,20] When abnormal movements are known to have been present soon after injury, whether unilateral or bilateral, they do not have the same significance, either as a localizing sign or as evidence of intracranial herniation, as when they develop as part of a progressive deterioration in responsiveness.

By the time operation takes place, most patients show some abnormality in motor responses. In the Glasgow series an intradural hematoma was associated with a greater frequency of motor dysfunction, both as an immediate consequence of injury (40%) and before operation (90%), than was pure extradural hematoma (22%, 82%). The side of the initial or greatest abnormality was contralateral to the clot in four out of five cases.

Pupil Changes

Pupillary signs are also much more significant when it is known that the pupils were previously equal in size and reacted normally. When there is dilatation of one pupil (or has been during the evolution of the clinical state of compression), then the side of this corresponds with the side of the hematoma in 90 percent of cases. However, even in the mid-70s almost a third of patients in Glasgow came to operation without there being any pupillary abnormality; as early diagnosis becomes the rule, particularly with CT scanning, fewer patients should develop pupil signs. It is vital to displace the notion that a fixed dilated pupil is one of the characteristic signs of an intracranial hematoma—it is a sign of the later stages of cerebral compression. A pupil may be unreactive after head injury for a number of reasons other than tentorial herniation.

161

Epilepsy

One or more fits occur in the first week after injury in 28 percent of patients with an acute hematoma, but in a third of cases the first fit is after surgical evacuation of the clot.[52,53] Only 2 percent of patients with extradural and 18 percent of those with intradural hematomas have fits before operation. Although a quarter of patients with early epilepsy will have had a hematoma, a fit is rarely the sole sign of a developing hematoma. However, the appearance of epilepsy in a patient not improving in other respects should raise the possibility of an intradural hematoma.

In practice, an early fit is more often a cause of diagnostic confusion, leading to the delayed recognition of an intracranial hematoma, than a useful clue to its presence. This is because the deteriorating responsiveness that is due to the hematoma may, when there has been a recent fit, be mistakenly ascribed to the postictal state; this situation may be further complicated by the depressant effects of anticonvulsant drugs.

Posterior Fossa Hematoma

These may present acutely after mild or severe injuries.[75] Deterioration may be rapid, with respiratory depression occurring without any pupillary change or motor signs. The clue is evidence of an occipital injury, such as scalp marks, stiff neck, or fracture. Delayed development, after several days, may be associated with more obvious focal signs of a posterior fossa lesion: headache and vomiting, papilledema, nystagmus, and cerebellar ataxia. There may be no deterioration of level of consciousness until shortly before autonomic signs of brain stem compression. Clots in the posterior fossa are apt to be associated with contrecoup lesions in the frontal and temporal lobes, and either the supra- or the infratentorial lesion may dominate the initial presentation.

Distinction between Extradural and Intradural Clots

The characteristic clinical features associated with the two main kinds of hematoma are summarized in Table 6. It is clear that no feature or combination of features provides a reliable guide to the kind of hematoma. Before operation this distinction depends upon neuroradiological investigations.

Table 6. Occurrence of various clinical features in patients with extradural or intradural hematomas

| | Proportion of Patients with Feature | |
	Extradural Alone	Intradural Alone or with Extradural
Age 40 yr	Two thirds younger	Two thirds older
Unconscious	Less than half	Two thirds
Lucid	Three quarters	One half–Two thirds
Unconscious at operation	One third–one half	More than two thirds
Epilepsy	2%	One in five

(From Teasdale and Galbraith[105])

162

Radiological Investigations

These range from skull x-ray to CT scanning. They may be of value in the early stages in indicating risk factors that increase the likelihood that a hematoma will (or has) developed, although it is not yet obvious clinically. Once it is clear that there is probably a mass, investigations are of value in confirming its presence and locating its position. Sometimes the patient is by this time so critically ill that investigation would entail unacceptable delay, as discussed later (p. 172).

Plain X-Rays

Most patients with an intracranial hematoma have a fracture.[27] This is found in 90 percent of extradural hematomas, the exceptions almost all being children.[73] The figure for intradural hematomas is about 70 percent, the exceptions being mostly in those patients over 60 years of age. The side of the fracture reliably indicates the side of an extradural hematoma; but about half of intradural hematomas are associated with a fracture on the other side of the skull. A fracture may also indicate whether a hematoma is likely to be frontal, temporal, parietal, or occipital—particularly an extradural hematoma; this is an especially useful clue to a hematoma in one of the less common sites, such as frontal or vertical or in the posterior fossa.

A depressed fracture was associated with an intracranial hematoma in 6 percent of cases according to one series,[9] but this occurred more often in children.[49] Half the clots were intracerebral, and the rest were almost equally divided between extradural and subdural.

Lateral shift of the pineal gland, seen on a well-centered axial anteroposterior (Towne's) view, is a useful clue to a laterally placed hematoma; but a central pineal does not exclude even a sizable subfrontal or subtemporal clot. Pineal calcification increases in frequency with age; many head injured patients therefore have no calcification, which also limits the value of this sign.

Angiography

The introduction of angiography resulted in an improvement in the diagnosis and management of traumatic intracranial hematomas.[35] Today it is still widely used because facilities for CT scanning are not universally available. The presence of an intracranial hematoma is recognized at angiography principally from displacement of the major cerebral vessels (p. 117). Diagnosis of the site of the hematoma depends upon interpretation of various patterns of shift and much less information is available than from CT scans. Surface hematomas other than in the lateral position can readily be missed on angiography (p. 117). Evidence of hydrocephalus on carotid angiography raises suspicion of a posterior fossa hematoma.

Computer Tomography

It is difficult to overestimate the difference that this technique has made to investigation of the patient suspected of having an intracranial hematoma. Not only does the CT scan reliably indicate the presence of an intracranial hematoma, but it conveys more information than any other investigation. The ease with

163

which it can be repeated has provided new insights into the evolution of intracranial hematomas.

In discussing computer tomography of intracranial hematoma it is convenient to consider collections on the surface (extradural and subdural hematomas) separately from the appearances of the intracerebral hematomas and associated brain damage, even though this distinction cannot always be made with certainty in every scan.

SURFACE HEMATOMAS. In the acute phase after injury both extradural and subdural hematomas show as a band of increased density between the brain and the skull. With an *extradural hematoma* there is a characteristic biconvex or lenticular area of increased density. Sometimes an extracranial hematoma and swelling of the scalp tissues can be seen (Fig. 5). Extradural clots in less typical sites, such as subfrontal or subtemporal areas, or in the posterior fossa, may be recognized only when approprite cuts are taken (Fig. 6). *Subdural hemorrhage* is also convex towards the skull, but its inner margin, conforming to the surface of the brain, is concave or half-moon shaped (Fig. 7). The relation between the CT appearances of subdural blood and the time elapsed since the injury presumed to be responsible for the bleeding has been studied by Sciotti and colleagues[91] and their conclusions are summarized in Table 7.

Decreased density is characteristic of chronic collections (Fig. 8) and is rarely seen in the acute phase after injury, but some surface hematomas have been reported as having the same density as the brain itself. This may be because recently shed blood has an EMI number similar to that of brain tissue, but it may also represent a reduction in the apparent density of a hyperdense hematoma as a result of computer overswing. This seems most likely to occur with extracerebral collections near the vertex, but can be compensated for by tilting the patient's head in the scanner so that the x-ray beam strikes the relevant area of the skull perpendicularly or by reconstruction of the scan in the coronal plane.

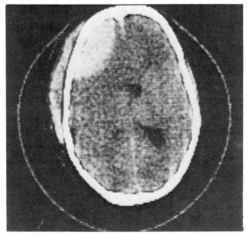

Figure 5. *Frontal extradural hematoma.* Nineteen-year-old male car passenger involved in a traffic accident and thrown through the windscreen. He was immediately and persistingly in coma. When first seen his left pupil was larger than the right, neither reacted, and he had abnormal motor responses on the right side. The scan, one and a half hours after injury, shows scalp swelling on the left side and a biconvex area of increased density in the left frontal region. There is marked ventricular shift to the right. Following evacuation of the hematoma by craniotomy there was immediate swelling of the brain, and the patient subsequently died. Postmortem showed cerebral infarction.

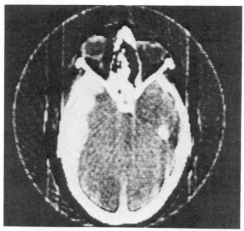

Figure 6. *Temporal extradural hematoma.* Thirty-nine-year-old woman who fell while "drunk." After a brief episode of unconsciousness, she recovered full consciousness, but 48 hours later deteriorated. At the time of the scan she was not obeying commands and had weakness of her right limbs. The left pupil was larger, but both reacted. The scan shows an extracerebral density in the left temporal fossa and displacement of the contents of the left orbit. The dense spot on the right side is caused by the upper surface of the petrous temple bone. Craniotomy, evacuation of clot, and control of bleeding from the anterior branch of the middle meningeal vessel were followed by good recovery.

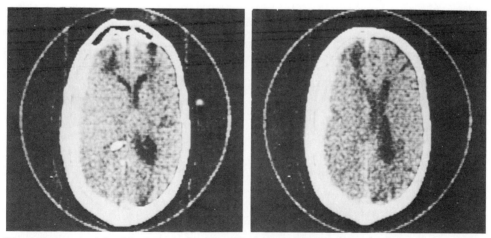

Figure 7. *Acute subdural hematoma.* Seventy-one-year-old male found drunk. Skull x-rays showed a left-sided fracture of the vault, and he was admitted to hospital. He recovered to a level of confused conversation, but the following day his consciousness deteriorated and he developed seizures. At the time of scanning, 36 hours after admission, he was localizing with his left arm but had a weakness of his right side. He opened his eyes to pain and groaned. The left pupil was larger than the right but both were reacting. The scan shows a band of increased density over the whole of the left hemisphere, shift of the ventricles to the right, and cortical atrophy on the right side. Craniotomy revealed a clotted subdural hematoma 1 cm to 1.5 cm thick covering the left hemisphere; the underlying cortex was diffusely contused.

165

Table 7. Appearances of subdural blood on computer tomography related to time after injury

CT Appearance	Time of Scan after Injury		
	7 days *n*	7–21 days *n*	22 days *n*
Hyperdense 30–45 EMI units	11	1	2
Isodense 14–29 EMI units	0	7	3
Hypodense 4–14 EMI units	0	2	16

(From Sciotti, Terbrugge, Melancon, et al.[91])

French and Dublin[23] have reported that if the CT scan shows a distinct surface band of increased density, then the extracerebral collection will be at least 1 cm thick (Fig. 9). Thinner collections may be more reliably detected by angiography, but if there is a significant hematoma the CT scan will show some ventricular shift.[28]

INTRACEREBRAL HEMATOMA. It is in clarifying the nature of an intracerebral swelling that computer tomography is most clearly superior to other investigations. The extent of intracerebral hemorrhage after head injury varies between wide extremes, from patchy contusional hemorrhage confined to the cerebral cortex, to large confluent areas of bleeding of considerable volume (Figs. 10 to 12).

Contusions of the frontal or temporal lobes, when scanned in the first 24 hours after injury, usually appear as areas of mixed density; the mottled or "salt and pepper" appearance[23] results from small areas, denser than normal brain, which correspond to contusional hemorrhages, being interspersed with less dense areas representing edema and necrosis. Such lesions are characterized as contusions rather than frank hematomas by the heterogenicity of the density changes. A day

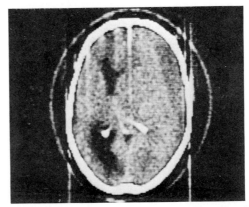

Figure 8. *Chronic subdural hematoma.* Sixty-eight-year-old man reported to have had 2 weeks of headache before his consciousness deteriorated. At the time of scanning he was in coma, with extension responses on the left side. Skull x-ray was negative, but the scan shows shift of the ventricles to the left and a band of reduced density over the surface of the hemisphere on the right side. A liquid subdural hematoma was drained through burr holes and eventually he made a good recovery.

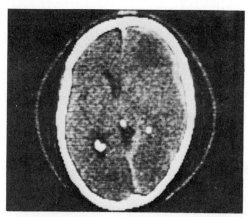

Figure 9. *Subdural hematoma and frontal contusion.* Thirty-six-year-old male admitted to hospital after being found drunk. He recovered consciousness, was discharged the following day, but 4 days later became disorientated, with mild weakness of the left arm and neck stiffness. The scan shows an extracerebral band of increased density in the right frontotemporal area and reduced density in the right frontal lobe, with shift of the ventricles to the left side. A 1-cm clotted subdural hematoma was removed. There were contusions of the frontal and temporal cortex, but no intracerebral hematoma was located.

or more after injury, homogeneous areas of reduced density are seen more commonly. From a single CT scan it is difficult to determine the extent to which such an area represents edematous, swollen, but largely intact brain, or is a mixture of "lucent" hemorrhage, infarction, and edema. Serial scanning has shown that small contusion hemorrhages can mature into large areas of reduced density.

Discrete intracerebral hemorrhages appear as homogeneous areas of increased

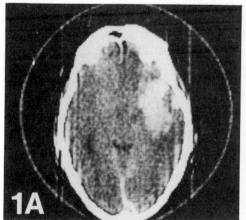
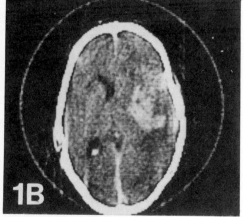

Figure 10. *Frontotemporal contusions and intracerebral hematoma.* Forty-five-year-old man who 6 months previously had a craniotomy for a subdural hematoma on the left side. He was readmitted to hospital after an epileptic fit, in which he struck his head. He recovered, but remained "drowsy." At the time of the scan, 24 hours later, he was opening his eyes to pain, obeying commands, and swearing. His pupils were equal and reacting but the left arm and leg were weak. The slices (**1A, 1B**) show a "fluffy" intracerebral area of increased density in the right frontotemporal area, extending to the surface of the hemisphere, with shift of the ventricles to the left. Craniotomy confirmed contusions of the temporal and frontal lobes; an intracerebral hematoma was evacuated from the temporal lobe.

167

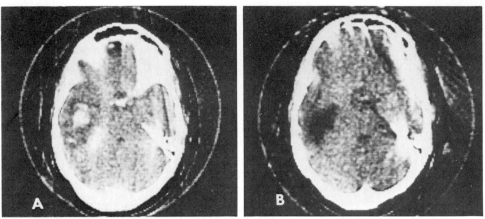

Figure 11. Sixty-five-year-old man who was found lying in a street, smelling of "alcohol." When stimulated by pain he opened his eyes, spoke, but did not obey commands. Scan **A** shows a left intratemporal hematoma. His ICP was only 10 to 15 mm Hg and he was managed conservatively. Within 3 days he regained full consciousness and made a good recovery. Scan **B,** 4 months later, shows an area of reduced density in the left temporal lobe.

density in scans taken in the first few days after injury. Hematomas resulting from trauma typically lie more superficially than those occurring spontaneously, which are usually found in the basal ganglia or the deeper part of the hemisphere. The smooth but irregular margin of a traumatic hemorrhage produces appearances described variously as "amoebic"[103] or "fluffy."[23] This may indicate that large

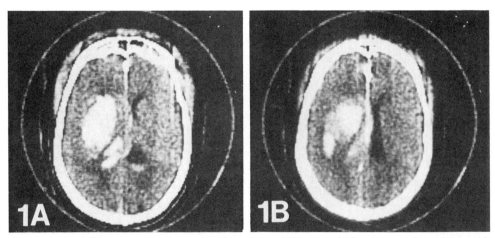

Figure 12. *Probable traumatic intracerebral hematoma.* Fifty-year-old female car driver whose vehicle hit a lamppost. She was immediately in coma and when first seen had abnormal flexion of the left side and was extending her right limbs; her pupils were nonreacting and the left was larger than the right. Shortly after admission she developed seizures. The scan (slices **1A** and **1B**), 5 hours after injury, shows an oval area of increased density deep in the left hemisphere, with blood in the left ventricle and shift of the ventricles to the right side. There is swelling in the scalp on both sides of the frontal region (she had a facio-maxillary fracture). A craniotomy was performed on the left side, where the cortex was seen to be contused, and the hematoma was aspirated through a cortical incision. She showed some improvement after operation but was never better than severely disabled and died 2 months after injury. The site of the hematoma is more characteristic of a spontaneous intracerebral hemorrhage, but the cortical bruising suggests that it was, in fact, traumatic.

168

hematomas develop as a result of smaller contusional hemorrhages becoming confluent. A ring of edema will usually be seen around a hematoma that is more than a day old, and some or all of the central area eventually loses its density, resulting in a hypodense lesion. When the entire clot takes on a low density, the appearances may be indistinguishable by present techniques from an area of edema or infarction and may even enhance after intravenous contrast so that an abscess is simulated.

RELIABILITY OF COMPUTER TOMOGRAPHY. When computer tomographic appearances are clear-cut, there is no difficulty in recognizing an intracranial hematoma, and reports indicate a high degree of reliability in head injured patients. Ambrose and colleagues found no false positive CT scans in a series of 300 head injured patients.[1] Tans referred to three false negative scans in 60 intracranial hematomas of either traumatic or spontaneous origin.[103,104] In fact, in none of the three cases was the scan considered to be normal; "negative" was merely a failure to identify with confidence that the intracranial lesion was a hematoma. Among 21 patients with traumatic hematomas, Svendsen encountered four cases in which computer tomography did not give any positive indication of the presence of a surface hematoma.[97] Three of these proved to have subdural hematomas of more than 10 day's maturity, with the clot largely liquified; one patient had an extradural hematoma, but this was only 4 mm in depth and the patient had a significant midline shift caused by an intradural lesion. Some of the patients had angiography and a hematoma was demonstrated in all, including two of the cases in which computer tomography did not demonstrate the lesion. Svendsen and colleagues concluded that, if midline shift was taken into account, no significant acute lesion was missed by CT.

We have studied the reliability of interpretation of CT scans by two neurosurgeons who reviewed the scans of 97 head injured patients previously treated by our unit, without access to names or clinical information.[28] A third neurosurgeon determined from the patients' case records and autopsy results whether a significant hematoma had been present at the time of the scan. There was complete agreement between the two surgeons about the presence or absence of a hematoma in 95 out of the 97 cases, and in all cases their diagnosis was correct. In the remaining two patients, whose scans were of poor quality, one or other of the surgeons felt uncertain about the diagnosis; his companion was, however, able to come to a firm opinion in both cases and again he was correct.

ESTABLISHING THE DIAGNOSIS OF AN INTRACRANIAL HEMATOMA

Knowing that hematomas almost always produce altered consciousness, sometimes focal signs in the limbs, and eventually inequality of the pupils, the question is to decide what degree of clinical suspicion justifies neuroradiological investigation, and what circumstances demand that exploratory surgery be performed, either with or without neuroradiological evidence. This entails discussion of differential diagnosis, and the balancing of priorities regarding further observation, investigation, or operation, according to the clinical state of the patient and the local facilities. In a patient who is in a general hospital 20 miles or more from a neurosurgical center, only mild clinical suspicion may justify moving the patient to that center—if only for further clinical observation in the first place. On the other hand, the patient arriving at the center by transfer and who is already decerebrate, with a fixed pupil, may be judged to be in too critical a condition for deferral of surgery even for the time needed to carry out neuroradiological investigations.

There are great variations in the rate at which patients deteriorate with intracranial hematoma—it may take many hours or days to pass from full consciousness to decerebrate coma; but it can all happen in half an hour. Where it is alleged to be very rapid, it is not uncommon to find, on scrutinizing the records, that there has been evidence of change over several hours before the final crescendo. In one study of over 300 patients in our unit, a third of patients transferred with intracranial hematoma had documented evidence of deterioration over 12 hours or more.[25] There were two explanations: *misdiagnosis* and *delayed diagnosis*. Two thirds of patients with evidence of prolonged deterioration were not thought initially to have had a head injury. In half of them impairment of consciousness was attributed to the effects of alcohol and the remainder were thought to have suffered a cerebrovascular accident. Eighty percent of both these groups later proved to have a fractured skull, although this was often not known during the early stages. In the final third of the patients in this Scottish study, when the case record was reviewed, there was evidence that although it was known that the patient had suffered a head injury, the deterioration was not recognized, or if it was its significance was not appreciated.

In their report from New York, Gallagher and Browder found that alcohol had obscured changes in consciousness in a third of a series of 167 patients with an extradural hematoma.[29] In 21 patients the hematoma was diagnosed only at postmortem; 8 of these patients had died in the "alcohol ward" without ever having been seen by surgeons. Although the other 13 patients had been in the neurosurgical department, the correct diagnosis was either not considered or was rejected when burr holes were negative.

Sometimes deterioration is due to other causes, either intracranial or extracranial. In one series of patients who "talked and died," 25 percent did *not* have a hematoma.[87] Other intracranial complications are edema and swelling, focal or general; meningitis; infarction; and fat embolism. Extracranial factors, particularly hypoxia and hypotension, can reduce responsiveness and may aggravate a focal deficit that was already present. Drugs may confuse the clinical picture—either the conscious state or the pupils. In all these circumstances, unless extracranial cause for deterioration is clearly present and can be remedied, the most important step is to seek an intracranial hematoma.

It is now essential to break the tradition that an intracranial hematoma is seriously suspected only when a patient is in coma, with a fixed dilated pupil. Indeed, there should be few such patients if proper observations are being made clinically, and if anticipatory steps are taken at the earliest suggestion of an intracranial hematoma. It should be remembered that remediable hematomas are not uncommon in patients who have been unconscious from the moment of injury.

CT scanning is the most reliable way to diagnose or exclude a hematoma and it is now becoming part of good medical practice to make every effort to secure a scan in any patient whose clinical state even raises the possibility of this complication. It is impractical to scan every head injured patient and guidelines about who should be scanned can be based upon the presence or absence of clinical abnormalities or a skull fracture. Several studies show that up to a half of patients who are in coma at some stage after head injury will have an intracranial hematoma (Table 8). French and Dublin[23] confirmed this observation and related the occurrence of abnormalities of CT scanning to the presence or absence of im-

Table 8. Intracranial hematoma in patients in coma after head injury

Source of Data	Total Cases in Coma	Hematoma or Mass Lesion
Pagni[81]	1091	53%
Turazzi[109]	240	48%
Hoff[42]	100	47%
French & Dublin[23]	214	49%
Becker[4]	160	39%
Collaborative Study[57]	1000	48%

paired consciousness and focal neurological signs (Table 9). Similar findings have also been reported by Zimmerman and associates.[113]

There is therefore a good case, whenever facilities are available, for investigating all patients in coma or with focal neurological signs. The value of investigating a patient without these features will depend upon whether he has suspicious symptoms such as headache, and for how long these have been present, and probably also upon whether or not there is a skull fracture. Scanning in the absence of neurological abnormalities rarely discloses a significant hematoma; in French and Dublin's study, in the 13 percent of patients in this group who did have an abnormality, none were considered to merit operation.

A negative scan soon after injury does not exclude the possibility that a new lesion may develop some days later, but this is uncommon.[93,98]

SURGICAL MANAGEMENT

There are close parallels between the approach of the surgeon to intracranial hematoma and to acute appendicitis. In both cases a fatal outcome may follow if operation is withheld, and both are potentially curable if operated on in time. In both, therefore, the rule is to explore if the diagnosis is even suspected. The similarity ends there, because exploring the abdomen for suspected appendicitis is both the most reliable way of confirming the suspected diagnosis and is also a safe procedure. On the other hand, intracranial exploration, especially by the nonexpert, or by burr holes even when done by a neurosurgeon, may fail to locate the hematoma, may allow only incomplete evacuation if the clot is found, or may even begin intracranial bleeding when the exploration has been negative. This is why there are so many discussions (not to say disagreements) about the indications for moving patients suspected of having an intracranial hematoma to a neurosurgical unit, about whether to undertake neuroradiology before operation (or even before transfer to the neurosurgeon if scanners are available in general

Table 9. Clinical findings and frequency of abnormality on CT scan

Clinical Findings		Abnormal CT Scan
Impaired Consciousness	Focal Signs	
—	—	13%
Present	—	35%
—	Present	50%
Present	Present	85%

(Data from French and Dublin[23])

171

hospitals), and about whether to use burr holes as an investigation as well as a means of initial treatment. The answers to these questions must depend on local circumstances (the geographical distribution of investigative and surgical expertise), and on the state of the patient.

The ideal to aim for is to suspect the possibility of an intracranial hematoma sufficiently early in its development to arrange CT scanning before there is a therapeutically critical condition. This may or may not entail moving the patient to the neurosurgical center at this stage, before the diagnosis is confirmed. When such a policy is pursued it is inevitable that some hematomas will be revealed in patients whose clinical state is so little affected that the question arises whether surgical evacuation is in fact required.

Operate or Observe?

It has been known for many years that some patients tolerate the presence of an intracranial hematoma and recover without its being removed. Occasionally such hematomas were discovered when intracranial surgery was undertaken some weeks after injury for other purposes—such as anterior fossa dural repair. Angiography also sometimes revealed a mass in a patient who was improving (or was static and satisfactory), and surgeons elected to let events take their natural course. Because CT scanning is undertaken much more readily than angiography ever was, it is inevitable that hematomas are discovered in patients who are not (yet) obviously in need of surgical intervention. Should it be assumed that unless these hematomas are removed the patients will inevitably develop signs of serious cerebral compression? Or is it safe to pursue an expectant policy in some cases, and if so, in what circumstances?

Our experience with a trial of nonoperative management, in a series of patients whose condition was not considered to justify immediate operation at the time of initial CT diagnosis, revealed that less than half did eventually need surgery.[106] Neither the patient's age, nor initial clinical responsiveness, nor the amount of lateral shift on the CT scan were reliable indicators of whether or not a hematoma would later require removal. The level of ICP within the next few hours after the scan did provide some indication of the prospects for success of conservative measures (Fig. 13). Now, when the ICP is persistently greater than 30 mm Hg, we recommend removal of the clot. Some patients with a pressure between 20 and 30 mm Hg will recover spontaneously, as will almost all of those whose ICP is under 20 mm Hg. Conservative management, however, is not without difficulties, anxieties, and complications, and more exact criteria for deciding upon a trial of conservative measures remain to be determined.

Operate or Investigate?

Deterioration in a patient with a clot may happen very rapidly indeed, and the inevitable "pilot error" of doctors and nurses on some occasions means that there will always be some patients whose condition becomes critical before investigations have confirmed the presence or location of an intracranial hematoma. It is a matter of fine judgment as to whether the delay involved in moving a patient to the neurosurgical unit, or that involved in carrying out neuroradiological investigations on the patient who has already reached the neurosurgeon, is justified. No rules can be given other than to emphasize the need to give due consideration to

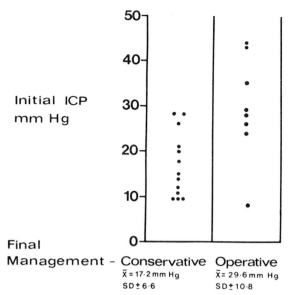

Figure 13. Base-line intracranial pressure following CT scan diagnosis of acute traumatic intracranial hematoma in 21 patients. In each case the clinician in charge decided that there was a good prospect of recovery without operation. The mean level of ICP was higher in the eight patients who subsequently deteriorated and required operation than in those in whom conservative management was successful. Only one patient with an initial ICP below 20 mm Hg came to operation 7 days later.[106]

the state of the patient, the rate of progress of his condition, and the expected further course in relation to the specific delay that transfer or investigation is likely to cause.

It might seem obvious that the sooner the patient is operated on the better, and this has led some surgeons to declare that the patient with a suspected hematoma should always be operated on immediately, wherever he is, and without investigation.[74] But surgical evacuation of an intracranial hematoma is often a difficult operation; in only a minority of cases is a simple extradural hematoma found in the classical site. Even in the hands of a neurosurgeon, blind burr hole exploration misses a third of hematomas (Table 10).

If a patient can be transferred to a neurosurgeon within an hour, this is probably always the best course; few general hospitals are able to have a surgeon "inside the head" within that time, because of unfamiliarity with this procedure and with the instruments required. The value of neuroradiology to the neurosurgeon is that

Table 10. Results of emergency exploration of severely head injured patients

Procedure	n	Result	n	Survived	
Exploratory burr holes	100	Positive	34	18	(53%)
		False Negative	19	4	(21%)
Angiography after burr holes	32	Positive	9	4	(44%)
		False Negative	1	—	

(From Hoff, Spetzler, and Winestock[42])

173

he can proceed directly to the hematoma—too often initial burr hole exploration fails to show anything but a tight brain, and the patient has then to go to the radiology department before returning to the operating room for exploration in the appropriate place. The overall delay involved has then been greater than if neuroradiology had been carried out in the first place. This is not to deny the need, on some occasions, to proceed directly to surgery, either in a general hospital or a neurosurgical unit. This will be justified only when a patient is already in an advanced state of deterioration, when there are usually good clues to the location of the hematoma, such as unilateral pupil dilatation, asymmetrical motor signs, and possibly a skull fracture.

Operation for Intracranial Hematoma

This is not a minor operation. Even if the patient is in coma it is unwise to begin without full anesthetic support, an intravenous line, and blood taken for cross-matching. The only exception is the patient thought likely to expire during the time taken to organize these precautions, which can usually be done while investigations are proceeding or the theater is prepared. These patients have high intracranial pressure and, therefore, are very vulnerable to incidents of respiratory obstruction, hypercarbia, or systemic hypotension. Their blood pressure may be normal or high because of the raised ICP, and once the hematoma begins to be removed the blood pressure may fall precipitously, especially if multiple injury has produced hypovolemia, the effects of which have been masked by the effects of raised ICP. In a child an extradural hematoma may itself be large enough to cause hypovolemia.

Exploratory Operation

The surgical approach will depend on whether or not neuroradiological investigations have revealed the exact site and extent of the lesion. When this has not been possible, simpler signs can help (Table 11). If the patient has a dilated pupil, the clot will be on the same side in over 90 percent of cases. A skull fracture that is on the same side as the dilated pupil strengthens this probability, and its location may indicate whether the clot is likely to be in an unusual position (frontal or occipital), or if it is temporoparietal, whether it is anterior or posterior in position.

Exploration begins with a burr hole low in the temporal region, just above the zygoma. This will detect an extradural hematoma in the temporal fossa and will also disclose, what in practice is a more common finding, a subdural hematoma or a burst lobe. Inexperienced surgeons often make this burr hole too high, near

Table 11. Side of hematoma and localizing features

Feature	Hematoma Side	
First or only dilated pupil	Ipsilateral	94%
Most abnormal motor response	Contralateral	82%
Skull fracture	Ipsilateral	66%

(From Teasdale and Galbraith[105])

174

the temporal crest. This may fail to disclose a hematoma in the temporal region and is also difficult to incorporate into a suitable bone flap.

If the initial temporal burr hole is negative, a second opening is made close to the fracture-line, or in the absence of a fracture, in the region of any scalp wound. The incision should, if possible, be made in such a site that it can be incorporated into the "question mark" flap. Neurosurgeons seldom choose to use a craniectomy, but for the non-neurosurgeon this offers a simple and respectable means of gaining sufficient exposure.

Operation for Known Extradural Hematoma

A "question mark" skin flap is best for the classical anterior temporal hematoma (Fig. 14), but if the hematoma is more posterior a "horseshoe" flap is adequate (Fig. 15). Hematomas in other sites will require whatever seems an appropriate flap, and the surgeon should always err on the side of generosity in size. Once a solid clot has been removed, extradural hemostasis is achieved; only in some cases is a major vessel still bleeding, and it can be clipped or cauterized. More often the dural surface is oozing and hemostatic gauze is needed for control.

Since about a third of extradural hematomas are associated with an intradural lesion, the next question is whether to open the dura. This should be done if preoperative CT scan has shown a definite intradural hematoma; or, in the absence of scanning, if the patient is known never to have talked since the injury, or if the dura is definitely blue and bulging. To open the dura unnecessarily, on the other hand, may allow damaging herniation of swollen brain.

Operation for Intradural Hematoma

If scanning indicates an intradural lesion, it should be assumed that there may be disruption of both frontal and temporal lobes—even under what may appear on the scan to be a "pure" subdural clot. Except when a circumscribed intracerebral clot has been seen (which may be removed through a local bone flap or a trephine), it is well always to turn a large frontotemporal bone flap, using the

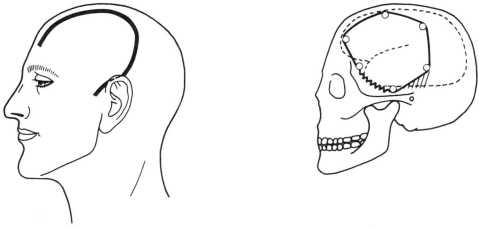

Figure 14. "Question mark" flap for acute traumatic intracranial hematoma.

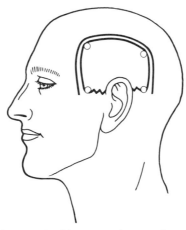

Figure 15. "Horse-shoe" flap for extradural hematoma in posterior temporal region.

question mark skin incision (Fig. 14). The backwards arch of the question mark above the ear is an important component in providing access to the full length of the temporal lobe and to the clot in the parietal region. The subdural clot is removed by suction and irrigation and then the extent of surface damage on the brain is assessed. Multiple contusions, showing the areas of hemorrhage beneath an intact pia-arachnoid, do not indicate that the underlying brain is necessarily irreparably damaged. If the pia-arachnoid is lacerated, and parts of the temporal or frontal lobes have become replaced by softened, necrotic brain intermixed with solid and liquid blood, these areas are probably best removed. The involved brain is likely to be irrecoverably damaged and may act as a source of compression to the remainder of the brain. Softened, necrotic brain is easily removed by gentle suction and irrigation; firmer, normal brain should not be removed unless a lobectomy is planned. This is sometimes the most appropriate procedure when the major portion of the lobe has been disrupted, especially if this is on the nondominant side. The surgeon should bear in mind in these circumstances the frequency of bilateral or diffuse damage. For this reason it is unwise to remove largely intact frontal or temporal lobes in order to provide an internal decompression in severely injured cases.

CLOSURE. Whenever possible, we close the dural incision and replace the bone flap. If the brain appears "tight" after removal of a subdural hematoma, we may leave the dura open in the temporal region. In extreme circumstances, when dural closure is difficult, it may be impossible to avoid leaving the dura open and removing the bone flap. Although this may temporarily have a beneficial effect upon brain tightness, it may also encourage brain swelling.[14,78] The brain herniates and this can compromise its blood supply and aggravate brain damage. Some surgeons have advocated performing hemicraniectomy,[86] bifrontal craniectomy,[10,60] or circumferential craniotomy on patients with severe intradural damage, arguing that this would provide extra volume within which brain swelling could be accommodated. The number of patients achieving an independent existence after such operations is very small.[13,15]

176

Posterior Fossa Hematomas

In an emergency situation it is probably safer to have the patient prone than in the sitting position. This is especially true when the hematoma has complicated injury to one of the major venous sinuses, for in this circumstance there is danger of air embolism. The possibility of having to elevate the head to reduce bleeding during operation must also be borne in mind. Access to the hematoma is gained by a standard suboccipital craniectomy. There is often a fracture of the occipital bone and care is necessary to avoid aggravating hemorrhage during removal of the bone fragments.

POSTOPERATIVE RECOVERY AND COMPLICATIONS

Postoperatively, patients require intensive monitoring in the same way as severely head injured patients without a surgical lesion (Chapter 6). During the postoperative period a number of complications may develop; these are often detected because there is further deterioration in the patient's condition, but are sometimes suspected when a patient fails to improve at the anticipated rate.

Rate of Recovery

It is uncommon for a patient in coma before operation to regain consciousness within the subsequent 6 hours. Indeed some of those previously talking before operation have still not recovered by this time, although most will soon do so. By the time 24 hours have passed a quarter of those in coma at 6 hours have recovered, including most of those who will eventually make moderate or good recoveries (Fig. 16). Pupil reactivity may take 2 or 3 days to return in a minority

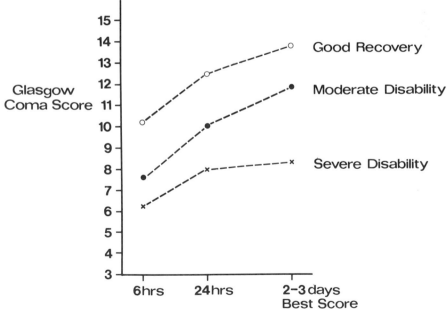

Figure 16. Rate of postoperative recovery in different outcome groups as shown by Mean Coma Score at 6 hours and 24 hours after operation, and the best level in the next 2 to 3 days.

of survivors, but in our experience, no patient whose pupils were still nonreacting 7 days after operation has recovered.

When a patient deteriorates or fails to improve in the postoperative period it is always necessary to decide whether this is evidence of persisting severe brain damage or an indication of the development of further remediable complications. This can best be settled by means of investigations.

Complications after Surgery

Incomplete Evacuation

This is rare but may happen for two reasons: a deliberate decision not to remove the full extent of an intracerebral lesion in case potentially functional brain may be sacrificed; or a failure to appreciate the full extent of a surface clot or an intracerebral lesion. Incomplete removal most often occurs when the initial surgery was performed outside a neurosurgical department, or if it was not preceded by neuroradiological studies.

Reaccumulation

Recurrent extradural or subdural bleeding in a volume sufficient to produce a significant space-occupying lesion is uncommon. However, swelling of the brain into the cavity left after removal of an intradural hematoma is usual. In interpreting postoperative studies that show persisting displacement of the brain, caution is necessary because continued shift is compatible with an apparently satisfactory rate of progress.[41]

New Hematomas

A new lesion is almost always an intradural hematoma, sometimes underlying the site of a previous extradural hematoma, but sometimes in an entirely different part of the brain. It is often an indication of the widespread nature of the brain damage, and this probably accounts for the unfavorable outcome of postoperative clots in the head injured patient. When the patient was in coma before the first operation, or when the preoperative CT scan suggested diffuse damage, monitoring intracranial pressure in the postoperative period is advisable. Persistently high ICP may provide an early indication of development of further mass effects and indicate the need for repeat CT scanning.

In the Glasgow series of hematomas about 10 percent of patients required a second operation, usually because of evidence of deterioration. The frequency of further operation was similar whether the initial surgery had been for an extradural or an intradural hematoma. However, in the case of extradural hematomas, the second operation was usually restricted to removal of further clot; among the intradural hematomas, half the second operations were for discrete clots, but almost as many were in order to perform a lobectomy, which in seven out of eight cases was of the right temporal lobe. The bone flap was left out at the second operation in more than half the cases with intradural hematomas. The effect of the second operation was to improve the patient in two thirds of cases, but this was marked only if there had been clinical deterioration immediately before the second operation.

Raised Intracranial Pressure

Intracranial pressure remains high (more than 20 mm Hg) after operation in a half of cases.[76] The cause of the elevation in a surprising proportion is either incomplete evacuation, a recollection, or a new lesion. The first step in management is to exclude these possibilities by an appropriate neuroradiological study. In many cases, however, there is swelling of one or both cerebral hemispheres. Sometimes this will be due to edema, but vascular engorgement is also possible and a block of CSF circulation may also be present (p. 59).

The methods of management that may be employed include drainage of CSF, osmotics, hyperventilation, and barbiturates. The value of these treatments is discussed in Chapter 9. The decision to institute treatment for raised ICP should not be taken just on the basis of its absolute level; the direction of any change and the clinical state of the patient are at least as important.

Low Intracranial Pressure

This is an enigmatic condition. It is suspected when, after removal of a surface hematoma, the brain apparently fails to re-expand and the patient makes little improvement. It is most often diagnosed following evacuation of chronic subdural hematoma, but may also follow removal of an acute intracranial hematoma, especially when the bone flap has been removed. Symptoms and signs attributed to CSF hypotension include headaches, nausea, dizziness, and focal neurological signs, including the signs of tentorial herniation. The most characteristic feature is that symptoms appear when the patient is sitting or standing and are relieved by lying down.

It seems useful to consider patients who have a large external decompression as a separate group. In the early postoperative period these patients usually show some swelling at the site of decompression, which resolves as the patient improves. Sometimes this is followed by marked indrawing of the area of decompression, but few patients develop symptoms that might be attributed to this. However, occasional cases have been described in which focal neurological signs have been closely related to an indrawn external decompression and have resolved soon after the bone flap was reinserted. It is probably worth considering replacing the bone flap at an early stage when a decompressed area has become indrawn, but without undue expectation for the relief of symptoms.

CSF hypotension is occasionally suspected in a patient who has not undergone surgery or at the most has had burr holes. There are three possible reasons: reduced production of CSF, increased reabsorption of CSF, or a traumatic CSF fistula. Convincing arguments for a disturbance of production or absorption of CSF are lacking, and the most convincing instances have been in patients with basal fractures and CSF leaks, as in the original description of this syndrome by Leriche.[64]

Single injections of fluid or air into the CSF pathways have only a transient effect upon CSF pressure and are not recommended for suspected CSF hypotension. Prolonged infusions of fluid have been complicated by infection. The simplest and probably most effective treatment is bed rest, in the head down position, and adequate hydration. When symptoms persist a CSF leak should be sought for.

Postoperative Epilepsy

Up to a third of patients with an intracranial hematoma have epilepsy in the first week, and in a third of these the first fit occurs only after surgery (p. 162). The importance of avoiding status epilepticus has been mentioned elsewhere. A more common problem is focal epilepsy after evacuation of an intradural hematoma. Such attacks may occur with great frequency, so that there is an almost continual focal seizure. This is often resistant to standard doses of anticonvulsants, and when this occurs it is preferable simply to ensure that adequate amounts are given to prevent generalized seizures. Total abolition of focal activity may be impossible without risking depression of consciousness and impairment of respiration.

Results of Treatment

There are numerous reports dealing with the outcome of series of patients with traumatic intracranial hematoma. The three series described by Jamieson and Yelland have become classic examples.[49-51] They contained large numbers of patients; the results were reported and analyzed in great detail; and the outcomes were exceptionally good in patients with extradural hematoma. Their results and those of some more recent studies are shown in Tables 12 and 13. However, most

Table 12. Extradural hematoma—results of operation

Source of Data	n	% with Intradural Lesion	% in Stupor or Coma	% Mortality (All Cases)
Jamieson and Yelland[49]	167	47	56	16
Jonker and Oosterhuis[58]	92	24	69	32
Kvarnes and Trumpy[62]	132	33	60	23
Glasgow 1974–1976[105]	55	27	59	23
Heiskanen[38]	80		56	16

(Modified from Teasdale and Galbraith[105])

reports refer only to mortality and there are considerable differences in these: comparisons are often difficult because of variations in the way that hematomas have been classified and in the ways and times the patients have been assessed. Several factors influence outcome and the interaction between these makes prognosis less simple than hitherto realized. In the following analysis, the information available from the Brisbane series is compared with results of a series studied in Glasgow between 1974 and 1976, analyzed by the Glasgow scales for early severity and ultimate outcome.

Extradural hematoma has a lower mortality and fewer survivors are disabled; if it is associated with intradural clot, then the outcome is less good (Table 14). Differences between the results for extradural hematoma may depend partly on whether cases of intradural damage are included or not, and on how this damage was recognized; this distinction has been much more readily made since CT scanning became available. Patients in Glasgow with pure subdural hematomas did no better than those with burst lobes, suggesting that subdural hematoma is usually associated with underlying brain damage, even when this is not obvious.

Table 13. Intradural hematoma—results of operation

Source of Data	Type	n	% in Stupor or Coma	% Mortality (All Cases)
Jamieson and Yelland[50]	Subdural	553	58	35
Jamieson and Yelland[51]	Intracerebral	63	49	25
Fell et al.[21]	Subdural/ intracerebral			
	<3 days	144	—	45
Rosenørn and Gjerris[90]	Subdural only:			
	acute<3 days	112	80	73
	subacute <3 weeks	37	24	27
Tandon et al.[102]	Temporal lobe			
	lesions	60	68	43
Glasgow 1974–1976[105]	All types			
	<2 weeks	125	66	41

(Modified from Teasdale and Galbraith[105])

In Brisbane the subdural hematomas had a better outcome; but more than half had been operated on more than a week after injury and probably included "chronic cases," thereby putting them in quite a different category. In both Glasgow and Brisbane pure intracerebral hematomas had a lower mortality than burst lobes.

The influence of age is important, as it is in patients without a hematoma. The worse outcome of older patients is much more marked with extradural hematoma; indeed, in Glasgow and Brisbane age had little effect on outcome from intradural hematoma below the age of 60 (Table 15). The overall effect of age and outcome is more difficult to interpret because hematomas are commoner in older patients, and older patients with hematomas more often have intradural clots, which are associated with a worse outcome.

Outcome is worse in patients operated on within 3 days of injury when compared with the outcome of patients coming to operation within the next 2 or 3 weeks (Table 16). Even within the first 3 days, outcome was worse in patients undergoing surgery within 24 hours of injury when compared with those operated on later. McLaurin and Tutor[72] observed a mortality of 73 percent within the first 24 hours, Jamieson and Yelland[50,51] 63 percent, and Fell and colleagues[21] 48 per-

Table 14. Type of hematoma and outcome

Type of Hematoma	Jamieson & Yelland[40–51]	Glasgow 1974–1976		
	Dead %	Dead/ Vegetative %	Severe Disability %	Moderate/ Good Recovery %
Extradural only	5	21	5	74
Extra + Intradural	27	33	10	57
Subdural only	22	49	15	36
Subdural + Intracerebral*	55	50	14	36
Intracerebral only	25	21	32	47

*Includes patients with "complicated" subdural and burst lobes.
(From Teasdale and Galbraith[105])

181

Table 15. Age and mortality of acute traumatic intracranial hematoma

	Jamieson & Yelland[49-51] Dead		Glasgow (1974-76) Dead	
	n	%	n	%
Extradural Hematoma	73	11	18	11
<20 years	87	18	15	40
20–40 years	7	29	20	25
>40 years				
Intradural Hematoma	188	39	34	38
<20 years	160	38	47	30
40–60 years	88	67	23	65
>60 years				

(From Teasdale and Galbraith[105])

cent; whereas, for patients with a 2 to 3 day interval between injury and operation, the mortality rates were 19 percent, 29 percent, and 21 percent, respectively.

Effect of State of Consciousness on Outcome

Mortality is much higher for patients who are in coma by the time they come to surgery, whether the hematoma is extradural or intradural (Table 17). More detailed analysis of the Glasgow series shows that the proportion of patients who are left severely disabled is not much affected by the state of the patient at the time of operation, but many more of the patients whose hematoma is evacuated before they are in coma make a satisfactory recovery.

Results of Posterior Fossa Hematoma

The outcome of patients with posterior fossa hematoma also depends upon their state before operation. Some patients present only some days or weeks after injury and often show features typical of any posterior fossa mass. In these cases the outcome may be extremely good. Although prognosis is bad in patients who present acutely and in deep coma, it is probably better than in the case of a

Table 16. Outcome of intradural hematomas operated upon at different times after injury

Interval between Injury and Operation	Jamieson & Yelland[49-51]	Glasgow (1974-76)
1–3 days	n=265	n=73
Dead	56%	47%
Severe/total disability	} 44%	18%
Moderate or good recovery		35%
3 days–2 to 3 weeks	n=155	n=52
Dead	14%	29%
Severe/total disability	} 86%	18%
Moderate or good recovery		53%

(From Teasdale and Galbraith[105])

Table 17. Influence on mortality of state of responsiveness before operation

	Jamieson & Yelland[49-51]	Glasgow (1974-1976)	
	% Dead	% Dead	% M/G Rec*
Extradural ± intradural			
Not in coma	1	3	91
In coma	27	53	39
Intradural			
Not in coma	10	9	70
In coma	54	63	21

*Moderate to good recovery.
(From Teasdale and Galbraith[105])

comparable patient with a supratentorial hematoma. Relief of pressure from a posterior fossa clot in a previously apneic patient can even be followed by a return of respiration. In such cases, perhaps because the cerebral hemispheres are only secondarily affected, the eventual outcome may be good.

Management and Outcome

There is evidence that a deliberate effort to achieve diagnosis, and so to operate on more patients before they are in coma, can improve the outcome. Jamieson and Yelland[46,49] showed this for extradural hematoma, but reported that this did not apply to intradural hematomas. In 1978 an expansion of neurosurgical facilities in Glasgow was coupled with a deliberate effort to transfer patients sooner, with the aim of reducing the mortality associated with extradural and intradural hematomas (Table 18). This policy led to the detection of more hematomas than in previous years, although there was no change in the size of the catchment population, nor in the incidence of head injuries, to account for this change. The modest improvement in results was not related directly to the introduction of CT scanning, because this had already been in use in Glasgow from 1974.

However, it is fair to ask whether CT scanning should (or can be expected to) improve the outcome of patients with intracranial hematoma. McKissock's successors in London concluded that the first two years of CT scanning in that unit had not noticeably improved results.[1] The results of extradural hematoma in Glasgow for the first 3 years of CT scanning (1974–1976) were similar to those published 15 years previously by McKissock. Any improvements in the results for intracranial hematoma will almost certainly be related in part to the earlier or more accurate diagnosis that scanning makes possible. But this benefit will be

Table 18. Comparison of results in two periods in Glasgow

Period	Extradural ± Intradural			Intradural Only		
	n	% in Coma	% Dead	n	% in Coma	% Dead
1974–1976	55	60	23	125	66	41
1978	38	55	18	82	52	36

realized only if appropriate organizational changes are made that ensure the early scanning of as many patients as possible who are at risk of developing this complication. This is discussed in the final chapter.

The statistics for intracranial hematoma probably provide the best audit of the level of provision of health care for head injuries in a community. These should include the diagnosis rate (per unit of population) of extradural and intradural hematoma, in life and at autopsy; the proportion of patients who reach the operating table at different intervals after injury; and the proportion who are in coma by the time they come to surgery.

FLUID COLLECTIONS IN THE SUBDURAL SPACE

Subdural Hygroma

In children, subdural effusions are a well-recognized entity, but in adults their status is more debatable. They are encountered in a variety of circumstances. There is least doubt about their significance when they are the cause of a space-occupying lesion in a deteriorating patient. Such collections usually consist of blood-stained CSF under pressure and are thought to arise because a tear in the arachnoid over the Sylvian fissure permits CSF to escape into the subdural space, with its return prevented by a valve-like mechanism. In one series of patients[39] the presentation was within a few hours or as long as 4 weeks after injury, but was commonest at the end of a week. These space-occupying hygromas measured between 75 and 200 ml, and in 10 out of 12 patients drainage of the hematoma, which was bilateral in half of the cases, was followed by improvement.

The significance of a subdural collection in other circumstances is less clear. Burr holes performed within a day of injury in a patient in deep coma from the time of injury occasionally disclose blood-stained CSF under low pressure in a subdural space. Benefit from drainage of this fluid is unlikely, as is also the case for collections disclosed when a CT scan is performed several weeks after injury in a patient who is not deteriorating.[23] Some of these late collections are found in patients complaining of headache and the fluid may then be xanthochromic, indicating a previous hemorrhage, but it is unclear whether the collection is responsible for the symptoms.

Chronic Subdural Hematoma

Up to half of adults with chronic subdural hematomas have no history of trauma. When there has been an injury it has often been a mild one; a subdural hematoma may even follow indirect force to the head, for example, whiplash injury. In some cases without a history of preceding trauma there is an identifiable cause such as a vascular lesion or a hemorrhagic diasthesis caused by disease or anticoagulants. It is usually presumed that the remaining cases are related to some unidentified injury. Cerebral atrophy, chronic alcoholism, and other factors that lower intracranial pressure predispose to subdural hematoma. Chronic subdural hematomas are rare after severe impact damage, possibly because the combination of brain damage and hematoma leads to diagnosis at an early stage.

Pathology

After an episode of subdural hemorrhage, organizational processes can be recognized histologically within 3 days. The cells originate from the dura and they spread first around the surface of the clot and then within it; eventually there may be only an area of dural pigmentation, a membrane on the inner surface of the dura, or a combination of these. Failure of complete cellular organization of the clot leads to the characteristic clinical finding: a collection of fluid of variable color and consistency, bounded by an outer membrane attached to the dura and an inner membrane lying on the arachnoid. The outer layer is the thicker, more vascular layer and may be the source of further hemorrhage into the cavity. The failure of some collections to resolve has not been explained satisfactorily: incomplete coagulation of the initial bleeding and excessive fibrinolysis have been suggested. Whatever the reason it seems likely that the fluid-filled space gradually enlarges and also can fluctuate in size, perhaps as a consequence of osmotic changes or as a result of repeated hemorrhage.

Age Incidence

There is an excess of subdural hematomas in older people. In most series the peak incidence is in the 50s and 60s, but the reduced numbers in older groups may only be a reflection of the smaller numbers at risk. Males predominate, in a ratio between 3 and 10 to 1.[11,66,69]

Localization

Ninety percent of hematomas are centered in the parietal area. The remainder can be found in frontal, temporal, or occipital regions, but hematomas are described in the posterior fossa, the interhemispheric fissure, the sellar region, and the spinal canal. A unilateral hematoma is more commonly found on the left side, but about one in seven cases are bilateral.

Clinical Features

Headache is a frequent but nonspecific complaint in a patient with a chronic subdural hematoma. The characteristic presenting features fall into three categories: personality disorders, paresis, and features of raised intracranial pressure (Table 19).[11] Personality disorders include impairment of consciousness and mental function. There may be apathy, confusion, tiredness, lack of concentration, and reduced performance; in some patients these are succeeded by increasing impairment of consciousness, although coma is unusual. Hemiparesis is observed in a half to three quarters of cases but is often on the same side as the collection. The finding of a hemianopia does not exclude the diagnosis of a chronic subdural hematoma, although it is certainly very uncommon.[69] Striking fluctuations in consciousness are traditionally regarded as a characteristic feature, but in many series they have been recorded only infrequently.

When there has been a definite preceding injury, there is generally a delay of 5 to 6 weeks before symptoms declare, and the relation between the two events is often uncertain. The presenting features can mimic a variety of other conditions,

Table 19. Features in 70 cases of chronic subdural hematoma

Average age	56 yr
History of head injury	57%
Bilateral hematomas drained	17%
Mental or personality change	33%
Coma	4%
Hemiparesis	
ipsilateral to hematoma	10%
contralateral to hematoma	24%
Papilledema	23%
Unequal pupils	1%
Fluctuation of symptoms or signs	30%

(From Cameron[11])

including psychiatric illness, brain tumor, and cerebrovascular disease, and distinction can rarely be made solely on clinical grounds.

Investigations

The most helpful investigation is a radioactive brain scan. An abnormality is present in more than 90 percent of cases and usually localizes the site of the hematoma. The increased uptake is usually easy to detect when the hematoma is unilateral. Difficulties can arise in bilateral collections, because of the symmetrical increased activity, and it is important to recognize also that a recent craniotomy produces an abnormal scan. In many patients the CT scan gives additional information about the site and size of hematoma and the extent of midline shift. However, the occurrence of collections that are isodense with the brain is now well recognized, and as a screening test isotope scanning is at least as valuable (p. 121).

Carotid angiography is probably the most reliable investigation in a patient with a chronic subdural hematoma, but its use now is restricted to occasional patients in whom there is doubt about the CT scan appearances. Little useful information is obtained from skull x-rays or EEG. In the first, this is because abnormalities are infrequent: a fracture is seen in only 2 to 6 percent of cases, and shift of the pineal gland is also uncommon. By contrast, although there is an abnormality in the EEG in up to 80 percent of patients with a chronic subdural hematoma, this is usually no more than nonspecific slowing; there is no record that is diagnostic for a subdural hematoma.

Treatment

The essence of treatment is to empty the subdural space of fluid. In adults this is generally achieved by means of one or two burr holes through which the blood is drained and the cavity irrigated. Many surgeons opt to drain the cavity via a catheter into a bottle for a few days.[100] This simple method is successful in more than 90 percent of cases; failure is likely only if the hematoma is clotted or is multilocular.[68] This is most likely to occur in cases presenting within the first 2 to 4 weeks of injury, and craniotomy may be required.

The success of conservative treatment of chronic subdural hematoma has been reported by Bender,[6] but a controlled trial of mannitol treatment showed that it was rarely effective and that surgery was always necessary. There seems little

186

indication for a trial of conservative management in chronic subdural hematoma because the surgery is so simple and the results almost invariably good; mortality is less than 5 percent and at least 90 percent of survivors make good recoveries.[11]

Subdural Hematoma in Infancy and Childhood

Infantile subdural hematomas are commonly considered a distinct clinical entity, separate from adult forms.[7,108] By the time of diagnosis the fluid within the subdural space commonly contains little blood, hence the alternative name for the disorder: subdural effusion. The fluid contains a substantial quantity of protein, which distinguishes it from CSF. The collection is nearly always bilateral, and the two sides communicate under the falx. In many cases a history of a clear episode of trauma is lacking; such cases may be related to birth injury, and the condition is commoner in male infants, perhaps because of their relatively larger head size. A number are due to injury inflicted by the child's parents, and about 10 percent of "battered children" have subdural hematomas. The essential features of the condition are no different when it follows meningitis or the rapid reduction of intracranial pressure by insertion of a shunt or when it is the result of a blood disorder. The presenting symptoms are nonspecific and the signs reflect the effects of an intracranial expanding process in the unfused skull. Papilledema is uncommon but intraocular hemorrhage occurs in almost half the patients. Many children are anemic.

Diagnosis is established by tapping the subdural space through the patent fontanelle. Attention to technique is important; if no fluid is present, brain damage may be caused, but failure to obtain fluid is possible even with quite large collections.[108] Aspiration is also the mainstay of treatment and is carried out daily so long as substantial volumes are being obtained (over 10 ml.). If the effusion fails to resolve within 1 or 2 weeks, a simple and effective measure is to shunt the fluid from the subdural space to the peritoneal cavity. External drainage, as for adult subdural hematoma (p. 186), has been used. A much more drastic measure is the removal of the membrane at craniotomy, but this has been abandoned as a routine measure.

Only half to two thirds of children with subdural effusions subsequently develop normally. About 1 child in 10 dies later, from repeated episodes of trauma. The quality of survival in the remainder is probably related more to the original illness and extent of associated brain damage than to the size or duration of the subdural effusion. About 10 percent of children are ineducable and 20 percent are educationally subnormal.[108] Hydrocephalus may occur and require treatment. Seizures are common but are unlikely to be solely caused by the previous effusion.

REFERENCES

1. Ambrose, J., Gooding, M. R., and Uttley, D.: *EMI scan in the management of head injuries.* Lancet i:847–848, 1976.
2. Antinnen, E. E., and Hillblom, E.: *On the apoplectic conditions occurring as delayed symptoms after brain injuries.* Acta Neurol. Scand. 32:103, 1957.
3. Baratham, G., and Dennyson, W. G.: *Delayed traumatic intracerebral haemorrhage.* J. Neurol. Neurosurg. Psychiatry 35:698–706, 1972.
4. Becker, D. P., Miller, J. D., Ward, J. D., et al: *The outcome from severe head injury with early diagnosis and intensive management.* J. Neurosurg. 47:491–502, 1977.

5. Bell, C.: *Surgical Observations*. Longman, London, 1816.

6. Bender, M. B., and Christoff, N.: *Non-surgical treatment of subdural haematomas*. Arch. Neurol. 31:73–79, 1974.

7. Blaauw, G.: "Subdural effusions in infancy and childhood." In Vinken, and Bruyn (eds.): *Handbook of Surgical Neurology 24*. North Holland Publishing Co., Amsterdam, pp. 329–341, 1976.

8. Bollinger, O.: *Uber traumatische Spat-Apoplexie; ein Beitrag zur Lehre von der Hirnerschutterung*. Festschr. Red. Virchow 70. Lebensjahr, Berlin 2:457–470, 1891.

9. Braakman, R., and Jennett, B.: "Depressed skull fracture (non-missile)." In Vinken, and Bruyn (eds.): *Handbook of Clinical Neurology 23*. North Holland Publishing Co., Amsterdam, pp. 403–415, 1975.

10. Browder, J.: *A resume of the principal diagnostic features of subdural haematoma*. Bull. N.Y. Acad., Med. 19:168–176, 1943.

11. Cameron, M.: *Subacute and chronic subdural haematoma*. J. Neurol. Neurosurg. Psychiatry 41:834–839, 1978.

12. Chambers, J. W.: *Acute subdural haematoma*. J. Neurosurg. 8:263–268, 1951.

13. Clark, K., Nash, T. M., and Hutchinson, J.: *The failure of circumferential craniotomy in acute traumatic cerebral swelling*. J. Neurosurg. 29:367–371, 1968.

14. Cooper, P. R., Hagler, H., and Clark, W. K.: "Decompressive craniectomy, intracranial pressure and brain oedema. An experimental study." In *Proceedings of IVth International Symposium on Intracranial Pressure*. Springer Verlag, New York, 1979.

15. Cooper, P. R., Rovit, R. L., and Ransohoff, J.: *Hemicraniectomy in the treatment of acute subdural haematoma*. Surg. Neurol. 5:25–28, 1976.

16. De Vet, A. C.: "Traumatic intracerebral haematoma." In Vinken, and Bruyn (eds.): *Handbook of Clinical Neurology 24*. North Holland Publishing Co., Amsterdam, 1976, pp. 351–368.

17. Drake, C. G.: *Subdural haematoma from arterial rupture*. J. Neurosurg. 18:597–601, 1961.

18. Echlin, F. A., Sordillo, S. U. R., and Garvey, T. Q.: *Acute and subacute chronic subdural haematoma*. J.A.M.A. 161:1345–1350, 1956.

19. Feldman, M. H.: *The decerebrate study in the primate. I. Studies in monkeys*. Arch. Neurol. 25:501–516, 1971.

20. Feldman, M. H.: *The decerebrate study in the primate. II. Studies in man*. Arch. Neurol. 25:517–525, 1971.

21. Fell, D. A., Fitzgerald, S., Moiel, R. H., et al.: *Acute subdural haematoma: review of 144 cases*. J. Neurosurg. 42:37–42, 1975.

22. Ford, L. E., and McLaurin, R. L.: *Mechanisms of extradural haematomas*. J. Neurosurg. 20:760–769, 1963.

23. French, B. N., and Dublin, A. B.: *The value of computerised tomography in the management of 1000 consecutive head injuries*. Surg. Neurol. 7:171–183, 1977.

24. Galbraith, S.: *Age distribution of extradural haemorrhage without skull fracture*. Lancet i:1217–1218, 1973.

25. Galbraith, S.: *Misdiagnosis and delayed diagnosis in traumatic intracranial haematoma*. Br. Med. J. 1:1438–1439, 1976.

26. Galbraith, S., Murray, W. R., and Patel, A. R.: *Head injury admissions to a teaching hospital*. Scot. Med. J. 22:129–132, 1977.

27. Galbraith, S., and Smith, J.: *Acute traumatic intracranial haematoma without skull fracture*. Lancet i:501–502, 1976.

28. Galbraith, S., Teasdale, G., and Blaiklock, C. T.: *Computerised tomography of acute traumatic intracranial haematoma: reliability of a neurosurgeon's interpretations*. Br. Med. J. 2:1371–1373, 1976.

29. Gallagher, J. P., and Browder, J.: *Extradural haematoma. Experience with 167 patients*. J. Neurosurg. 29:1–12, 1968.

30. Gillingham, F. J.: *The importance of rehabilitation*. Injury 1:143–147, 1969.

31. Gjerris, F., and Schmidt, K.: *Chronic subdural haematoma. Surgery or mannitol treatment*. J. Neurosurg. 40:639–642, 1974.

32. Gradwohl, R.: *Legal Medicine*. ed. 2. Williams & Wilkins, Baltimore, 1968, p. 318.

33. Gurdjian, E. S., and Thomas, L. M.: "Traumatic intracranial haemorrhage." In Feiring (ed.):

Brock's Injuries of the Brain and Spinal Cord. ed. 5. Springer-Verlag, New York, 1974, pp. 203–282.

34. Gurdjian, E. S., and Webster, J. E.: *Head injuries —Mechanism, Diagnosis and Management.* Little, Brown and Co., Boston, 1958, p. 276.

35. Hancock, D. O.: *Angiography in acute head injuries.* Lancet ii:745–747, 1961.

36. Harris, P.: "Acute traumatic subdural haematomas." *Proceedings of an International Symposium.* Churchill Livingstone, Edinburgh, 1971, pp. 321–326.

37. Hase, V., Reulen, H. J., Meinig, G., et al.: *The influence of the decompressive operation in the intracranial pressure and the pressure-volume relation in patients with severe head injuries.* Acta Neurochir. 45:1–13, 1978.

38. Heiskanen, O.: *Epidural haematoma.* Surg. Neurol. 4:23–26, 1975.

39. Hoff, J., Bates, E., Barnes, B., et al.: *Traumatic subdural hygroma.* J. Trauma 13:870–876, 1973.

40. Hoff, J., and Gauger, G.: *Arterial subdural haematomas of unusual origin.* J. Trauma 15:528–531, 1975.

41. Hoff, J., Grollmus, J., Barnes, B., et al.: *Clinical arteriographic and cisternographic observations after removal of acute subdural haematoma.* J. Neurosurg. 43:27–31, 1975.

42. Hoff, J., Spetzler, R., and Winestock, D.: *Head injury and early signs of tentorial herniation.* Western J. Med. 128:112–116, 1978.

43. Hooper, R. S.: *Observations on extradural haemorrhage.* Br. J. Surg. 47:71–87, 1959.

44. Hooper, R.: "Indications for surgical treatment." In Vinken, and Bruyn (eds.): *Handbook of Clinical Neurology 24.* North Holland Publishing Co., Amsterdam, 1976, pp. 637–667.

45. Iwakama, T., and Brunnagraber, C. V.: *Chronic extradural haematomas. A study of 21 cases.* J. Neurosurg. 38:488–494, 1973.

46. Jamieson, K. G.: *Extradural and subdural haematomas. Changing patterns and requirements of treatment in Australia.* J. Neurosurg. 33:632–635, 1970.

47. Jamieson, K. G.: "Epidural haematoma." In Vinken, and Bruyn (eds.): *Handbook of Clinical Neurology.* North Holland Publishing Co., Amsterdam, 1976, pp. 261–279.

48. Jamieson, K. G.: "Posterior fossa haematoma." Ibid. pp. 343–348.

49. Jamieson, K. G., and Yelland, J. D. N.: *Extradural haematoma. Report of 167 cases.* J. Neurosurg. 29:13–23, 1968.

50. Jamieson, K. G., and Yelland, J. D. N.: *Surgically treated traumatic subdural haematomas.* J. Neurosurg. 37:137–149, 1972.

51. Jamieson, K. G., and Yelland, J. D.N.: *Traumatic intracerebral haematoma. Report of 63 surgically treated cases.* J. Neurosurg. 37:528–532, 1972.

52. Jennett, B.: *Early traumatic epilepsy. Incidence and significance after non-missile injuries.* Arch. Neurol. 30:394–398, 1974.

53. Jennett, B.: *Epilepsy and acute traumatic intracranial haematoma.* J. Neurol. Neurosurg. Psychiatry 38:378–381, 1975.

54. Jennett, B., and Carlin, J.: *Preventable mortality and morbidity after head injury.* Injury 10:31–39, 1978.

55. Jennett, B., Murray, A., Carlin, J., et al.: *Head injuries in 3 neurosurgical units. Scottish Head Injury Management Study.* Br. Med. J. 2:955–958, 1979.

56. Jennett, B., Murray, A., MacMillan, R., et al.: *Head injuries in Scottish hospitals.* Lancet ii:696–698, 1977.

57. Jennett, B., Teasdale, G., Braakman, R., et al.: *Prognosis in series of patients with severe head injury.* Neurosurgery 4:283, 1979.

58. Jonker, C., and Oosterhuis, H. J.: *Epidural haematoma. A retrospective study of 100 patients.* Clin. Neurol. Neurosurg. 78:233–245, 1975.

59. Kalyanaram, S., Ramamoorthy, K., and Ramamurthi, B.: *An analysis of 2000 cases of head injury.* Neurol. India 18:3–11, 1970.

60. Kjellberg, R. N., and Prieto, A., Jr.: *Bifrontal decompressive craniotomy for massive cerebral oedema.* J. Neurosurg. 34:488–493, 1971.

61. Klonoff, H., and Thompson, G. B.: *Epidemiology of head injuries in adults: a pilot study.* Can. Med. Assoc. J. 100:235–241, 1969.

189

62. Kvarnes, T. L., and Trumpy, J. H.: *Extradural haematoma. A report of 132 cases.* Acta Neurochir. 41:223–224, 1978.

63. Laudig, G. H., Browder, J., and Watson, R. A.: *Subdural haematoma—a study of 143 cases, encountered during a five year period.* Ann. Surg. 113:170–188, 1941.

64. Leriche, R.: *De l'hypotension due loquide cephalo-rachidien dans certaines fractures de la base du crane et de som traitment par l'injection de serum sous la peau.* Lyon Chir. 17:638–640, 1920.

65. Lewin, W.: *The Management of Head Injuries.* Balliere, Tindall and Cassell, London, 1966.

66. Loew, F., and Kivelitz, R.: "Chronic subdural haematomas." In Vinken, and Bruyn (eds.): *Handbook of Clinical Neurology 24.* North Holland Publishing Co., Amsterdam, 1976, pp. 297–327.

67. Loew, F., and Wustner, S.: *Diagnose, Behandlung und Prognose der traumatischen Hamatoma des Schadelinneren.* Acta Neurochir. (Wien) Suppl. 8, 1960.

68. Maurice-Williams, R. S.: *Superimposed chronic subdural hygromas. Report of 2 cases.* J. Neurosurg. 43:623–626, 1975.

69. McKissock, W., Richardson, A., and Bloom, W. H.: *Subdural haematoma. A review of 389 cases.* Lancet i:1365–1369, 1960.

70. McKissock, W., Taylor, J. C., Bloom, W. H., et al.: *Extradural haematoma. Observations on 125 cases.* Lancet ii:167–172, 1960.

71. McLaurin, R. L., and Ford, L. E.: *Extradural haematoma. Statistical survey of 47 cases.* J. Neurosurg. 21:264–271, 1964.

72. McLaurin, R. L., and Tutor, F. T.: *Acute subdural haematoma. A review of 90 cases.* J. Neurosurg. 18:61–67, 1961.

73. Mealey, J.: *Acute extradural haematoma without demonstrable skull fractures.* J. Neurosurg. 17:27–37, 1960.

74. Mendelow, A. D., Karmi, M. Z., Paul, K. S., et al.: *Extradural haematoma: effect of delayed treatment.* Br. Med. J. 1:1240–1242, 1979.

75. Miles, J., and Medlery, A. V.: *Post fossa subdural haematomas.* J. Neurol. Neurosurg. Psychiatry 37:1373–1377, 1974.

76. Miller, J. D., Becker, D. P., Ward, J. D., et al.: *Significance of intracranial hypertension in severe head injury.* J. Neurosurgery 47:501–516, 1977.

77. Morin, M. A., and Pitts, F. W.: *Delayed apoplexy following head injury (traumatische Spat-Apoplexie).* J. Neurosurg. 33:542, 1970.

78. Nakatani, S., Koshino, K., Kondo, T., et al.: *Measurement of brain interstitial fluid pressure on acute head injury patients.* Neurol. Med. Chir. 19:7, 1979.

79. O'Brien, P. K., Norris, J. W., and Talin, C. H.: *Acute subdural haematomas of artefactual origin.* J. Neurosurg. 41:435–439, 1974.

80. Ommaya, A. K., and Yarnall, P.: *Subdural haematoma after whiplash injury.* Lancet ii:237–239, 1969.

81. Pagni, C. A.: *The prognosis of head injured patients in a study on coma with decerebrate posture. Analysis of 471 cases.* J. Neurosurg. Sci. 17:4, 1973.

82. Paul, M.: *Haemorrhages from head injuries.* Ann. R. Coll. Surg. Engl. 17:69–101, 1955.

83. Philips, D. G., and Azariah, R. G. C.: *Acute intracranial haematoma from head injury: a study of prognosis.* Br. J. Srug. 52:218–222, 1965.

84. Pia, H. W., Abtahi, H., and Schonmayer, R.: "Epidemiology classification and prognosis of severe cranio-cerebral injuries: a computer assisted study of 9038 cases." In Frowein, Wilcke, Karimi-Nejad, et al. (eds.): *Advances in Neurosurgery 5.* Springer Verlag, Berlin, 1978, pp. 31–35.

85. Ramamurthi, B.: "Acute subdural haematoma." In Vinken, and Bruyn (eds.): *Handbook of Clinical Neurology 24.* North Holland Publishing Co., Amsterdam, 1976, ppo. 275–296.

86. Ransohoff, J., Benjamin, M. V., Gage, E. L., et al.: *Hemicraniectomy in the management of acute subdural haematoma.* J. Neurosurg. 34:70–76, 1971.

87. Reilly, P. J., Adams, J. H., Graham, D. I., et al.: *Patients with head injury who talk and die.* Lancet ii:375–381, 1975.

88. Richards, T., and Hoff, J.: *Factors affecting survival from acute subdural haematoma.* Surgery 75:253–258, 1974.

190

89. Rose, J., Valtonen, S., and Jennett, B.: *Avoidable factors contributing to death after injury*. Br. Med. J. 2:615–618, 1977.

90. Rosenørn, J., and Gjerris, F.: *Long term review of patients with acute and subacute subdural haematomas*. J. Neurosurg. 48:345–349, 1978.

91. Sciotti, G., Terbrugge, K., Melancon, D., et al.: *Evaluation of the age of subdural haematomas by computerised tomography*. J. Neurosurg. 47:311–315, 1977.

92. Shuloff, L. A., Rivet, R. R., and Maroon, J. C.: *Severe head injuries. A retrospective review of 100 consecutive cases*. J. Indiana State Med. Assoc. 65:739–746, 1972.

93. Snoek, J., Jennett, B., Adams, J. H., et al.: *Computerised tomography after recent severe head injury in patients without acute intracranial haematoma*. J. Neurol. Neurosurg. Psychiatry 42:215–225, 1979.

94. Sparacio, R. R., Khatib, R., Chiu, J., et al.: *Chronic extradural haematoma*. J. Trauma 12:435–439, 1972.

95. Steadman, J., and Graham, J. G.: *Head injuries: an analysis and follow-up study*. Proc. R. Soc. Med. 63:23–28, 1970.

96. Suzuki, J., and Takaku, A.: *Non-surgical treatment of chronic subdural haematoma*. J. Neurosurg. 33:548–553, 1970.

97. Svendsen, P.: *Computer tomography of traumatic intracerebral lesions*. Br. J. Radiol. 49:1004–1012, 1976.

98. Sweet, R. C., Miller, J. D., Lipper, M., et al.: *Significance of bilateral abnormalities on the CT scan in patients with severe head injury*. Neurosurgery 3:16–21, 1979.

99. Tabbador, K., and La Morgese, J.: *Complication of a large cranial defect*. J. Neurosurg. 44:506–508, 1976.

100. Tabbador, K., and Shulman, K.: *Definitive treatment of chronic subdural haematoma by twist-drill craniotomy and closed system drainage*. J. Neurosurg. 46:220–226, 1977.

101. Tallala, A., and Morin, M. A.: *Acute traumatic subdural haematoma: a review of 100 consecutive cases*. J. Trauma 11:771–776, 1971.

102. Tandon, P. N., Prakash, B., and Banerji, A. K.: *Temporal lobe lesions in head injury*. Acta Neurochir. 41:205–221, 1978.

103. Tans, J. Th. J.: *Computed tomography of intracerebral haematoma*. Clin. Neurol. Neurosurg. 79:285–295, 1976.

104. Tans, J. Th. J.: *Computed tomography of extracerebral haematoma*. Clin. Neurol. Neurosurg. 79:296–306, 1976.

105. Teasdale, G., and Galbraith, S.: "Acute traumatic intracranial haematomas." In *Progress in Neurological Surgery 10*. Karger, Basel, 1981.

106. Teasdale, G., Galbraith, S., and Jennett, B.: "Operate or observe? ICP and the management of the 'silent' traumatic intracranial haematoma." In Shulman, Marmarou, Miller, et al. (eds.): *Intracranial Pressure IV*. Springer-Verlag, Berlin, 1980, pp. 36–38.

107. Thomas, L. M., and Gurdjian, E. S.: "Intracranial haematomas of traumatic origin." In Youmans (ed.): *Neurological Surgery 2*. Saunders, Philadelphia, 1973, pp. 960–968.

108. Till, K.: *Subdural haematoma and effusion in infancy*. Br. Med. J. 3:400–402, 1968.

109. Turazzi, S., Alexandre, A., and Bricolo, A.: *Incidence and significance of clinical signs of brainstem traumatic lesions*. J. Neurosurg. Sci. 19:215–222, 1975.

110. Venes, J. L., and Collins, W. F.: *Bifrontal decompressive craniectomy in the management of head trauma*. J. Neurosurg. 42:429–433, 1975.

111. Voris, H. C.: *The diagnosis and treatment of subdural haematomas*. Surgery 10:447–456, 1941.

112. Wood-Jones, F.: *On the grooves upon the ossa parietalia commonly said to be caused by the arteria meningea media*. J. Anat. Physiol. 46:228, 1912.

113. Zimmerman, R. A., Bilaniuk, L. T., and Gennarelli, T.: *Computed tomography of shearing injuries of the cerebral white matter*. Radiology 127:393–396, 1978.

CHAPTER 8

Open Injuries

When the skull is penetrated there is a risk of intracranial infection, and the management of such injuries is largely directed towards minimizing that risk. However, it is not always obvious that an injury is open; moreover infection may be delayed for months or years, so that its association with a preceding injury may not be suspected. For these reasons it is impossible to assess how often open injuries that have been overlooked or inadequately treated in fact develop infective complications. Military experience, when initial surgery is sometimes inevitably delayed, leaves no doubt about the serious consequences of neglecting such injuries. But in civilian life, difficulty in diagnosis sometimes results in such injuries being unsuspected, and some of these patients present later with established infection.[14]

Open injuries caused by nonmissile accidents are conveniently classified into compound depressed fractures of the skull vault and fractures of the skull base. Scalp lacerations without an underlying depressed fracture may technically be considered to constitute open injuries, and their treatment is also discussed here. By the same token, closed depressed fractures are contrasted and compared with those that are compound. Injuries caused by high velocity missiles are dealt with separately, because they often present quite different problems; low velocity puncture wounds that penetrate the skull are regarded as a variety of depressed fracture.

DEPRESSED FRACTURES OF THE SKULL VAULT

A fracture is considered to be significantly *depressed* if the inner table fragments are depressed by at least the thickness of the skull. A depressed fracture is *compound* if there is an associated scalp laceration, whether or not the dura is torn. Some surgeons apply the term compound *penetrating* only to those injuries associated with dural tearing. Series of depressed fractures from Glasgow, Oxford, and Rotterdam[1] have been shown to be strikingly similar (Fig. 1), and the aggregated series of 1000 patients (90% with compound fractures) forms the basis of most of the statistics in this chapter. The findings correspond closely to previous smaller series reported from Finland,[8] Germany,[26] and Australia.[10]

193

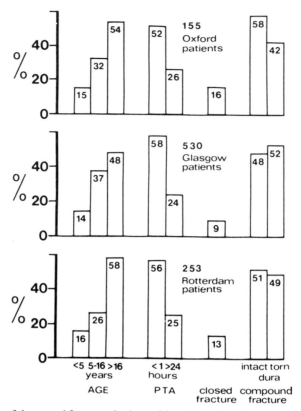

Figure 1. Features of depressed fractures in three cities. (From Braakman and Jennett[2])

Cause of Injury (Table 1)

In Western industrialized countries about half the cases are due to road accidents. In adults almost a third of depressed fractures occur at work and are often due to falling objects; protective helmets would prevent most of these. Assault with a variety of weapons accounted for 15 percent of adult fractures in Europe, where firearms are not as readily available as in North America. Hammers, axes, chisels, screwdrivers, and golf clubs figure frequently; both victim and assailant are frequently under the influence of alcohol (p. 10). When injury has been caused by assault there is often a reluctance to seek medical aid, because this entails

Table 1. Causes of depressed fractures[12]

	<16 years (444)		≥16 years (495)	
Road accident	221	50%	219	44%
Work	6	1%	142	29%
Assault	18	4%	76	15%
Home	144	35%	40	8%
Sport	55	12%	18	4%

194

giving details about what happened and may attract unwanted attention; this accounts for some instances of delayed diagnosis and consequent infection.

About half the patients are under 16 years of age, and for them falls in and around the house, or during formal sports or unorganized play, largely replace assault and work as the reasons for injury, in those injuries not caused by road accidents. Younger children are prone to puncture wounds from sharp toys, knitting needles, or sticks, which are either fallen against or brandished about during informal and innocent play.

Degree of Brain Damage

Depressed fracture caused by nonmissile injury is usually associated with only focal brain damage, and many patients therefore never lose consciousness, or do so only briefly. In our series half of the patients were reported by witnesses never to have lost consciousness at all, and only 25 percent had more than 24 hours of PTA. Focal neurological signs (of cerebral hemisphere dysfunction) occurred in only 20 percent of cases, because the fracture is often remote from eloquent areas of the brain; in half of these the signs had resolved 6 months later. Half the compound fractures had dural tearing, and this was associated with a higher incidence of prolonged PTA and of focal signs (Table 2). Dural tearing was quite often found also when closed fractures were operated on, but as only the most markedly depressed closed fractures are usually submitted to surgery (p. 200), it is not possible to estimate the true frequency of dural tearing with this type of injury. That signs of focal brain damage are only marginally less common in closed than in compound fractures also suggests that brain damage may be considerable under a closed depressed fracture. Children less often show signs of brain damage, and this is not wholly accounted for by the somewhat lower incidence of compound fractures and of dural tearing in the younger age groups.

Diagnosis

As well known and common as this injury is, the diagnosis is not infrequently overlooked initially. Scalp lacerations are common in accident/emergency departments, forming a feature of 40 percent of all head injury attendances in the

Table 2. Interaction of features of compound depressed fractures[12]

Frequency of Focal Signs	Focal Signs		P
Dura intact	3/40	8%	<0.01
Dura torn	33/97	34%	
PTA<24 hours	12/76	16%	<0.01
PTA>24 hours	27/72	33%	
Frequency of PTA>24 hours	PTA>24 hours		
Dura intact	64/411	16%	<0.001
Dura torn	145/414	35%	
No focal signs	94/538	17%	<0.001
Focal signs	72/148	49%	

Scottish study;[27] it may therefore seem unrealistic to regard every one of them as a potential depressed fracture. Only occasionally is it obvious on clinical inspection that there is a depressed fracture, because bone fragments, or brain, or CSF can be seen in the wound. Even careful examination of the wound may fail to reveal the true state of affairs: because of the mobility of the scalp, the laceration may not lie directly over the fracture; and even if a fracture line is seen, the contour of the outer table is often well preserved, even when there is marked depression of the inner table of the skull.

X-rays are therefore usually needed to diagnose a depressed fracture. A single film may indicate depression, particularly if a fragment of "double density" bone is seen (Fig. 2). However, depression may be obvious only when two films are taken at right angles (Fig. 3); sometimes only a tangential view is diagnostic.

Early Complications

Unless there are complications most patients recover rapidly and completely. Some 10 percent of the Glasgow series[21] were complicated from the beginning by involvement of one of the venous sinuses with the fracture: this makes elevation hazardous, because of the risk of serious bleeding. Infection developed owing to inadequate initial management of 10 percent of cases, and the details of this are discussed below. In 6 percent an intracranial hematoma was found, usually in cases with dural tearing; in more than half the hematoma was intracerebral, with or without subdural clot. These complications were associated with an increased

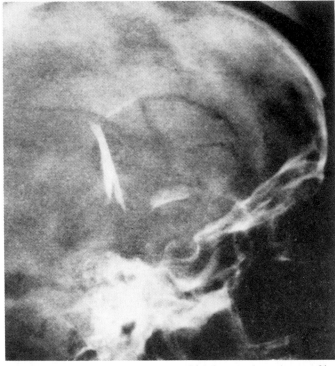

Figure 2. "Double density" of depressed fragment, which is seen through part of intact vault. (From Jennett[13])

196

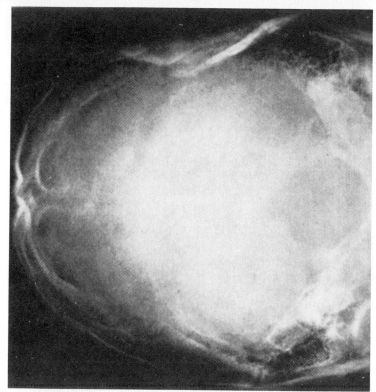

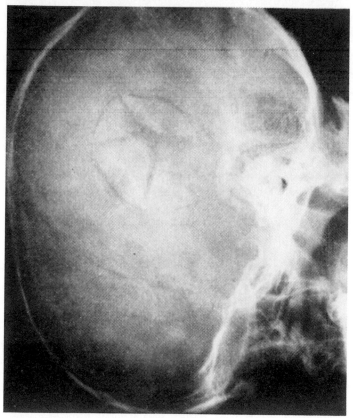

Figure 3. Depression may be obvious only on one of two films taken at right angles to each other. (From Jennett[13])

197

Table 3. Consequences of complications[21]

	n	Death (%)	Lasting Neurological Signs (>6 months) (%)
Venous sinus involvement	46	4	20
Infection	38	11	24
IC hematoma	28	11	25
Uncomplicated	296	1	11

mortality, and with more frequent occurrence of neurological signs persisting for more than 6 months (Table 3). Early epilepsy complicated 10 percent of 947 cases (Table 4). It was no more common after compound than after closed fractures; nor did dural tearing or focal signs increase the risk in compound fractures.

Infection

This is more common in civilian life than might be expected; rates of 6, 8, 10, and 12 percent have been reported from three European[1,21] and one Australian city.[10] This compares poorly with the incidence of 1 percent finally achieved by United States military surgeons in Korea and Vietnam dealing with combat wounds.[6,7] The rate was much higher (41%) earlier in the Korean war before the policy was established of rapid evacuation to base neurosurgical units where formal debridement could be carried out.[19] Inadequate debridement was the commonest reason in one civilian series[14] for patients reaching the neurosurgeon with infection already established; the usual explanation was that a depressed fracture had not been suspected, so that the case was treated as a simple scalp laceration. This happened more often when the patient had never been unconscious, presumably because in these circumstances both the patient and his doctors regarded the injury as having been only trivial (Table 5). Indeed some of these patients had not consulted a doctor at all immediately after injury; others had attended an accident/emergency department but had been sent home after suture of the scalp laceration, usually without an x-ray of the skull.[14]

When infection occurred after adequate surgery, as occasionally happened, this was always confined to the wound. By contrast, two thirds of those infected before proper wound toilet had been carried out developed meningitis or brain abscess, or both.

Table 4. Early epilepsy after depressed fracture

	n	%
White et al.[28]	6/54	11
Stowsand and Geile[26]	15/122	12
Hendrick and Harris[9]	30/300	10
Cabral and Abeysuriya[4]	30/310	10–12
Jamieson and Yelland[10]	16/322	5
Jennett[12]	96/947	10

Table 5. Initial unconsciousness and diagnosis of depressed fracture[14]

	n	Never Unconscious (%)	P
Missed diagnosis	36	67	<0.01
Correct diagnosis	323	41	
Infection	24	71	<0.01
No infection	335	42	

Treatment

While skin closure should be carried out as soon as is practical, this should be deferred until definitive debridement is possible, preferably by a neurosurgeon. As long as the surrounding skin is shaved, cleaned, and covered there need be no rush to surgery, providing this can be done within the first 24 hours. If there is shock, or certain kinds of associated injuries (p. 246), these must take precedence over the skull fracture. If a bone fragment is thought to be lodged in a major venous sinus, then it may be inadvisable to elevate the fracture at all, particularly if the overlying wound is fairly clean; in that event local debridement of the wound may be accepted. Should it be deemed necessary to elevate such a fracture, usually because there is extensive contamination with dirt or because a large bone fragment is markedly depressed, then adequate blood must be available for transfusion before embarking on surgery.

General anesthesia is usually used, but it may be possible to do the necessary surgery under local anesthesia if associated injuries (e.g., maxillofacial or chest injuries) make it advisable to avoid inhalational agents. Having thoroughly cleaned the soft tissues of the wound, the depressed fragments must be tackled. Sometimes a piece is loose and can be lifted out, which gives access to any others there may be. More often the outer table is impacted or overriding, and a burr hole must be put in beside the depressed fragment, then bone nibbled away until the fragment can be lifted out. A dural tear must be carefully sought, but if none is found and the dura is not blue and bulging (suggesting a subdural hematoma), it should not be opened. If it is already open, then badly lacerated brain and any in-driven material should be sucked away. Small dural tears can be sutured and defects made good with patches of pericranium. In the potentially infected, recent wound it is probably unwise to use any form of artificial dura.

Views differ about the advisability of replacing larger bone fragments as a mosaic or loose jig-saw. Surgeons with military experience find it difficult to relax the rule that every bit of bone must be removed, as was recommended in Korea[19] and in Vietnam.[7] But there is now good evidence that the replacement of bone fragments in civilian injuries is not associated with an increased risk of infection, provided that the fragments are not grossly contaminated and that debridement has not been delayed for more than 24 to 36 hours (Table 6). The fragments can be washed in saline or antiseptic before replacement, but are better not wired unless

Table 6. Infection after surgery for depressed fracture

	Glasgow[14]		Rotterdam[1]		Ann Arbor[15]		New Orleans[23]	
Bone removed	6/135	4.4%	6/56	10.7%	—	—	—	—
Bone replaced	6/166	3.6%	5/109	4.6%	2/79	2.5%	7/110	6.4%

they are very unstable, because the foreign body may encourage infection. The alternative is to close the bone defect by acrylic cranioplasty, but this itself is associated with a significant incidence of delayed infection; once this occurs, it usually requires sacrifice of the plate before it can be controlled. For this reason it is seldom wise to carry out primary cranioplasty (at the time of initial debridement), even though cranioplasty will entail readmission to hospital and a second operation. Since the practice of primary replacement of bone fragments was adopted we have reduced the need for cranioplasty to less than a third of the former rate.

Antibiotics

In the early part of the Korean campaign debridement was deliberately delayed, but full doses of antibiotics were given; the infection rate was 41 percent. However, Jennett and Miller[14] found that in civilian patients whose debridement had been delayed, the infection rate was even higher (68%) in those who had not been admitted to hospital than in those who had (32%); the latter can be assumed to have had antibiotics. If debridement has to be delayed, or can only be partially completed (e.g., because of venous sinus involvement), then antibiotics should be given, both topically and systemically. Penicillin (or erythromycin if the patient is sensitive to penicillin) is probably the most suitable, and there is certainly no case for wide-spectrum agents. If adequate and early debridement has been carried out and local antibiotic spray used, it is doubtful whether systemic antibiotics are either required or justified. Antitetanus toxin should be given.

Elevation of Closed Depressed Fracture

Relieved of the need to operate to prevent infection, the surgeon can find it difficult to decide which closed fractures should be elevated. Cosmetic considerations may justify operation, particularly in pond (ping-pong) frontal fractures in young children. The thin, cardboard-like bone that sustains such deformity can usually be equally easily remodelled by the surgeon to near its original contour.

It used to be believed that a depressed fragment might lead to epilepsy, from continued pressure on the brain or by the formation of a cicatrix. However, there is evidence to show that the risk is no greater in unelevated closed fractures than in those operated on (Table 7). The low rate for unelevated compound fractures may be because these included many with relatively mild depression or with fragments in the venous sinuses (the reasons why they were not elevated).

When a depressed fragment is associated with limb weakness or other signs appropriate to the fracture site, then surgeons often recommend elevation, although this seldom leads to rapid return of neurological function. Both in this instance and in the case of traumatic epilepsy, the presumption is that the brain damage sustained at the moment of maximum skull distortion is what determines

Table 7. Late epilepsy after depressed fracture[12]

	Closed		Compound	
Not elevated	3/34	9%	5/87	6%
Elevated	3/47	6%	89/524	17%

the sequelae rather than the continued presence or pressure of a bone fragment on the brain.

Late Epilepsy

The risk of this complication is 15 percent for depressed fracture as a whole, but the rate ranges from 3 percent to over 70 percent according to various features of the injury. About 40 percent of patients with depressed fracture are only marginally more likely to develop epilepsy than are those with other injuries, and these patients can be identified by the methods described in Chapter 11.

BASAL DURAL TEARS

A CSF leak clearly indicates that there has been dural tearing, but it is not the only evidence that can point to this important diagnosis. Nor are all dural fistulae associated with leakage of CSF; and cessation of rhinorrhea does not necessarily indicate healing of the dura. Meningitis is not uncommon in patients who have had no known escape of CSF, as well as in those in whom it has been quite transitory. The surgeon's concern should therefore be with the diagnosis and management of *a basal dural tear,* rather than the treatment of a CSF leak. Four kinds of evidence can point to this pathological condition: (1) CSF leak from nose or ear, (2) aerocele, (3) meningitis, and (4) appropriately placed fractures. The first three provide proof of a dural fistula, while a fracture can indicate only a high probability of dural tearing; this can occur, however, without radiological evidence of fracture.

Anatomy

The interface between air sinuses and the basal dura varies considerably from one individual to another (Fig. 4). It is less extensive in children, in whom the sinuses are smaller. Caldicott and associates[5] have shown that, although the proportional distribution of the various pneumatized cavities varies with age, there is a significant risk of CSF fistulae even in young children (Fig. 5). While the *frontal sinuses* do not develop a relationship to the anterior fossa until 4 years of age or more, the *cribriform plate* is ossified (and therefore brittle) by 2 years of age; by the third year the *ethmoidal sinuses* are relatively as large as in adults. The *sphenoidal sinus* is the last to develop and is not sizable until the age of 10. The middle ear cleft is large at birth and the tegmen tympani already rigid but thin. The *mastoid air cells* are very small at birth, but by 5 years are extensive and are related to the dura in the posterior fossa, medial and lateral to the internal auditory meatus.

CSF Rhinorrhea

This occurs in about a quarter of patients with an anterior basal fracture; sometimes the fistula is through the tegmen tympani into the cavity of the middle ear, and CSF reaches the nose via the eustachian tube. In 60 percent the rhinorrhea begins in the first few days after injury, and in more than half of these the leak lasts for only 2 or 3 days. Rhinorrhea beginning later may be due to resolution of hematoma and of brain swelling close to the fracture site; sometimes it follows

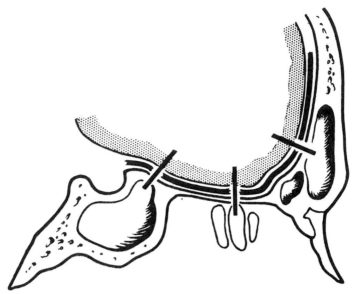

Figure 4. Relationship of air sinuses to base of skull, with common sites for dural tearing. (From Jennett[13])

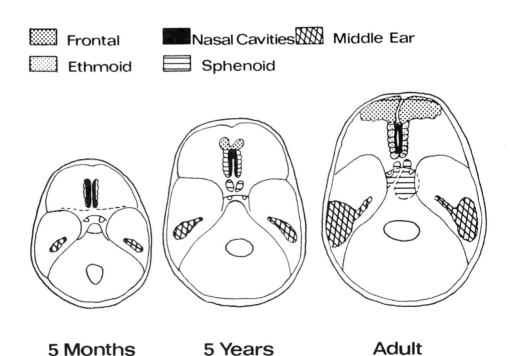

Figure 5. Development of air sinuses and middle ear cavity, in relation to base of skull. (From Caldicott, North, and Simpson[5])

202

reduction of nasal or facial fractures; occasionally it appears for the first time only weeks or months after injury.

The diagnosis may not be obvious because in the supine patient the fluid may mostly be swallowed. An alert patient may report a salty taste, or the observant nurse may notice a wet patch on the pillow; but a free flow of fluid may happen only when the head is dependent or on one side (such as may occur during positioning in the radiology department for skull x-rays).

If enough fluid can be collected to analyze, then the demonstration of reducing sugar will confirm that it is CSF—but with such a profuse leak the diagnosis is seldom in doubt. Dextrostix in the nose is unreliable, as normal nasal secretions may give a positive reaction. Allergic rhinorrhea can be difficult to distinguish, but there is much less sugar and there may be eosinophils in the deposit. Dyes (phenolphthalein or indigo-carmine) or isotopes (^{99m}Tc or ^{24}Na) injected by lumbar puncture or into the ventricle may be detected in the nasal cavity and so confirm the diagnosis. Isotopes are particularly useful in localizing the *site* of the leak; patties or pledglets are placed in the various recesses of the nasal cavity and the differential radioactive counts may indicate where the CSF is likely to be coming from. This is much more accurate than scintiphoto or scintiscan pictures taken after isotope injection.

CSF Otorrhea

This occurred in only 7 percent of 300 basal skull fractures in one report.[25] Although the leak is often profuse, it almost always dries up in 5 to 10 days.

Aerocele

This occurs in almost a third of patients with rhinorrhea,[25] but how often it is seen depends on how carefully it is looked for. In more than a third of one series, air appeared more than 48 hours after injury, a previous x-ray having shown no air;[24] only half of the 41 cases in that series had rhinorrhea. Air is usually in the subdural or subarachnoid spaces (or both), often in the frontal region or in the basal cisterns; one in five has air in the ventricles and a similar proportion air in the brain substance. The best method of showing air is also the easiest, a brow-up lateral view with the x-ray beam horizontal (p. 103). Even restless or uncooperative patients will usually lie still long enough in this natural position for a diagnostic film to be made. A fluid level can then usually be detected, and fluid may also be shown in one of the sinuses (Fig. 6).

Evidence of Fractured Base

X-rays of the skull base are neither easy to obtain nor to interpret in the early stages after head injury. Stereoscopic views and tomograms are unwise because they are unlikely to be successful at this stage. However, routine skull and sinus views, including the brow-up lateral, may show obvious fractures, opaque sinuses, and perhaps intracranial air or a fluid level in one of the sinuses. Even if a fracture is not seen, the appearance of periorbital hematoma, particularly if bilateral, or of bruising behind the pinna over the mastoid process should be taken as evidence of a fractured base until this can be excluded (p. 100). About a quarter of patients

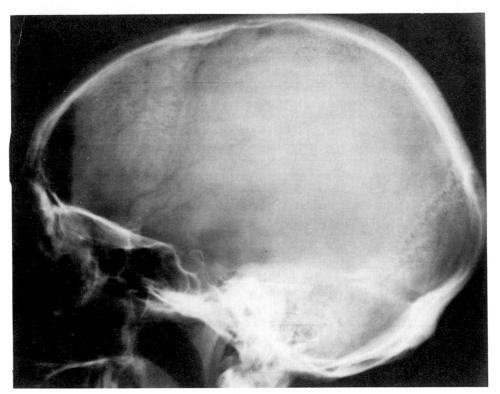

Figure 6. Aerocele shown on brow-up lateral film.

with fracture of the skull also have fractures of the facial bones. Only later, when operative procedures are under consideration, is it appropriate to undertake special investigations to define accurately the fracture line likely to be associated with a dural tear; the latter may be suspected if there is a broad fracture line or if a flake of bone is angled up towards the dura. In about 25 percent of cases of CSF leak or of meningitis, no fracture is recognized radiologically; in some of these a fine crack is found at operation, but in others the assumption is that avulsion of filaments of the olfactory bulb from the cribriform plate has been enough to form a fistula.

Meningitis

The risk of meningitis cannot be assessed because many cases of dural tearing, even with CSF leakage, go undetected. It may not be as high as the estimate of 25 percent that has been made by several neurosurgeons,[17,22] because neurosurgical units attract the more severe fractures and patients with aerocele or those who have had meningitis. On the other hand, those who claim that meningitis seldom occurs in spite of a conservative attitude to basal fractures have not published evidence of systematic follow-up of large numbers of such cases. Meningitis may first develop long after injury, and as the injury may have been relatively mild, no connection may be suspected. Not only does the original surgeon remain unaware of the meningitis, but the physician treating this complication often knows nothing of the head injury. Even early meningitis may go undiagnosed, and a recent review of autopsies in a neurosurgical unit revealed several patients with meningitis that had been unsuspected during life. Another factor influencing the meningitis rate is whether appropriate antibiotics in adequate dosage have been given for a long enough period. This may account for discrepancies between reports in the 1950s and those based on more recently selected cases. Several of the latter put the risk, when there has been a CSF leak, at 10 percent or less.[3,16,18] In the large series of aeroceles reported by North, 15 percent developed meningitis; but the fistula was probably repaired in many of these cases before infection could occur.

Indeed, this is a problem in assessing reports of the incidence of meningitis, in that it is likely that a number of patients with profuse rhinorrhea or broad fractures (as well as those with aeroceles) are repaired relatively soon after injury. The data on the efficacy of prophylactic antibiotics are even more confused. Certainly meningitis can develop in spite of antibiotics, but many factors that influence the situation cannot be allowed for: unusual organisms, the density or character of the flora in that particular patient's nasal cavity, and the concentration of antibiotics achieved in CSF in the face of a profuse leak, among others. The commonest organism is pneumococcus, which is found in more than half the cases; others are listed in Table 8. When the middle ear is involved, gram-negative organisms, sometimes more than one, are often found.

Recurrent meningitis is a feature of some cases, and neurosurgeons have reported several series of such patients. Three or four attacks are not unusual. There may be long intervals (years) between one attack and the next, and there is usually no continuing CSF leak during this period (if there was, then surgical repair would probably have been advised). Different organisms may sometimes be found in successive episodes of meningitis in the same patient, but the pneumococcus is by far the most commonly incriminated in cases of recurrent meningitis.

Table 8. Organisms reported in 147 cases of traumatic meningitis*

Pneumococcus	61%
Hemophilus inf.	12%
Streptococcus	9%
Meningococcus	8%
Stephylococcus	6%
Other	4%

*Cases are from larger series in literature.

Management of Basal Dural Fistulae

This is one of the controversial areas in head injury care. It is perhaps the only commonly occurring condition in which North American neurosurgeons tend to be more conservative about recommending operative intervention than their British colleagues. The aim of management is to reduce the risk of meningitis. How difficult it is to assess this risk has already been explained; it follows that the need for, and the success of, surgical repair is equally difficult to evaluate.[11,16]

Meningitis

Preventive measures against this complication should be taken as soon as a basal tear is even suspected. That means not only in patients with an obvious CSF leak from nose or ear, or with a definite radiological fracture, but also in those who have bilateral orbital hematoma, a middle-third fracture of the face, or a retromastoid bruising. Treatment with antibiotics should be for at least a week if no leak or aerocele is detected; when there is a leak, the drug should be continued for a week after it has ceased.

As the pneumococcus is the commonest organism, penicillin is the most rational choice. Many surgeons also give sulfonamides, which penetrate the inflamed blood-brain barrier; but bacteriologists argue against using a bacteriostatic and a bacteriocidal combination and may recommend chloramphenicol. In children the threat of hemophilus may justify ampicillin, but in general wide-spectrum antibiotics are to be avoided, because of the risk of breeding resistant pathogens. It is wise to take nasal (and aural if indicated) swabs in order to find out an individual patient's flora—in the event of meningitis developing this may enable appropriate change of medication without waiting for new cultures.

A review of the published meningitis rates with and without prophylactic antibiotics is difficult to interpret, because the selection of patients was probably different in separate series. However, two large series of cases collected in single units have shown a lower rate of meningitis with adequate prophylactic treatment (Tables 9 and 10). In cases of recurrent meningitis there are instances of a further attack developing within a day or so of discontinuing long-term prophylactic antibiotics. Factors other than antibiotics that may influence the incidence of meningitis have already been referred to.

Table 9. Effect of prophylactic antibiotics on the incidence of meningitis

MacGee et al.[18]	Rhinorrhea		Otorrhea		Total	
Antibiotics	1/17	6%	0/24	0	1/41	4%
No antibiotics	1/6	17%	1/11	9%	2/17	12%
P		NS		NS		NS
Literature (MacGee)						
Antibiotics	40/196	20%	5/88	6%	45/284	16%
No antibiotics	1/27	4%	1/33	3%	2/60	3%
P		<0.05		NS		<0.02

Dural Tear

WHICH PATIENTS NEED REPAIR? When a CSF leak persists for more than a week, or there is an aerocele, or there has been an attack of meningitis, it is generally agreed that surgical repair of the tear is needed to provide permanent protection against meningitis. That cessation of rhinorrhea cannot be equated with dural healing is obvious from the occurrence of late and even recurrent meningitis, long after the leak has stopped, or sometimes in patients who have never reported a fistula at all. Operative findings indicate that a small hernia of brain can plug the hole in the dura; this stops the leak but it also prevents dural healing, and does not appear itself to act as an effective barrier against organisms.

206

Table 10. Meningitis in first week (no repair) (Glasgow[16])

	Rhinorrhea		Otorrhea		Total
Adequate chemotherapy	0/76	0	1/19	5%	1/95
Inadequate chemotherapy	7/42	17%	5/12	42%	12/54
P	<0.001		<0.05		<0.001

In the absence of absolute indications (meningitis, aerocele, or continuing leak) the selection of patients for dural repair must depend on balancing the probable risks—of meningitis on the one hand and of bifrontal exploration on the other. A broad fracture line, an angulated spicule of bone, or rhinorrhea persisting for more than a week is each a relative indication of this kind. Their corollaries are not valid, because infection can occur without a radiologically identified fracture and without any reported rhinorrhea. If there is a fracture of the middle third of the face, this should be reduced sooner rather than later, because rhinorrhea often stops after reduction and does not recur. Some surgeons recommend spinal drainage of CSF, in the belief that the tear will then have a better chance of healing because the flow of fluid through it is stemmed. An opposing view is that contaminated air may more readily enter the head from the nose, through the fistula, if the intracranial pressure is unduly low.

WHEN TO REPAIR? Only when a fractured base is associated with a compound vault fracture that has to be repaired immediately will the question arise of a dural repair soon after injury. Even then it is probably wiser to postpone it and to limit the initial surgery to the vault fracture. In all other cases, even when there is continuing rhinorrhea, operation is best deferred for 2 to 3 weeks, especially if the patient is in coma or confused. Exploration too soon after bifrontal contusions can result in aggravation of the local brain damage, with postoperative edema and swelling, and marked deterioration of the patient's condition.

HOW TO SEAL THE TEAR. First the tear must be found. If a single fracture is seen that is compatible with the likely source of the leak, then the site may be obvious. Often the matter is in doubt but associated features may help; anosmia suggests involvement of the cribriform plate or the ethmoidal sinuses; profuse rhinorrhea or involvement of the optic nerve or of external ocular movements suggests a tear into the sphenoidal sinus. Dural tears are often bilateral, and it is seldom possible to be sufficiently certain before surgery to recommend only unilateral exploration. The possibility of a eustachian nasal leak from a petrous fracture must be remembered.

Intradural exploration is the most reliable way to identify small tears, which may be recognized by the small funnel or hernia of brain going down into the defect; small tears may be felt rather than seen as a probe is gently run over the suspected area and reveals a roughness in comparison to the gliding smoothness of intact dura. When no defect can be found, some surgeons recommend air insufflation up the nose and watching for the bubbles—like spotting the puncture in a bicycle tire.

The patient's own fascia is the best repair. Enough can often be cut from the periosteum of the frontal bone flap, but if a larger piece is needed, then fascia lata from the thigh can be used. Sutures are probably not necessary, but a generous overlap should be allowed (0.05 cm). Dural substitutes and tissue glues have also been used recently.[23]

OTHER OPEN INJURIES

Puncture Wounds

The most deceptive open injuries are those due to assaults with sharp instruments, such as scissors or screwdrivers, or to falls (often in children) against sticks or sharp toys. If the puncturing agent has already been removed, it may be difficult to believe that penetration of the skull has occurred. This is particularly so if the wound of entry is in the eyelid or sclera, beyond which the orbital roof needs little force to fracture it. The only safe course, if there is any doubt, is to explore and debride as an open injury.

Scalp Wounds

In the Scottish study 40 percent of attenders at accident departments had a scalp laceration, many of them without underlying fracture or any initial impairment of consciousness. There seems little doubt that these patients would not have come to hospital but for blood from their scalp. There are more than the average proportion of assaults and of injuries connected with alcohol, and this compounds the problem. Although most of these injuries are relatively clean, and owing to the vascular nature of the scalp will heal satisfactorily even if sewn up casually (as all too often they are), there are among patients with scalp lacerations a few with underlying depressed fractures. If these are overlooked there is a real danger of intracranial infection.

It is therefore wise to have clear rules for dealing with scalp lacerations, which must include shaving of the hair all round. All should be adequately inspected and debrided, with proper light and after infiltration of local anesthetic. Whether an x-ray is required, and whether it is done before or after scalp closure, must depend to some extent on local circumstances. If in doubt, always x-ray; and if possible, do so before scalp closure.

Missile Injuries

Missile or gunshot wounds vary from high velocity rifle bullets to the lead slug or pellet of an air-gun.[6,7,19] The damage done depends on the velocity and the mass of the missile when it strikes the head, so that the factor of range also counts. The term "high velocity" is usually reserved for bullets that exceed the speed of sound, 1050 ft/sec; modern rifles have a muzzle velocity greater than 2500 ft/sec. Passage through the brain induces instability in the flight of a rifle bullet and this accentuates the brain damage that it causes; this also explains why the bone at exit often fractures widely, and why there is more extensive scalp damage than at the site of entry. A low velocity bullet, on the other hand, may traverse the brain, leaving an exit wound little bigger than the missile itself. Missiles may cause tangential, guttering wounds; they may penetrate and remain within the intracranial cavity; or they may traverse the skull. In penetrating injuries, bone fragments may be found at a distance from the retained missile.

Consciousness may be retained, even after penetrating injuries that traverse the brain completely, but rapid deterioration—from edema rather than hematoma—is not uncommon. The principles of maintaining a clear airway and of avoiding hypotension, hypoxia, and hypercarbia are even more important after missile injury because any of these adverse factors may trigger off edema and engorgement. The wound track in the brain should be explored and cleaned as soon as possible, removing all bone fragments; the missile itself is less likely to cause delayed infection and need not be followed into dangerous areas of the brain. The dura and scalp should be closed. X-rays the following day are needed to confirm that there are no retained bone fragments.

The prognosis after missile injuries is usually more obvious than after blunt injuries. Those in deep coma on arrival seldom if ever survive; and only one in five of those in coma but still reacting to pain survive. Those who remain conscious should recover well, although they may have focal neurological signs from local brain damage. The late epilepsy rate after missile injuries is high, about 45 percent developing fits within 5 years of wounding (p. 284).

REFERENCES

1. BRAAKMAN, R.: *Depressed skull fracture: data, treatment, and follow-up in 225 consecutive cases.* J. Neurol. Neurosurg. Psychiatry 35:396–402, 1972.

2. BRAAKMAN, R., AND JENNETT, B.: "Depressed skull fracture (non-missile)." In Vinken, P. J., and Bruyn, G. W. (eds.): *Handbook of Clinical Neurology.* vol. 23. North Holland Publishing Co., 1975, pp. 403–415.

3. BRAWLEY, B. W., AND KELLY, W. A.: *Treatment of basal skull fractures with and without cerebrospinal fluid fistulae.* J. Neurosurg. 26:57–61, 1967.

4. CABRAL, S. A., AND ABEYSURIYA, S. C.: *The management of compound depressed fractures of the skull.* Ceylon Med. J. 14:105–115, 1969.

5. CALDICOTT, W. J. H., NORTH, J. B., AND SIMPSON, D. A.: *Traumatic cerebrospinal fluid fistulas in children.* J. Neurosurg. 38:1–9, 1973.

6. HAGAN, R. E.: *Early complications following penetrating wounds of the brain.* J. Neurosurg. 34:132–141, 1971.

7. HAMMON, W. M.: *Analysis of 2187 consecutive penetrating wounds of the brain from Vietnam.* J. Neurosurg. 34:127–131, 1971.

8. HEISKANEN, O., MARTTILA, I., AND VALTONEN, S.: *Prognosis of depressed skull fracture.* Acta Chir. Scand. 139:605–608, 1973.

9. HENDRICK, E. B., AND HARRIS, L.: *Post-traumatic epilepsy in children.* J. Trauma 8:547, 1968.

10. JAMIESON, K. G., AND YELLAND, J. D. N.: *Depressed skull fractures in Australia.* J. Neurosurg. 37:150, 1972.

11. JEFFERSON, A., AND REILLY, G.: *Fractures of the floor of the anterior antral fossa. The selection of patients for dural repair.* Br. J. Surg. 59:585–592, 1972.

12. JENNETT, B.: *Epilepsy after Non-Missile Head Injuries.* ed. 2. Heinemann, London, 1975.

13. JENNETT, B.: *An Introduction to Neurosurgery.* ed. 3. Heinemann, London, 1977.

14. JENNETT, B., AND MILLER, J. D.: *Infection after depressed fracture of skull. Implications for management of nonmissile injuries.* J. Neurosurg. 36:333–339, 1972.

15. KRISS, F. C., TAREN, J. A., AND KAHN, E. A.: *Primary repairs of compound skull fractures by replacement of bone fragments.* J. Neurosurg. 30:698–702, 1969.

16. LEECH, P.: *Cerebrospinal fluid leakage, dural fistulae and meningitis after basal skull fracture.* Injury 6:141–149, 1974.

17. LEWIN, W.: *Cerebrospinal fluid rhinorrhoea in closed head injuries.* Br. J. Surg. 42:1, 1954.

18. MacGEE, E. E., CAUTHEN, J. C., AND BRACKETT, C. E.: *Meningitis following acute traumatic cerebrospinal fistula.* J. Neurosurg. 33:312–316, 1970.

19. MEIROWSKY, A. M.: "Compound fractures of the convexity of the skull." In Coates, J. B., and Meirowsky, A. M. (eds.): *Neurological Surgery of Trauma.* U.S. Government Printing Office, Washington, D.C., 1965, pp. 83–101.

20. MILLER, J. D.: "Infection after head injury." In Vinken, P. J., and Bruyn, G. W. (eds.): *Handbook of Clinical Neurology.* vol. 24. North Holland Publishing Co., Amsterdam, 1976, pp. 215–230.

21. MILLER, J. D., AND JENNETT, W. B.: *Complications of depressed skull fracture*. Lancet ii:991–995, 1968.
22. MORLEY, T. P., AND HEATHERINGTON, R. F.: *Traumatic cerebrospinal fluid rhinorrhoea and otorrhoea, pneumocephalus and meningitis*. Surg. Gynecol. Obstet. 104:88–98, 1957.
23. NADELL, J., AND KLINE, D. G.: *Primary reconstruction of depressed frontal skull fractures including those involving the sinus, orbit and cribriform plate*. J. Neurosurg. 41:200–207, 1974.
24. NORTH, J. B.: *On the importance of intracranial air*. Br. J. Surg. 58:826, 1971.
25. ROBINSON, R. G.: *Cerebrospinal fluid rhinorrhoea, meningitis and pneumocephalus due to non-missile injuries*. Aust. N.Z. J. Surg. 39:328–334, 1970.
26. STOWSAND, D., AND GEILE, G.: *Cerebrale symptome bei impressions frakturen der schadelkonvexitat*. Deutsche Zeitschrift fur Nervenheilkund 189:330–344, 1966.
27. STRANG, I., MACMILLAN, R., AND JENNETT, B.: *Head injuries in accident and emergency departments at Scottish hospitals*. Injury 10:154–159, 1978.
28. WHITE, J. C., LIU, C. T., AND MIXTER, W. J.: *Focal epilepsy. II. Epilepsy secondary to cerebral trauma and infection*. N. Engl. J. Med. 239:1, 1948.

CHAPTER 9

Management of Head Injuries in the Acute Stage

All head injuries require an initial assessment and a diagnosis reached about the kind of injury sustained—diffuse or focal, mild or severe, closed or open, with or without extracranial injuries or complications. All patients have then to be monitored for evidence of developing complications that may call for treatment; a minority will need an operation, either because there are open injuries (p. 199) or because there is an intracranial hematoma (p. 174). None of these statements is controversial, and it is only the details of techniques that vary from clinic to clinic or from country to country.

In the management of milder injuries (those in which the patient is already talking) opinions may differ about how closely and for how long they need be observed—and whether or not this requires admission to hospital. But in the case of the patient in coma after head injury there is wide variation between the practice of different doctors and hospitals. All agree on the need to avoid secondary brain damage, but not on what regimen is appropriate to achieve this in various circumstances. One difficulty in dealing with management is that the state of patients in the first few hours after head injury can change rapidly; a patient's responsiveness may improve so that the initial impression of severity has to be revised, or a patient whose initial state gives no cause for alarm may deteriorate into coma. It is therefore unwise to adopt too rigid a routine for the management of severe head injury; there is no substitute for intelligent assessment of each individual's problems and for having a system that can respond to his changing needs.

MANAGEMENT BEFORE HOSPITAL

The head injured patient who is in coma has two major needs before admission to hospital: the maintenance of an effective airway and the institution of monitoring of responsiveness. Ambulance personnel should therefore be trained in maintaining an oropharyngeal airway, in the administration of oxygen, and in the assessment of consciousness. However, when a head injury is accompanied by multiple injuries, the situation is more complex and may call for more sophisticated skills and facilities. MacKay estimated that 43 percent of fatally injured riders or vehicle occupants might have had a greater chance of survival if medical treatment had been available at the scene within 10 minutes of the accident.[59] It has been suggested that 15 percent or more of road traffic accident victims die at the scene from factors that were potentially reversible by trained personnel.[22] In patients who reach hospital in coma it is common to find severe systemic dysfunction that can threaten the brain, such as hypoxia, hypotension, or anemia.[41,66] These are particularly frequent after multiple injury.

The response to these needs varies widely. In some places it has been possible to organize what amount to mobile intensive care units, staffed by highly trained personnel, sometimes including doctors. In other, often rural situations, a primary care physician is the first responder. In yet other places there have been efforts made to translate to civilian circumstances the undoubted benefits of helicopter transport from the battlefield. The debate about the effectiveness of various systems and their economic feasibility is unresolved. The system in the United Kingdom depends upon an efficient emergency communication system linking the public with emergency serivces by "999" telephone call system, the provision of regionalized ambulances and designated hospitals with accident services, and the training of ambulance personnel in the initial care of the injured patient. Surveys of patients evacuated by this system suggest that few of those with head injury who die before arrival at hospital could have been saved, no matter how much had been done.[36] Most have an overwhelming degree of brain damage, such as laceration of the brain stem, or irrecoverable chest injuries.

INITIAL HOSPITAL MANAGEMENT

Immediate resuscitation may have to take precedence over formal assessment—for example, clearing the airway, ensuring adequate ventilation, or correcting profound hypotension. But as soon as possible answers should be sought to four questions:

1. Is it a head injury and only a head injury? Uncertainty about whether a head injury has in fact been sustained can arise in two circumstances: in the patient known to have struck his head but who appears to have fully recovered; and in a patient who has no clear story of injury when brought to hospital unconscious or confused. For the first patient the question is whether delayed intracranial complications are possible, and the answer usually depends upon an x-ray demonstrating a skull fracture or, less usefully, upon a history of post-traumatic amnesia. In the second patient the question is whether his evident brain dysfunction is wholly or partly due to the head injury. Fits, cerebrovascular accidents, or alcoholic collapses may frequently be a source of diagnostic difficulty, and each can also result in a head injury. The evidence of witnesses can be crucial, but if there is doubt, altered consciousness should be regarded as being due to a head injury and appropriate action taken. A third of moderate or severely head injured patients have injuries in other places, and these may be overlooked because the patient does not complain of them.

2. Is there evidence of diffuse or focal brain damage? The extent of altered consciousness reflects the severity of diffuse brain damage (p. 90) and patients should be classified soon after injury according to whether they are then talking, and if so whether they are orientated and have a clear memory of the accident and of everything since. If the patient is not talking, it is likely that he has diffuse brain dysfunction and there is a need to chart the level of responsiveness and determine whether the patient is getting worse or better. Focal neurological signs indicate local damage and it can be important to detect these and separate the effects of focal damage from those of depression of overall responsiveness. Thus, dysphasia is sometimes wrongly interpreted as mental confusion; hemiparesis may be missed if there are associated limb injuries, but on the other hand, immobility caused by a limb fracture or brachial plexus injury may be wrongly interpreted as a sign of focal brain damage. Early detection of cranial nerve palsies, particularly pupillary signs, is important, because if first noticed later they may be interpreted as evidence of progressive cerebral compression.

3. Is the patient improving or deteriorating? Changes in responsiveness provide the most reliable evidence of alterations in the patient's intracranial state. It is vital when the patient is first seen, therefore, to discover whether there has been an alteration in the level of responsiveness since the time of injury. Ambulance personnel, police, or any other witnesses must be actively sought and questioned. Their evidence should be clearly recorded, and indeed many record systems now make specific provision for the observations of ambulance attendants. In the patient who is improving it is obvious that the process of recovery has already begun, while in the deteriorating patient the reason must be urgently sought (p. 170).

4. Is there a skull fracture and is it an open injury? The prevention and early diagnosis of complications depends upon anticipation; knowledge of the existence of a skull fracture and of its location can be invaluable evidence of the potential for intracranial hematoma and infection. Most often the fracture will be diagnosed from a radiograph, but clinical signs may be the only evidence of a basal fracture (p. 100).

PRIMARY CARE OF MILD INJURIES

For the talking (and usually walking) patient, after the initial assessment of conscious level, of CNS signs and examination for other injuries, three measures may be necessary: repair of any scalp wound, skull radiography, and continuing observation.

Scalp Lacerations

A scalp laceration was present in 40 percent of one large series of patients attending hospital soon after injury.[82] The majority of these are relatively minor and effectively managed by simple closure. Occasionally, with extensive lacerations, particularly in the atherosclerotic patients, bleeding may be extensive and may even require transfusion. Wounds with skin loss may require skin grafting or transposition of a flap and are best managed in combination with a plastic surgeon.

That most lacerations are simple does not excuse inadequate management. The first step is inspection; unless the wound is in the forehead, this requires that the hair be cut short around the wound; the surrounding skin should be shaved, unless it seems more likely that this will inflict extra damage. The skin should be cleaned with an antiseptic detergent, then treated with an antiseptic such as 0.5 percent chlorhexadine in 70 percent spirit, and finally allowed to dry; final cleansing of the wound can be completed after it has been infiltrated with local anesthetic. If the wound is extensive and through the full thickness of the scalp, it is justifiable to explore it with a gloved finger, but this cannot be taken as a reliable way of excluding a depressed fracture. Foreign bodies and devitalized tissue (including blood clot) should be removed, but skin edges need be trimmed only when ragged or badly bruised, and then as sparingly as possible. When skin has been lost or excised and tension prevents easy closure, it is helpful to undermine the galea aponeurotica with scissors. An area of skin loss can be converted into a long S-shaped wound in order to achieve skin closure.

If the wound is superficial, and the galea intact, the scalp can be closed by a single layer of sutures or by means of adhesive strips. The latter, however, are not suitable if the galea has been lacerated for any distance; then the ideal is a closure in two layers, the deeper being inverted sutures through the galea. On the other hand, a single full-thickness suture can be used to close a scalp laceration that involves the aponeurosis if the wound is only an inch or two long or is contaminated or severely contused.

Skull X-ray and Continued Observation

Views differ considerably about the need for skull x-rays in a mildly injured patient and also about how continued observation is best arranged. The origins of debate lie in the contrast between the many patients in whom an x-ray or observation might be desirable and the small number of patients who actually show abnormalities or develop complications. The criteria thus come to depend both upon the circumstances of the individual case and upon the overall strategy of management, a topic more fully discussed elsewhere (p. 343).

ESSENTIAL SUPPORT OF THE UNCONSCIOUS PATIENT

Essential Support

The intracranial events that follow head injury are repeatedly emphasized in this book. All patients who are unconscious, no matter how briefly, run the risk of respiratory obstruction. When the head injury is associated with multiple trauma, there are the additional risks of hypoxia, hypotension, and other systemic events that can harm the recently damaged brain. Unconscious patients must be afforded the care proper to this state and attention to the head injury itself initially takes second place to ensuring that the body is well perfused with adequately oxygenated blood. Once this has been achieved it is then safe to explore the precise nature and severity of the head injury and its specific treatment.

Airway

The unconscious patient is at risk even during partial airway obstruction. After head injury this may be due to the tongue falling backwards, but there may also be aspiration of vomitus, secretions, blood, CSF, or foreign bodies, and occasional patients will have injuries to the respiratory passages. The risk begins at the roadside and steps should be taken to anticipate and to prevent it from the time the patient is first seen, during transport in the ambulance, in the admitting accident and emergency department, and in particular within the corridors and elevators of the hospital, in the radiology department when the patient undergoes an investigation, and even in the ward itself. All too often it is when the patient has reached hospital that insufficient attention is paid to the airway,[94] particularly when a patient is being urgently referred from a nonspecialist unit to a neurosurgical center.[78]

214

Establishing a Clear Airway

Initially the mouth or pharynx should be cleared of foreign bodies, vomitus, and dentures by the use of a finger. Suctioning considerably assists the initial steps in obtaining a clear airway, and it may be necessary to repeat it at frequent intervals to remove bronchial secretions or saliva. To maintain a clear airway it may be necessary to employ one or other of a variety of different measures: positioning the patient; maintenance of an oropharyngeal or nasopharyngeal airway; endotracheal intubation; and tracheostomy. Sometimes the appropriate measure is obvious: in a patient in deep coma with atonic jaw muscles immediate endotracheal intubation is appropriate, even if this proves to be necessary only as a temporary measure. In general it is best to employ the most simple measure that is effective, but it is also better to decide what this is as soon as possible, than to persist with a succession of ineffective measures, in the course of which the patient's condition may worsen.

With the patient supine, the oropharyngeal passages can be kept patent temporarily by exerting forward pressure behind the angle of the jaw. This has the advantage of allowing access to the chest and abdomen for initial examination and other procedures.

Maintaining an Airway during Continued Coma

POSITION AND OROPHARYNGEAL AIRWAY. Skilled nursing with the patient in the semiprone position and with intermittent nasopharyngeal suction may be adequate even for several days of coma—particularly in children. An oropharyngeal airway prevents the tongue from falling backwards (Fig. 1), and the stomach can be kept empty by intermittent aspiration through a nasogastric tube.

ENDOTRACHEAL INTUBATION. It is a good rule that if the patient will tolerate a tube he needs one. On the other hand, inexpert attempted intubation, which provokes coughing and which causes a rise in ICP, can only be harmful, so that the decision to intubate must take account of the skill of the inserter and the likely ease of the maneuver.

In the patient tolerating a tube, the question is how long he will need it, because as time passes (day by day), the risks of chest infection and laryngeal damage increase. This latter risk can be minimized by using a small tube (less than 10 mm internal diameter in men and 9 mm in women), with low pressure cuffs, and by ensuring that there is not repeated gagging or coughing, causing abrasion of the tube against the mucosa (Fig. 2).

Views differ as to when, in the event of continued coma, an endotracheal tube needs to be replaced by tracheostomy—which brings its own complications, particularly in children. With proper attention to detailed care, modern endotracheal tubes may be safely tolerated for a week or so in adults and for several weeks in children.

TRACHEOSTOMY. Ten years ago most patients in coma after head injury had a tracheostomy, often performed soon after injury. Nowadays most units do this less often and very seldom on the first day—when an endotracheal tube is almost always adequate (unless there are extensive maxillofacial or neck injuries). Tracheostomy, however, may be considered necessary soon after injury in patients with chest injuries of such severity that prolonged ventilation can be anticipated. Even in the latter it has been suggested that over-enthusiasm for ventilator therapy,

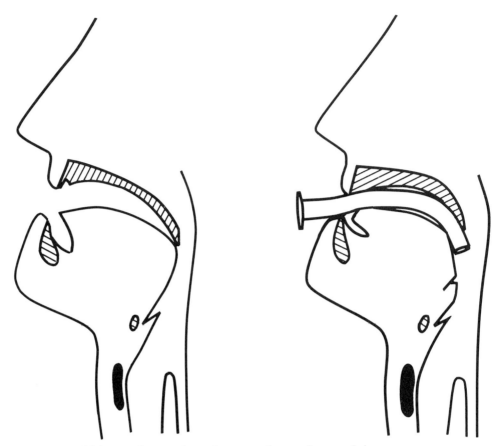

Figure 1. Establishment of patent airway by means of an oropharyngeal airway.

with the high incidence of tracheostomy, may actually increase morbidity and mortality.[90]

Tracheostomy is most often carried out as an elective procedure when endotracheal intubation has to be prolonged beyond what is judged to be a safe period. The operation should be performed under optimal conditions whenever possible (and this may mean in an operating theatre) with good lighting and good equipment; it is easier in a patient who already has an endotracheal tube. The tracheal incision should be low, leaving at least one or two rings of the trachea; if this is not done, the destruction of cartilage around the tube, which is an inevitable occurrence, either as a consequence of pressure or of tube movement, may involve the cricoid and lead to subglottic stenosis. Some advocate stitching a flap of the anterior trachea to the skin edge to facilitate changing of the tube. Tracheostomy has no specific advantages over endotracheal intubation, and its extra hazards include infection, surgical emphysema, and vascular injuries.

SUCTION. Suction is required in the management of many head injured patients, and in all those who require endotracheal intubation or tracheostomy. It should be carried out under sterile conditions. The catheter should have side suction holes; if a tube with only an end opening is used it may damage the mucosa during

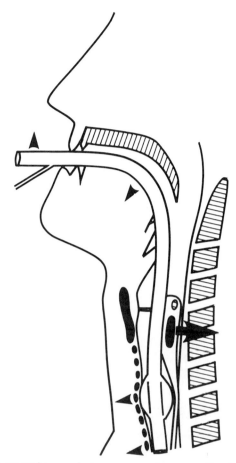

Figure 2. Sites of pressure exerted on respiratory passages by conventional endotracheal tube. (Modified from Lindholm and Grenvik[52])

suction. A patient is at risk of temporary interference with ventilation; this can lead to a rise in intracranial pressure as a result both of raised intrathoracic pressure and cerebral vasodilatation. For these reasons suction should be carried out only briefly and intermittently, and should be preceded by the administration of 100 percent oxygen for 5 minutes, and also by an analgesic or sedative. Moreover, reflex bradycardia and even a cardiac arrest may occur; patients who prove susceptible to these events should be given atropine.

Air reaching the trachea is normally fully saturated with water vapor in the nose or mouth; humidification of inspired air is therefore important in an intubated patient in order to prevent drying out of the airway secretions and impairment of mucociliary transport. An ultrasonic nebulizer is usually employed. The fluid thus administered will be lost again in the expired air; in calculating the overall fluid balance, the normal net loss by respiration is not applicable.

BRONCHOSCOPY. When humidification, physiotherapy, and tracheal suction fail to prevent retention of secretions and atelectasis, flexible fibreoptic bronchoscopy may be useful. In a ventilated patient, the procedure can be carried out without interrupting respiration. Recent models make it possible to remove obstructing secretions under direct vision; in up to 80 percent of patients improvement can be shown radiologically, but precautions are necessary to prevent adverse effects upon respiratory and cardiovascular function.[53]

Breathing

Inadequate ventilation—hypoventilation and respiratory failure—is uncommon in severely head injured patients. But hypoxemia is common and may not be recognized unless it is sought for. Clinical signs of hypoxemia may be lacking, and an apparently effective, even hyperventilatory breathing pattern may not be producing satisfactory oxygenation and may indeed be a response to hypoxemia.

Respiratory dysfunction should be suspected in all unconscious head injured patients, and it has been suggested that use of the nomenclature of the anesthesiologist and pulmonary care physician is a mandatory skill for the neurosurgeon.[91] The causes of respiratory dysfunction can conveniently be divided into central and peripheral types (Fig. 3).[23]

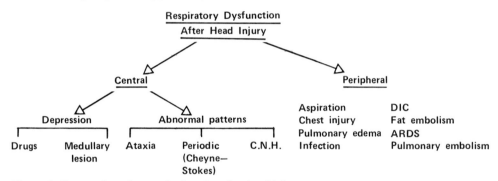

Figure 3. Causes of respiratory dysfunction after head injury.

Central Respiratory Dysfunction

The respiratory pattern of brain damaged patients may vary greatly and abnormal patterns are common. Respiratory function may be impaired when there are prolonged periods of apnea, which may occur at regular intervals (Cheyne-Stokes breathing) or irregular intervals (ataxic breathing). Irrespective of the rate of respiration and the duration of periods of apnea, it is the net effect upon blood gases that is important, rather than any particular duration or frequency of abnormality. Hyperventilation is often seen in head injured patients. It is usually a response to hypoxia; true neurogenic hyperventilation is rarely if ever seen. Even when hyperventilation is associated with a satisfactory level of arterial oxygen content, it has been suggested that it may be harmful because of the work associated with breathing. But before the oxygen consumption of breathing approaches even 10 percent of the resting whole-body consumption (with normal lungs), ventilation must reach 70 liters/min., and the minute volume of brain damaged patients even with a breathing frequency of over 30 is unlikely to be more than 30 liters.

Excessive intake of alcohol or drug overdose often coexists with head injury

218

and may be responsible for respiratory abnormalities; the typical pattern is of decreased tidal volume and respiratory rate and elevated $PaCO_2$.

Peripheral Respiratory Dysfunction

Aspiration is common after head injury; loss of the protective pharyngeal reflexes, decreased gastric motility, and regurgitation are all liable to occur even in a patient who is unconscious for only a short period after the injury. Later there may be an increase in respiratory rate, decreasing tidal volume, increasing hypoxemia, and widespread abnormalities in the chest x-ray. Eventually the respiratory distress syndrome may supervene.

Chest trauma is common in severe head injury, particularly when the patient has been a victim of a road traffic accident. The addition of a head injury to a major chest injury worsens outcome, and the converse is also true. A major chest injury can involve any one or all of four components: pulmonary contusion; chest wall injury (flail chest); cardiovascular injury (rupture of the aortic valve cusps, traumatic myocardial infarction, rupture of the aorta); and tracheal and bronchial injury. The individual disorders interact to result in respiratory insufficiency (Fig. 4).

Pulmonary edema in a multiply injured patient may have a variety of causes. The frequency and even the existence of neurogenic pulmonary edema have been debated. Unequivocal examples are rare and are seen more often after sponta-

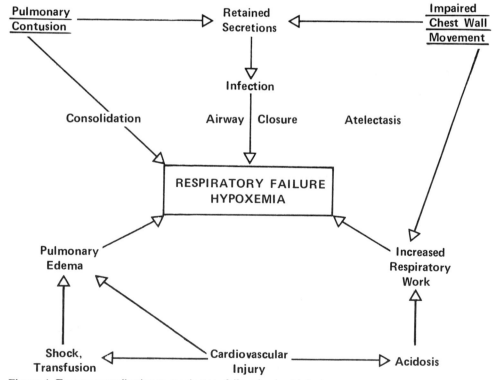

Figure 4. Factors contributing to respiratory failure in chest injuries.

neous intracranial hemorrhage than after head injury. There are copious, frothy, blood-stained secretions that fill the airways; inspiratory pressures are greatly increased because pulmonary compliance is low. Tachycardia and elevation of central venous pressure are usual, and diffuse rales and bronchospasm can be heard in the chest. A chest x-ray shows mottling spreading out from the hila of the lungs, but this cannot be detected until lung water is increased by at least 50 percent. The exact pathophysiological mechanisms involved in neurogenic pulmonary edema are still unclear; a massive sympathetic discharge, resulting in increased arterial, left atrial, and pulmonary artery pressures, has been postulated,[88] but the syndrome has been difficult to reproduce experimentally.[35,72]

Frank pulmonary edema is the final and obvious disaster in a progressive process of accumulation of fluid in the lungs. It has been reported that this may occur to lesser degrees in association with brain damage;[18] this could be a cause of reflex hyperventilation, of decreased lung compliance, and possibly of hypoxemia.[85]

Disseminated intravascular coagulation can occur in head injured patients and may be an important factor in some kinds of respiratory dysfunction. Pulmonary capillary microthrombosis was found in a quarter of a series of patients dying after head injury.[15] Intravascular coagulation should be suspected when respiratory distress is associated with a falling hematocrit, abnormal coagulation mechanisms, and copious bloody secretions from the lungs. An early sign of this complication is low alveolar (end-tidal) PCO_2 relative to arterial PCO_2, indicating increased alveolar dead-space.

Fat embolism shows its classic picture 24 to 52 hours after an injury. A patient who has shown little or no signs of brain damage becomes restless and delirious and deteriorates into coma over the next few hours and may even show focal neurological signs. There is often fever and respiratory dysfunction. The lungs are probably damaged by the fatty acids released from the fat globules, and the physiological abnormalities are not merely a consequence of microvascular obstruction. There is edema, hemorrhage, and emphysema, which combine to give a "snow storm" appearance on the chest x-ray. Hypoxemia may be the main cause of the cerebral dysfunction, and the role of cerebral fat embolism is uncertain. In the brain the picture is of perivascular petechial infarction in a multifocal pattern. The differentiation from the development of an intracranial complication can be extremely difficult. A petechial hemorrhagic rash over the chest, hemorrhages in the conjunctiva and fundus, and increasing respiratory difficulties point to fat embolism being responsible.

Pulmonary embolism can be difficult to diagnose in the unconscious patient. The signs include tachycardia, respiratory asynchrony, unexplained hypoxia, and reduced compliance and increased alveolar arterial (A-a) PCO_2 gradient, which indicates increased alveolar dead-space. Only with a massive embolus are there clinical and electrocardiographic signs of right ventricular dysfunction. The radiological signs include effusions and infiltrates, but these do not appear until 12 to 36 hours after the event and can be difficult to recognize in the chest x-ray of a supine comatose patient.

The Adult Respiratory Distress Syndrome (ARDS) or Shock Lung includes severe abnormalities of gas exchange and intrapulmonary shunting. The syndrome usually develops 3 to 4 days after multiple injury and has three characteristic phases:

1. The arterial PaO_2 is reduced, $PaCO_2$ is reduced, but the chest x-ray is normal.
2. There is restlessness, respiratory distress, and diffuse shadowing on chest x-ray.
3. Consciousness becomes impaired, arterial PCO_2 rises; finally, there is acidosis and generalized opacification on the chest x-ray ("white out").

Pulmonary function studies show several abnormalities. An increased proportion of the cardiac output does not exchange with alveolar air (intrapulmonary shunt). Also, an increased proportion of the tidal volume does not exchange with pulmonary blood. Thus there is ventilation-perfusion mismatching in both senses (increased physiological dead-space). The functional residual capacity is reduced and pulmonary compliance is increased. Many factors can be responsible for the syndrome (Table 1). The incidence of the syndrome appears to be reduced by avoiding excessive infusion of noncolloidal solutions during resuscitation, by careful monitoring and control of hemodynamic function, and by early mechanical ventilation. The importance of neurogenic factors was suggested by Moss,[69] but is still unknown. Some head injury patients who have no evident pulmonary damage and no major extracranial injuries do show ventilation-perfusion disorders.[95]

Table 1. Factors contributing to adult respiratory distress syndrome (shock lung)

Chest Injury	Heart failure
Shock	Uremia
Sepsis	Pancreatitis
Disseminated intravascular coagulation	Oxygen toxicity
Aspiration	Burns
Transfused microemboli	XS crystalloid transfusion
Raised ICP	Pulmonary edema

Management of Respiratory Dysfunction

The aims in management of respiratory dysfunction are simply to maintain adequate oxygen exchange in the lungs and to avoid carbon dioxide retention. Some patients, after initial resuscitation is completed, are normoxic, but achieve this only at the price of tachypnea, increased work of breathing, and hypocapnia. The last may be of such a degree to raise concern about the effects of vasoconstriction upon blood supply to the brain, and some believe that spontaneous hypocapnia should be corrected by paralysis and mechanical ventilation; others believe that hypocapnia may be beneficial, and indeed it is often induced deliberately in order to control intracranial hypertension (p. 225).

The level of arterial PO_2 for adequate delivery of oxygen to the body cannot be defined without considering also the oxygen-carrying capacity of the blood and the cardiac output. In the absence of circulatory disorders, cerebral metabolism is not affected (in experimental conditions) until very low levels of PaO_2 are reached (p. 48), but this depends upon adaptive responses by the cerebral circulation. In the severely head injured patient these responses are likely to be impaired, and most would agree that measures should be taken to prevent PaO_2

from falling below 70 to 80 mm Hg. Experimentally, ischemic neurons may recover function when PaO_2 is raised *above* normal,[7] but the clinical value of hyperoxygenation is not clear.

The measures that can be used to prevent or reverse hypoxia include those that ensure an adequate airway, as described above. After initial resuscitation, continuing physiotherapy, suctioning, and humidification are important in preventing and treating hypostatic pneumonia and atelectasis.

Oxygen should be given to all unconscious patients (100%, 10–12 liters/min) until results of blood gases are known. Thereafter, the concentration should be reduced appropriately; if it is necessary to maintain a very high concentration of inspired oxygen in order to prevent hypoxemia, this indicates severe lung dysfunction and it may be necessary to consider mechanical ventilation. Prolonged use of high levels of inspired oxygen can be toxic to the lung.

SPECIFIC MEASURES. Sometimes, specific treatments may be appropriate. Respiratory depression owing to drugs can be reverted by appropriate antagonists, for example, naloxone hydrochloride in the case of narcotic overdose. In the patient with chest trauma, drainage of hemothorax or pneumothorax may be necessary as an urgent measure. The insertion of a chest drain is particularly important if positive pressure ventilation is contemplated, as this may provoke a tension pneumothorax. Crushed chest injuries have usually been managed by prolonged, positive pressure ventilation, but as an alternative, a vigorous regimen of fluid restriction, diuretics, steroids, frequent pulmonary toilet, and intercostal nerve block may reduce the need for ventilation and so avoid the attendant morbidity and mortality.[90] Drugs that may be employed in pulmonary edema include frusemide (Lasix), dopamine, and aminophylline, and, possibly, alpha-adrenergic blocking drugs. Disseminated intravascular coagulation is treated with replacement of the appropriate factors and possibly by heparin. A variety of treatments have been proposed for fat embolism, including steroids, amophylline, alcohol, heparin, and dextrans, but the most important steps are to ensure that hypoxia is corrected and that before making this diagnosis, intracranial complications are excluded.

Mechanical Ventilation

One of the reasons for the controversy about the benefits of controlled ventilation in severe head injuries is that several different objectives are sometimes confused. These objectives include maintenance of an airway, ensuring adequate ventilation (normal $PaCO_2$), ensuring adequate oxygenation (PaO_2), controlling intracranial pressure, and treating chest injuries or complications.

No one disputes the importance of keeping the airway clear, but intubation is not in itself an indication to employ controlled ventilation. Similarly, inadequate ventilation and oxygen exchange may require assisted ventilation, but this need not mean hyperventilation nor need it always entail paralysis and controlled ventilation.

Methods of Ventilation

Mechanical ventilators can be cycled in response to pressure or volume. The most widely employed method is time-cycled, volume-preset, determining the volume of gas delivered to the patient. Ventilation can then be adjusted in order to alter the PaCO$_2$. It is important that the ventilator is simple and that the staff responsible for management fully understand the particular model that they use. Problems are more likely to be the result of the operator than the ventilator, and familiarity gives confidence. Frequent and accurate blood gas analyses and regular radiological examination are important in indicating the efficiency of ventilation and the need for adjustment. Disconnection in the patient circuit is an all too common event and an alarm system is essential.

Triggering of the ventilator by the patient is sometimes useful when ventilation is being discontinued. The patient's inspiratory effort alters pressure in the respirator tubing and activates the cycle. Its value lies in its depending upon the patient's own respiratory drive to produce ventilation.

Intermittent mandatory ventilation (IMV) has similar advantages[51] and is increasingly used. Essentially the technique allows a mechanically ventilated intubated patient to take spontaneous breaths in between mandatory artificial inflations. The proportion of ventilation provided by spontaneous and mandatory respirations can be varied and the frequency of mandatory ventilations is progressively reduced as adequate spontaneous respiration develops. The method is particularly useful in patients who will not tolerate an abrupt discontinuation of mechanical ventilation and transfer to a T-tube system. A further development is mandatory minute volume (MMV), in which the circuit supplies the patient with preset volume per minute. Some or all of this is taken by the patient breathing spontaneously; any deficiency is supplemented by the ventilator.

Patterns of Ventilation

During spontaneous respiration the airway pressure fluctuates from positive to negative (Fig. 5). In the simplest form of positive pressure respiration, after the

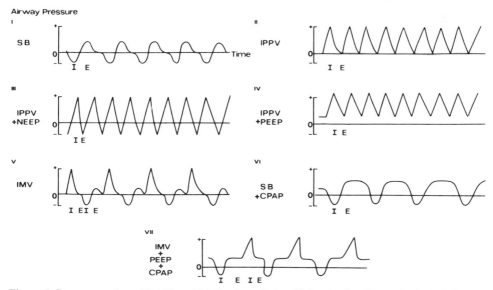

Figure 5. Pressure cycles with different kinds of ventilation (I=inspiration; E=expiration). I) Spontaneous breathing (SB); II) intermittent positive pressure ventilation (IPPV); III) negative end expiratory pressure (NEEP); IV) positive end expiratory pressure (PEEP); V) intermittent mandatory ventilation (IMV); VI) continuous positive airway pressure (CPAP).

223

inspiratory period, the pressure falls passively to atmospheric by the end of expiration. In recent years a number of refinements to these cycles have been described, which are aimed at improving treatment of pulmonary failure, but which may have important effects upon intracranial pressure.

Negative end-expiratory pressure (NEEP) assists venous return and may lower intracranial pressure,[77] but it is not widely used.[62] Positive end-expiratory pressure (PEEP) provides a continuous distension pressure, minimizes atelectasis, and may also impede the exudation of fluid into the alveoli in pulmonary edema. Although PEEP may be effective in correcting hypoxemia that has been resistant to other methods, the continuous positive pressure in the airways may have disadvantages: alveolar capillary flow may be reduced, venous return and cardiac output can fall, and $PaCO_2$ rises. Barotrauma may result in entry of air into the lung spaces or even the circulation. PEEP is therefore inadvisable in patients with emphysema or hypovolemia or other cardiovascular instability. It has been reported that PEEP produces a rise in intracranial pressure, especially in patients with reduced intracranial compliance,[3] but others have found that this does not occur if the patient is kept 30° head up.[24] The state of the lungs may also be important in determining the extent that airway pressures affect intracranial pressure. If a choice has to be made, the correction of systemic hypoxia usually takes precedence over minor effects upon intracranial pressure.

A combination of IMV and PEEP may permit management of some chest injuries without recourse to full controlled ventilation. Continuous positive airway pressure (CPAP) may be employed to prevent alveolar collapse as controlled ventilation is discontinued. It is even possible to have a combination of IMV, PEEP, and CPAP!

Patient Cooperation

When ventilation is employed in a patient with adequate spontaneous respiratory drive, synchronization of the patient with the machine may present considerable difficulties. Central respiratory depressants can be used; diazepam, morphine, chlorpromazine, and phenoperidine have been employed. These drugs have the advantage that they do not make the patient completely inaccessible to neurological examination. Coughing, straining, and fighting against the ventilator, however, raise intracranial pressure and should be avoided; these events may also increase the tendency to laryngeal damage. If adequate patient-ventilator synchronization cannot be achieved, it is preferable to employ long-acting neuromuscular blocking agents.

Ventilation Parameters

The patient should be ventilated with an air/oxygen mixture. In the first few hours 100 percent oxygen can be used; thereafter, an effort should be made to reduce the oxygen concentration (FIO_2) below 50 percent. Positive end-expiratory pressure can be applied up to a maximum of 10 cm of water. A respiratory rate of 10 to 15 is usually satisfactory; the tidal volume should usually be 10 to 15 ml/kg body weight, but this should be adjusted to achieve the desired $PaCO_2$.

Suction should be carried out at intervals, but each episode should not be prolonged beyond 15 seconds. During physiotherapy it is permissible to tilt the patient's head down for up to 10 minutes to assist clearing of secretions. It has been suggested that a preliminary bolus of thiopentone may help prevent an increase in intracranial pressure during physiotherapy.[68]

The patient's blood pressure should be maintained as close as possible to normal; if he becomes hypotensive it is necessary to seek for some cause before attributing it to the effects of the positive pressure ventilation. Fluid intake should be carefully monitored.

Ventilation as Treatment for the Damaged Brain

Advantages

That respiratory abnormalities are common in head injured patients and that hypoxia and hypercapnia are bad for the injured brain cannot be seriously contested; nor is there debate about the need for ventilation when measurements have shown that defined abnormalities are present and have been resistant to other forms of treatment. One view is that because abnormalities are so common, it is better electively to intubate and to ventilate all patients with a specified degree of impairment of consciousness rather than to await the development of abnormalities.[63] Control and toilet of the airway are more secure, percentage of inspired O_2 can be more readily regulated, sedatives and analgesics can be used as necessary, the work of breathing is relieved, shivering is abolished, decerebrate rigidity is depressed, and the hazards of a convulsion are minimized.

Disadvantages

Against the advantages have to be set the disadvantages of controlled ventilation: the interference with assessment of the patient; the demands upon staff and facilities; and the possible complications and technical failures. Complications include atelectasis, pulmonary infection, adverse effects upon cardiovascular function and possibly upon intracranial pressure, and the hazards associated with intubation or tracheostomy. Lung compliance may decrease, alveolar dead-space ventilation may increase, and cardiac output can be reduced. There is little evidence that can be used to determine whether mechanical ventilation per se exerts a beneficial effect upon the outcome of severe head injury; most studies have related to the effects of *hyper*ventilation.

Hyperventilation in the Management of Head Injury

There is general agreement that spontaneous hyperventilation and hypocapnia are common in severely head injured patients,[43] but there is still considerable debate about the usefulness of inducing controlled hyperventilation.

Advantages

Hyperventilation causes cerebral vasoconstriction in the normal brain, and it is therefore possible that the reduction in cerebral blood volume will result in a lowered intracranial pressure. After head injury, however, the reactivity of the cerebral blood vessels to altered levels of $PaCO_2$ is reduced as compared with normal; moreover, when a change in blood flow does occur in response to a change in $PaCO_2$, there is subsequently a gradual adaptation to the new conditions and over a period of several hours both CSF pH and cerebral blood flow return towards previous levels. Nevertheless, hyperventilation often does lower raised intracranial pressure after head injury. In one recent study,[39] responses were seen in 9 out of 16 head injured patients; the maximum reduction of intracranial pressure was usually seen within 10 minutes of initiating hyperventilation, but in more than half the patients intracranial pressure returned to control levels within at the most 80 minutes. Also, intracranial pressure always returned to control levels after hyperventilation was stopped. In another study in which 16 patients with intracranial pressures of greater than 20 mm Hg were hyperventilated, the pressure fell in ten cases but subsequently rose in eight.[71] When hyperventilation was discontinued in patients with a pressure above 20 mm Hg, the level usually increased but then returned to baseline within 2 hours. Hyperventilation may affect intracranial compliance, but these changes are usually in parallel with those in intracranial pressure. Clearly, when an elevated pressure has become established, hyperventilation has an inconsistent and often only transient effect.

Hyperventilation has been observed to improve cerebral autoregulatory status after brain damage, but the importance of this is not clear. Hyperventilation has also been held to readjust the distribution of blood flow within a focally damaged brain by vasoconstricting the vessels outside the damaged area and thus promoting an increase in flow within the latter. The evidence that this actually occurs in the head injured brain is scanty. There is more evidence that focal areas of hyperemia are reduced during hyperventilation[12] but the significance of this observation is also unclear. There is much evidence for the presence of a metabolic acidosis in the CSF and cerebral tissue after head injury (Table 2), and of a correlation between CSF acidosis and spontaneous hyperventilation, and the implication is that the latter is often a compensatory mechanism, with the function of returning cerebral pH to normal. In clinical practice controlled hyperventilation will usually increase CSF pH,[29] but extreme hyperventilation per se can increase CSF lactate concentration.[14]

Table 2. Ventilation and hyperventilation for head injury

Pros	Cons
Ventilation	
Corrects hypoxia	Costs in resources
Prevents hypoxia (?)	Complications/failures
Prevents airway obstruction (?)	Intubation/tracheostomy
Prevents hypercapnia (?)	Unrecognized hypercapnia
Reduces work of breathing	Low energy cost of breathing
Reduces abnormal motor activity	Loss of clinical signs
Hyperventilation	
Decreases ICP	Increase in cardiac output
Improves regional distribution of CBF	Possible ischemia owing to vasoconstriction
Corrects cerebral/CSF acidosis	Possible increase in CSF lactate and aggravation of biochemical abnormalities
	Adverse effects upon lungs

Disadvantages

There are several disadvantages in hyperventilation. The increase in CSF lactate seen during extreme hyperventilation may be an indication of cerebral tissue hypoxia. Hyperventilation can increase total oxygen consumption, but a greater concern is the possibility of severe vasoconstriction. When $PaCO_2$ is reduced below 20 mm Hg, biochemical signs suggesting hypoxia develop, and these changes can be reversed by inhalation of hyperbaric oxygen.[73] Corroborative evidence for deleterious effects caused by hyperventilation comes from observations of the development of EEG slow wave activity, which can be reversed by hyperbaric oxygen.[11] It is also possible that the respiratory alkalosis may directly interfere with metabolic processes. In several experimental studies of focal cerebral ischemia, the beneficial effects of hypocapnia upon lesion size or recovery has been unconvincing. Indeed, the adverse metabolic effects of ischemia were accentuated in one study.[61] Mechanical hyperventilation has been shown experimentally to deplete pulmonary surfactant and thus further enhance the liability to alveolar collapse.[20]

Results of Ventilator Treatment

Evidence that patients treated by controlled ventilation or by hyperventilation do in fact do better is difficult to evaluate because of variations in methods of assessment and because different groups of patients were studied. Particularly difficult to substantiate are claims of good results from centers that include patients subjected to controlled ventilation from the earliest stage after injury. It is a common experience that brain damage may appear to be more severe than it actually is if assessment is made too early before resuscitation is complete. It is impossible to judge how many such patients may have been included in a series of patients treated by controlled ventilation from the time of admission to hospital, and it is certainly invalid to compare results of such series with one made up only of patients selected for ventilation treatment because of the persistence of certain abnormalities despite conventional measures or when the patient has been in persisting coma for several hours.

Krenn and associates[47] reported on 44 head injured patients who were allocated at random to ventilation at normocapnia or to spontaneous breathing. There were 4 deaths among the 24 ventilated cases, and 1 in the 20 spontaneously breathing. This difference is not significant, but does suggest a trend toward *higher* mortality in treated patients.

Few studies of patients treated with or without ventilation are available in which methods of assessments are sufficiently consistent to permit comparisons. Gordon's initial report[27] indicated a fall in mortality from 33 to 10 percent and he subsequently reported two successive series treated at the Karolinska Hospital.[28] Between 1959 and 1967, when only a small minority of the 201 patients were treated with hyperventilation, mortality was 32 percent. In subsequent years hyperventilation was employed and mortality was 17.5 percent. Rossanda and colleagues and others have also reported beneficial effects from hyperventilation.[80] In the collaborative study, by contrast, ventilation was not associated with improved outcome (Table 3).[42]

Unfortunately no randomized controlled study of the effects of hyperventilation after head injury has been reported. Such a study has been carried out in

Table 3. Comparison of outcomes of patients with severe head injury treated with or without ventilation

Coma Score (Best in 1st 24 hours)	Nonventilated			Ventilated		
	n	D/V	%	n	D/V	%
3,4,5	174	131	75	105	92	88
6,7	277	106	38	150	92	61
>8	238	42	18	39	21	54

(Data from Jennett et al.[42])

patients suffering from stroke and showed no benefit to the patients treated by hyperventilation.[10]

Most neurosurgeons (as distinct from anesthetists) probably prefer to use controlled ventilation very selectively and would base the decision to ventilate on the answers to the following questions:

1. Is controlled ventilation necessary to maintain adequate| ventilation (i.e., is $PaCO_2$ high during spontaneous breathing when airway is clear)?

2. Is controlled ventilation necessary to achieve normal arterial oxygenation?

3. Is controlled ventilation necessary to hyperventilate the patient in order to reduce $PaCO_2$ and therefore reduce ICP?

4. Is controlled ventilation necessary because of associated injuries or complications?

To apply such a system in terms of practical decision-making requires prior agreement of the limits of abnormality that can be tolerated without recourse to controlled ventilation. These should include the duration of the abnormality and whether it persists in spite of defined measures, such as a clear airway, oxygen-enriched inspired air, and, in the case of raised intracranial pressure, the completion of necessary intracranial surgery.

CIRCULATION

Hypotension may have disastrous effects upon a recently injured brain but is very rarely a consequence of injury to the brain. In a series of 70 cases dying in a neurosurgical unit, there was only one patient with hypotension (BP<90 mm Hg systolic) that could be ascribed only to brain damage.[38] In the same study, in a series of 400 head injured patients admitted to a general surgical unit, there was also only one patient whose hypotension could not be explained; bleeding was present in 11 other hypotensive cases and blood loss caused the death of three patients. Possible causes of shock after head injury are shown in Table 4. Blood loss from the head injury itself sufficient to cause shock is rare, but can occur as a complication of extensive scalp lacerations in a very young child with an extradural hematoma; when a depressed fracture of the vault tears the sagittal sinus; or when a basal fracture involves a major vessel.

Profuse hemorrhage from a scalp wound is rarely cause for concern, but there are occasional extensive lacerations, often in elderly patients, when persisting arterial bleeding can lead to significant blood loss. Such hemorrhage can usually be controlled by a firm pad or dressing; another method is to close the wound with through and through sutures without further preparation; definitive wound toilet and repair can be carried out once the blood volume has been restored.

Table 4. Causes of hypotension after head injury

Extracranial
1. Hypovolemia
   a) Loss of blood/fluid
   b) External/concealed
2. Chest injury
   a) Cardiac injury
   b) Tamponade
   c) Hemothorax
   d) Tension pneumothorax
3. Associated spinal injury
4. Septic shock

Cranial (uncommon)
1. Extensive scalp injury
2. Subgaleal or extradural hematoma in an infant
3. Compound fracture involving major venous sinus (vault or base fracture) or artery (basal fracture)

Hurried attempts to pick up a bleeding point with forceps have little to recommend them, although eversion of the scalp by means of forceps applied to the galea is an important method of controlling bleeding during operations. In infants an extradural hematoma can be associated with sufficient blood loss to produce dangerous circulatory depletion. If an attempt is made to evacuate the clot before the blood volume has been at least partially replenished, disastrous hypotension may develop during operation, owing to the release of brain stem compression (which may have been producing a hypertensive response), together with the additional blood loss caused by surgery.

Profuse hemorrhage from a major venous sinus can be controlled by a pressure dressing and head-up tilt. If bleeding ceases, the area that was bleeding should not be disturbed at operation until a sufficient amount of the surrounding bone has been removed to enable repair or ligation to be achieved without a further disastrous bleed.

Monitoring

When a head injury is not complicated by multiple injuries, it is usually sufficient to assess cardiovascular function and the adequacy of the circulating blood volume by clinical means, but this is not adequate in the gravely ill casualty with multiple injuries and impaired consciousness. Hoffman stated that road accident victims with multiple injuries still frequently die of hemorrhage,[36] and in these circumstances more invasive and direct methods of monitoring circulatory functions are therefore justified.

Central venous pressure measurements can provide useful information about right heart filling, but also have limitations and complications.[44] A catheter should be inserted into the bladder in order to monitor urinary output and hence the adequacy of renal perfusion; when there is pelvic trauma, a suprapubic catheter may be required. A suitable artery—usually the radial—should be cannulated percutaneously. This permits direct measurements of arterial pressure and also facilitates frequent arterial blood gas measurements. The right side of the heart and pulmonary artery can be cannulated by means of a cannula inserted into a peripheral vein.[87] This technique can be valuable in the early management of severe trauma when there is need to guide blood replacement in the presence of a failing heart, but even in the hands of those with adequate experience in the technique there are potentially serious complications, and this technique is justified only in selected patients.

Transfusion

The advantages and disadvantages of different fluids as replacements are a matter of some controversy. However, it is undeniable that some part of the replacement for profound blood loss should be blood, even when the potential drawbacks of massive transfusions are considered. These include the possibility of a reduction in temperature, unless the blood is adequately warmed; the increased oxygen affinity of stored blood (owing to its loss of 2:3 diphosphoglyceric acid), which impedes delivery of oxygen to the tissues; the presence of aggregates of cell fragments, protein strands, platelets, and other particles that may obstruct the pulmonary vascular bed and lead to adult repiratory distress syndrome (p. 220) and that require the use of a microfilter; and the depletion of platelets and clotting factors, which can lead to a coagulation disorder. The dangers of a fall in pH and the developments of hypocalcemia have probably been overemphasized; bicarbonate and calcium need not be given routinely but only as indicated by blood gas measurements and ECG changes (prolonged Q-T interval in hypocalcemia).

Some of the replacement for blood loss may be given in the form of plasma protein solution (half life 4 to 14 days) or plasma substitutes such as dextrans, or gelatin or starch solutions. With each there is a very small risk of an allergic reaction, but the hemodilution that they provide may be beneficial; the lowered viscosity improves blood flow, and tissue oxygenation may be best served by a hematocrit of about 30 percent.[30]

GENERAL MEDICAL CARE

Fluids, Electrolytes, and Nutrition

The alterations in fluid and electrolyte balance and in metabolism that occur in response to injury or starvation are well recognized. The metabolic changes reported in head injured patients seem to be similar to those that follow trauma elsewhere in the body;[60] this is surprising because hypothalamic and endocrine factors are important in the mediation of these responses, and more than 40 percent of fatal head injuries have damage in this region. Diabetes insipidus is probably the most common specific disorder resulting from hypothalamic injury, but even this is rare. Other endocrine disorders have been recorded: an elevated cortisol level with loss of diurnal rhythm and with impaired regulation; a paradoxical rise of growth hormone during hyperglycemia;[46] and hypothyroidism.[19,60]

Fluid and Electrolyte Balance

After injury there is retention of salt and water and excretion of potassium. Characteristically, there is greater retention of water than sodium, resulting usually in mild hyponatremia (Na 130–135 mEq/liter), but this does not indicate a deficit of total body sodium. Aldosterone is involved in the retention of sodium, and antidiuretic hormone in the retention of water. Another important factor is a redistribution of blood flow between the cortex and medulla of the kidney; this may be exacerbated by circulatory abnormalities. The increased potassium loss is due to both the effects of aldosterone and the release of potassium from cells as a result of protein catabolization.

MAINTENANCE FLUID AND ELECTROLYTE THERAPY. An intake of between 1500 and 2000 ml/24 hours is probably optimum for the average adult. In the first 3 or 4 days after injury, fluid is best given intravenously as a dextrose/saline combination. After this time, if the patient remains in coma, the nasogastric route should be employed whenever possible. By then the risks of aspiration will have lessened and the need to supply a more substantial amount of calories and other food sources will have become important.

It is not necessary to set up intravenous lines on a restless head injured patient soon after injury, unless there are associated injuries calling for such administration. In any event a slight degree of dehydration may reduce the risk of cerebral edema, and certainly overloading with fluid must be avoided.

FLUID/ELECTROLYTE IMBALANCE. In a series of head injured patients studied in Vancouver[86] there was often an increase in osmolality in the blood on admission, and this increase paralleled the level of blood alcohol. Electrolyte abnormalities subsequently developed in about a third of those patients who had head injuries sufficiently severe to have produced coma for at least an hour, and in two thirds who were unconscious for more than a day; hyponatremia and hypernatremia occurred about equally frequently, and in some cases the electrolyte abnormalities did not appear for more than a week after injury.

Hyponatremia. Extreme hyponatremia (Na<130 mEq/liter) is abnormal and usually reflects excessive fluid intake. Sometime inappropriate excessive secretion of antidiuretic hormone may be responsible, in particular in patients with basal fractures; hyponatremia can also result from mechanical ventilation and as a complication of severe sepsis.

The urine is often hypertonic, with a sodium greater than 25 mEq/liter. Despite this finding it is important to recognize that total body sodium is not reduced and the term "cerebral salt wasting," which has been applied to this syndrome, is usually inappropriate. The relatively high sodium level in the urine is probably a result of the suppression of aldosterone secretion that occurs as a response to the overhydration and expansion of circulating volume. Occasionally, this eventually may result in a true sodium depletion.

Severe hyponatremia produces impairment of cerebral function, and this can lead to a misdiagnosis of an intracranial complication of head injury. When the syndrome has been present for several days, it may be necessary to attempt to improve the patient's condition by the use of hypertonic intravenous saline. Ordinarily, the mainstay of management is to restrict fluid intake to 800 ml or less per day.

Hypernatremia and Hyperosmolality. Hypertonicity is also usually due to a disorder of water balance, and the explanation is usually found in inadequate intake. The patients most at risk are not those in coma, who will usually receive fluids by infusions or nasogastric tube. Instead, it is the patient who is confused and uncooperative and who will not swallow sufficient food or fluids, yet who will not tolerate a nasogastric tube, who develops hypernatremia. Such patients may have disturbance of their thirst mechanisms. In occasional patients hypertonicity is due to excessive fluid loss (e.g., from diabetes insipidus), excessive use of osmotic agents for the control of intracranial pressure, or excessive protein feeding, which leads to the release of large quantities of nitrogen and possibly to nonketotic hyperglycemia. The common factor in all cases is a reduction in circulating volume, which stimulates aldosterone secretion, resulting in relative retention of sodium over fluid. This accounts for the syndrome having been termed "cerebral salt retention." The management of hypertonicity depends upon identifying and, if possible, treating the cause; and upon rehydration by nasogastric or intravenous route.

Nutrition of the Head Injured Patient

How much feeding a head injured patient needs depends upon what balance is struck between the *reduction* in energy utilization, which occurs because of the combination of starvation and enforced bedrest, and the *increase* in energy expenditure, which is part of the metabolic response to injury. In starvation, 80 to 90 percent of energy requirements are provided by release from fat stores of free fatty acids; ketone bodies may be formed after several days, and these can provide much of the brain's energy requirement. The other main source of energy is muscle protein, but the net result of the metabolic adaptation to starvation is to conserve body protein. By contrast, the response to injury is an accelerated protein catabolism, which provides the liver with substrates for the increased gluconeogenesis necessary to supply the glucose demands of injured tissues. The hypermetabolism after injury is associated with glucose intolerance and insulin resistance.

The degree of accelerated tissue catabolism after injury is proportional to the severity of injury, but it may be prolonged and exacerbated by complications such as infection. The changes are also enhanced when injury occurs in a patient whose metabolic state is already poor, as may be the case in the alcoholic or elderly patient. It is not clear whether head injury per se influences the metabolic response to injury: early suggestions that injuries in specific locations may *reduce* the nitrogen loss have not been substantiated; indeed, it has been suggested that severe brain damage may actually *increase* the metabolic response to trauma.[33] In practice, the patient's nutritional needs usually depend more upon the extent of associated injuries than the severity of the head injury, although the latter determines how long it will be before he can take responsibility for feeding himself.

In the patient who has only a head injury, the increased metabolic demand owing to the injury may be offset by the energy-sparing effects of starvation and bedrest, so that the total energy requirements may be little different from normal. A fast of 2 or 3 days may therefore be of little clinical significance. During this time the daily fluid therapy will usually include 1.5 to 2 liters of 4 to 5 percent dextrose with saline, and this supplies only 250 to 400 calories per day. It becomes important to provide nutrition after 3 or 4 days; this is also the stage at which it is usually possible to change from parenteral to intragastric administration. Whenever possible, feeding should be carried out via the alimentary tract; only when this is not tolerated, or when specific reasons preclude its use, is it necessary to resort to intravenous regimens.

Feeding by nasogastric tube is easy, safe, effective, and cheap, provided that it is carried out properly. There are advantages in using a fine bore (8-fg) Ryle's tube, or alternatively a long intravenous type of catheter can be introduced into the stomach.[2] The feed may be administered as a continuous drip or as a bolus given by a nurse every 1 to 2 hours. The continuous drip technique saves nursing time and probably causes less diarrhea. The stomach should be aspirated every 4 hours.

When starting nasogastric feeding it is customary to use a combination of milk and water, 30 to 100 ml/hour. Once this is tolerated the appropriate feed is given half-strength for a day before full feeding commences. Unless there are multiple injuries it is probably sufficient to supply 2000 to 3000 calories per day, with a calorie-nitrogen ratio of 180:1. In severely catabolic patients, daily requirements may be several thousand calories. The simplest source of nutrition is a liquidized ward diet. However, this tends to be extremely viscous and may be difficult to administer; also, its precise constitution may not be known. An alternative is to use a combination of commercially available foodstuffs, and Allison[2] has recommended a combination of 250 g *Calorine* (Scientific Hospital Supplies Limited) with 300 g *Complan* (Glaxo Limited). This is made up into 3 liters with water and will supply 2070 calories/day and 60 g of protein.

Apart from the pulmonary hazards of incorrect administration of the feed and of regurgitation, there are few complications. Hyperglycemia may occur when large amounts of carbohydrate are given, because of the glucose intolerance that follows injury. Glycosuria will provide early warning of this, and when hyperglycemia is severe, insulin may be necessary. The blood urea may increase if renal function is poor, if food restriction is excessive, or if too low a ratio of carbohydrate to nitrogen is given. Gastrointestinal problems are infrequent; nausea or vomiting can be helped by metoclopramide (10 mg three times a day), while codeine phosphate (30 mg daily) usually stops diarrhea.

Hematological Disorders After Head Injury

Anemia

Hemoglobin often falls in severely head injured patients, and usually by more than can be accounted for by water retention. The cause of the anemia is not clear, but it has been suggested that there may be red cell aggregation and intravascular clotting with subsequent lysis of the cells.

Platelet Function

Thrombocytopenia is common after trauma. Platelet aggregation may be transiently abnormal, and both increased and decreased aggregation have been observed. Mildly head injured patients do not have significant alterations of platelet function, but in more severe injuries platelet function may be impaired, aggregation being less when coma is deeper.

Clotting Mechanisms

After injury there is characteristically a sequence of changes in blood coagulation and fibrinolysis; a phase of hypercoagulability in the first few hours after injury is followed by hypocoagulability, which may last for several days.[15] Fibrinolytic activity is increased along with the coagulability, but is subsequently inhibited. Several authors have observed hypercoagulability in the early stage after head injury,[4,70] raising the possibility that excessive disseminated intravascular coagulation might occur, and that it might be responsible for some of the physiological abnormalities in severely head injured patients. Brain tissue is rich in thromboplastic material, and release of this from the damaged brain may activate coagulation. Other factors may be injury to vessel walls in the brain and a neurogenically determined effect, perhaps mediated by increased circulating catecholamine levels. Later, the hypocoagulability may be mainly due to the impairment of platelet function, and this may reduce the likelihood of thromboembolic complications.

Disseminated Intravascular Coagulation

Disseminated intravascular coagulation (consumption coagulopathy, defibrination syndrome) can be regarded as a pathological process in which the patient's plasma is converted into serum, rendering him liable to excessive bleeding. The essential features of this syndrome are the conversion of fibrinogen to fibrin within the circulation. In addition, there is agglutination of platelets and red cells, and stickiness of granulocytes. The characteristic hematological findings are a low fibrinogen concentration, an increased level of breakdown products of fibrin and fibrinogen (FDP), and the presence of fibrin monomers. The last is the most crucial evidence, and its detection depends upon the ability of ethanol or protamine to cause the monomers to polymerize into fibrin, so causing gelation (Fig. 6).

Multiple injuries are a potent cause of this disseminated intravascular coagulation, but it is likely that head injury per se may also cause abnormalities in coagulation,[93] because the incidence of abnormalities appears to be related to the severity of the head injury, as judged by impaired consciousness and brain stem function. Van der Sande and colleagues[92] found coagulation tests to be abnormal

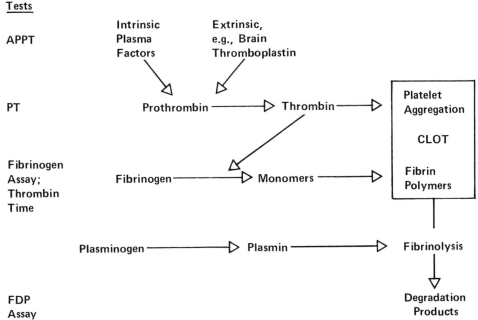

Figure 6. Simplified outline of coagulation and fibrinolytic pathways. APPT=activated partial thromboplastin time; PT=prothrombin time; FDP=fibrin degradation products.

in 18 percent of mildly head injured patients with normal consciousness, in 41 percent of patients with impaired consciousness, and in every patient in coma. Ethanol gelation tests in this study were positive in 12 of 150 patients, although only 3 of these showed abnormal bleeding tendencies. Other consequences of diffuse intravascular coagulation include obstruction of the microcirculation from fibrin deposition, causing pulmonary, renal, and cerebral dysfunction. Intravascular coagulation may be an important component of fat embolism.

Heparin is the usual treatment for clinically evident disseminated intravascular coagulation: by preventing the deposition of fibrin, it causes fibrinogen levels to rise so that the secondary hematological abnormalities resolve. Administration of fibrinogen alone, without heparin, may be ineffective. There has been understandable reluctance to use heparin in head injured patients in view of the risk of precipitating intracranial hemorrhage. Just how real this risk is is not clear; the possibility that heparin might actually improve neurological function and outcome is at present no more than an intriguing possibility.

Other Aspects of General Medical Care

Impaired consciousness and coma deprive a person of the ability to respond to a variety of simple dangers. Loss of these volitional or reflex protective responses can lead to complications resulting in preventable eventual disability. The steps taken to protect the patient from these risks vary from center to center, and local practice is largely derived from empirical experience and common sense.

The eyes may need to be taped closed and lubricated periodically (e.g., with methylcellulose) to prevent corneal damage from abrasion or drying out. Limbs should be put through as full a range of movements as possible several times a day in order to prevent contractures. Chest physiotherapy, in combination with postural drainage, is extremely important. The immobilized patient needs to be turned every 2 hours and his skin rubbed and protected against pressure sores. By contrast, some restless aggressive patients can harm themselves, their family, or their attendants unless they are restrained. When it is necessary to restrain a patient in bed, bandages can be tied over plentiful padding on the wrists and ankles or a simple body jacket can be used. The bladder will usually empty reflexly. Bed linen will need to be changed frequently when there is incontinence in order to minimize the risk of pressure sores. Persisting spasms of extension rigidity can make nursing more difficult. Nitrazepam 25 to 40 mg three or four times a day has been reported to be helpful; the application of ice-packs to the limbs will also reduce muscle tone.

Fever

Pyrexia in a severely head injured patient is often simply evidence of infection; occasionally it results from damage to the hypothalamus. It is well known that extreme hyperpyrexia can be lethal. Lesser degrees can also be harmful because intracranial compliance is reduced and intracranial pressure may rise, while at the same time metabolism is stimulated, and the net result may be ischemic damage.

In the head injured patient the commonest site of infection is within the respiratory tract. The risk is increased with each day that coma persists and when a tracheostomy is necessary. Urinary tract infections are probably next in fre-

235

quency. Pyrexia may also be due to infection of a wound, either in the scalp or, more often, elsewhere in the body. Intracranial infection is usually the sequel of a delay in treating a compound fracture of the vault or base of the skull. Fever is a feature also of fat embolism and of deep vein thrombosis.

The debate about the value of prophylactic antibiotics is unresolved. They should be given to all patients with a clinical cerebrospinal fluid leak (e.g., penicillin and sulphadimidine) or as indicated for tetanus prophylaxis. Otherwise we give antibiotics only when infection has been confirmed, and then use one with as narrow a spectrum as possible. The overall incidence of gram-negative infection can be reduced by avoiding broad spectrum antibiotics.[74] Extreme fever should be prevented by cooling once the temperature has reached 102 to 103°F. A variety of measures can be used: sponging with cold water; covering with a damp sheet over which air is blown by means of an electric fan; intravenously infusing cold fluids; and reducing shivering with chlorpromazine. Cooling blankets and rooms in which the ambient temperature can be reduced to about 10°C are sometimes useful.

The first step in a patient with a fever is a careful clinical examination of the chest, abdomen, legs, and any wounds. Cultures of sputum and urine should be obtained routinely at 2- or 3-day intervals and blood cultures as indicated by a spike of temperature. Examination of the CSF is important if the injury was complicated by a fracture, if a craniotomy has been performed, or if intradural pressure measurements have been carried out. A patient in whom a hematoma has been removed or excluded can have a lumbar puncture, but CSF should otherwise be obtained by ventricular tap—remembering that the bacteriological findings may differ in the two sites.

Gastrointestinal Bleeding

Severe bleeding in the gastrointestinal tract occurs in less than 10 percent of even severely head injured patients, but may be more common in those taking steroids. The source may be a discrete ulcer (Cushing's ulcer) or, probably more commonly, an acute erosive gastritis. Fibreoptic endoscopy establishes the cause of the bleeding in the majority of patients. Initially management is conservative, but if there is persisting hemorrhage it is important to encourage surgeons to undertake operation on the same grounds as in a non-head injured patient. Medical treatment is of uncertain value in established hemorrhage, but recently introduced antagonists of histamine H-2 receptors appear to have a role in the prophylaxis of erosive gastritis. The drug currently employed is cimetidine in a dosage of 200 mg intravenously, 4 to 6 hourly up to a maximum of 2 g/day. Antacids are probably of less value; they have to be given very frequently and in high doses to be effective.

MANAGEMENT OF EARLY EPILEPSY

There is good evidence from studies in Glasgow[40] that epilepsy during the first week after injury is distinctly different from late epilepsy; this is now widely accepted as the appropriate definition of early epilepsy. One or more *early* fits occur in 5 percent of patients admitted to hospital with nonmissile head injuries. Early epilepsy is more common after some kinds of injury; in adults it seldom occurs except in association with prolonged PTA, depressed fracture, or intracra-

236

nial hematoma. It occurs more commonly in young children, and only in them does it complicate trivial injuries. Hendrick and Harris[34] found 5 percent of a large series of patients under 15 years of age had early epilepsy; but 7 percent of those under 5 years and 11 percent of those with injuries in the first year of life (excluding birth injuries) had it. Therefore the overall incidence of 5 percent will be exceeded in children's hospitals, and in neurosurgical departments, which selectively admit more severe or complicated injuries.

In 60 percent of patients with early epilepsy the first (sometimes the only) fit occurs within 24 hours of injury; in rather less than half of these the epilepsy is within an hour of injury. Two thirds of patients have more than one early fit; 10 percent develop status epilepticus, but the rate is twice as great as this in children under 5 years. About 40 percent of patients have generalized fits without a recognizable focal component; in another 40 percent only focal motor twitching occurs, without any generalized seizures, a form of epilepsy seldom encountered after the first week.

Significance of Early Epilepsy

When epilepsy occurs soon after injury it may be of diagnostic importance in regard to intracranial complications (p. 162); or it may itself threaten to cause additional brain damage, if it is inadequately controlled. Its other significance is for the future, because it increases the risk of late epilepsy (p. 284).

Hazards of Status Epilepticus

Status carries considerable hazards, particularly in young children, in whom it occurs twice as often as in patients over 5 years of age. Severe hypoxic brain damage owing to inadequately controlled status was one of the avoidable causes of death identified in a series of fatal injuries that had initially been judged relatively mild, in terms of impact damage (p. 339). Even in those who survive an episode of status in childhood there is the possibility of persisting brain damage; when epilepsy has followed head injury it is sometimes difficult to ascribe relative significance to the original injury, to epilepsy, and to other early post-traumatic complications.

Prophylaxis and Treatment of Early Epilepsy

There can be no argument about the need to give anticonvulsants to any patient who has already had a fit. On the other hand there is need to avoid the possibility of confusing the clinical monitoring of the recently injured patient by giving large doses of depressant anticonvulsants, except when status epilepticus is regarded as a real threat. In a third of cases there is only one early fit, and in 40 percent no generalized convulsion ever occurs. It is necessary, therefore, to maintain a sense of proportion, remembering that probably no harm comes of seizures that remain at the focal motor level. A regimen such as this would be appropriate:

1. *After the first fit* give phenytoin (Diphenyldantoin, Epanutin, Dilantin) 200 mg followed by 100 mg 6 to 8 hours later, orally (or by nasogastric tube).

2. If a further *generalized fit* occurs, consider intramuscular phenytoin, up to 0.8 g as a loading dose (50 mg per minute, monitoring heart rate during investiga-

tion). Further dosage can be by nasogastric tube; if absorption is improved, further IV doses can be given. Whatever route is used, blood levels should be checked and used to regulate dosage (10–20 μg/ml is the therapeutic level). An alternative is phenobarbitone 60 mg every 8 hours, or sodium valproate (Epilim) 200 to 300 mg every 12 hours.

3. If *status epilepticus* has developed, or repeated generalized fits persist, it is an urgent matter to control the situation, because the consequences may be serious, particularly with a recently damaged brain. In these circumstances the disadvantages of using drugs that obscure clinical monitoring are outweighed by the threat of further brain damage, and if necessary other means of excluding intracranial complications must be relied on (ICP pressure measurements, CT scanning).

Diazepam (Valium) is the most widely used drug of first choice, but hypotension is a side-effect to be alert to and ready to counter. Initially 10 mg intravenously coupled with 10 mg intramuscularly should be given. If this is ineffective a continuous intravenous drip is used, up to 40 mg per hour in solution of 50 to 100 mg in 500 ml of glucose saline. This solution is unstable, and a newly mixed bottle should be made up every 6 hours.

Clonazepam (Rivotril) can be given at 1 mg in 1 ml intravenously, or as an infusion (3 mg in 250 ml of saline or dextrose, or a mixture). Injections must be mixed just before use and infusion solutions made up every 12 hours.

Clormethiazole (Heminevrin) is used in solution of 50 mg/ml, giving 40 to 100 mg intravenously over 3 to 5 minutes; it can also be given as a continuous intravenous infusion.

Phenytoin is often effective, given intravenously up to 250 mg initially followed after 30 minutes by a further 150 mg; but cardiac arrhythmias can occur, so the injection rate must not exceed 25 to 50 mg per minute. It precipitates free acid when mixed with intravenous solutions, and a drip infusion cannot therefore be used. Intramuscular dosage is up to 200 mg every 6 hours.

Should these measures prove ineffective, then a thiopentone (Pentothal) drip may be required; in that event it is probably wise to paralyze and ventilate the patient for 1 or 2 days, while maintaining adequate phenytoin dosage. Even though clinical seizures are suppressed, the EEG will indicate when seizure activity in the brain has subsided.

Phenobarbitone is not an appropriate drug for status—it is not very effective, and it accumulates and causes respiratory depression. Nor is valproate, carbamezapine, or mysoline useful.

4. *In patients who have not (yet) had a fit* there may be a case for prophylactic anticonvulsants if the patient is in a high-risk category. Some regimens for the management of severe head injuries include routine phenytoin; for example, Becker and associates give 100 mg every 8 hours. However, the incidence of early epilepsy after combat injuries in Vietnam was not significantly reduced by the routine administration of 3 to 400 mg intramuscular phenytoin within 6 to 7 hours of wounding.[9] This is not surprising considering that so many fits occur on the first day, indeed in the first hour; moreover, after oral or intramuscular administration, attainment of therapeutic levels may not occur for some time and perhaps not at all if the dose is not related to body weight.

The pharmacokinetics of phenytoin have been studied by Young and colleagues[96] with a view to devising a reliable regimen. In order to attain an effective plasma concentration (10–20 μg/ml) rapidly after recent injury, their recommendation is intravenous administration of 11 mg/kg body weight, followed by intra-cannular injection until oral administration is possible. However, most physicians prefer to repeat IV dosage, if necessary, monitoring the blood levels. No results have yet been reported of the reduction of *early* seizures in a large series of patients at risk, but it has been claimed that if this regimen of prophylaxis is instituted, there is a significant reduction in fits during the first year (excluding the first week).

TREATMENT OF RAISED INTRACRANIAL PRESSURE AND THE DAMAGED BRAIN

No one doubts that the prospects for recovery after severe head injury are immediately improved by dealing with adverse factors such as airway obstruction, shock, respiratory dysfunction, and intracranial hematoma. It is less certain what can be done to promote recovery of the brain, or to prevent further secondary damage, once hypoxia and hypotension have been corrected and intracranial mass lesions have been adequately treated surgically. It is when patients remain in coma after all this primary management has been completed that questions arise about the efficacy of a number of other measures. These reputedly act upon the mechanisms underlying various pathophysiological processes leading to second-ary brain damage—ischemia, edema, destructive biochemical reactions, and, less specifically, upon raised intracranial pressure and also upon brain shift and distor-tion. These measures mostly have several effects and these may not always be beneficially additive. For example, reduction of edema may lower ICP and so increase CBF; but reduced ICP may promote the accumulation of edema, as may an extreme increase in CBF. It is wise to consider what particular process is expected to be advantageously influenced by different therapeutic techniques, when considering their possible benefits. Often the complexity of the situation is such that the matter cannot be resolved, and this explains the continued uncer-tainty about the clinical value of methods for which there appears to be a sound theoretical basis.

Raised Intracranial Pressure

There is always a reason for an increased intracranial pressure. The first thing to do when a patient is discovered to have a high level of ICP is to consider what the cause might be, and whether it can be eliminated by some specific measure. This may be as simple as a change in position or the adjustment or clearing of an airway, or it may mean the evacuation of a hematoma. Sometimes no specific cause can be found, and it must be presumed that the raised pressure reflects "swelling" of damaged brain or interference with CSF dynamics.

Then the choice lies between any one of several methods: drainage of CSF; hyperventilation; osmotic agents; diuretics; steroids; or cerebral depressant drugs. Some of these agents may be of value as a means of temporarily reducing ICP, thereby "buying time" until more definitive treatment can be carried out. With each treatment the ICP is reduced by decreasing the volume of one or more of the intracranial components. Some of the measures may also affect those pro-cesses within the damaged brain that ultimately result in "swelling," and thus have specific benefits other than by an influence upon ICP.

239

CSF Withdrawal

Reducing the volume of the cerebrospinal fluid is a simple and almost universally effective method of lowering a raised level of intracranial pressure, whatever its cause. Withdrawal of as little as 1 or 2 ml of CSF can have a marked effect, but it usually lasts for only a few minutes. To achieve a more prolonged reduction of intracranial pressure, repeated withdrawal or continuous drainage must be carried out. This method can, of course, be employed only in patients who have a ventricular catheter in place, and continued drainage can be difficult because the ventricular walls may collapse and obstruct the catheter. When a progressive pathological process is present, rises in pressure can be prevented only by increasingly frequent withdrawals of larger volumes of CSF, the very circumstance in which obstruction of drainage is likely. Obstruction of the catheter is less likely if drainage is carried out to a constant level of pressure of 10 to 15 mm Hg. This can be done in conjunction with continued monitoring of pressure by leading a line from one aperture of the transducer to a drainage bottle and adjusting the height of the latter according to the level of pressure recorded.

Osmotic Agents

The reduction in intracranial pressure which is produced by the intravenous infusion of a hyperosmotic agent depends upon the establishment of an osmotic gradient between the plasma and the brain. This osmotic gradient results in a shift of water from brain to blood and thus a reduction in pressure. Although an increase in plasma osmolality of 30 mosmoles above the normal level of 295 may be required to alter a *normal* intracranial pressure, a rise by 10 mosmoles is almost always enough to reduce *raised* pressure.

The most commonly used osmotic agent is mannitol (molecular weight 180) given as a 20 to 25 percent solution. Solutions of 30 percent urea (molecular weight 60) and 10 percent glycerol (molecular weight 92) have also been used: the equivalent strengths of these solutions will contain more molecules than in the case of mannitol, but this advantage is offset because their smaller molecular weight permits more rapid equilibration in the brain. Neither urea nor mannitol is metabolized, both being excreted unchanged in the urine; glycerol is metabolized rapidly and has a high calorific effect.

There are several possible disadvantages in the use of osmotic agents, particularly when prolonged therapy is considered. The first is that the effect of a single dose lasts for only 3 to 4 hours at the most, because brain and plasma equilibrate. The osmotic gradient dissipates and, because new intracellular osmoles appear, the brain adapts to plasma hyperosmolality by increasing cellular osmolality. Repeated treatment becomes increasingly difficult, since reduction of raised intracranial pressure is achieved only by raising plasma osmolality higher and higher, and this can have serious side-effects, which include severe systemic acidosis and renal failure.[17] When mannitol is discontinued in these circumstances, intracranial pressure usually rises very quickly. Such a rebound increase in intracranial pressure can also appear with smaller doses, but is not common. The effects of mannitol depend upon the presence of an intact blood-brain barrier and the water that is removed may come mainly from relatively normal parts of brain, making it at least theoretically possible that extravasation of mannitol into the edematous area might only increase the edema. This view is probably too

240

simple because it overlooks the possibility that edema may be present in areas with an intact barrier. That this can occur can be shown experimentally in animals with a cryogenic lesion of the cortex: the barrier is disrupted only in the affected area of the cortex, but the edema fluid spreads into the white matter. Studies with tracers such as Evans blue have shown that the barrier remains intact in the white matter, although this is the site of maximum edema. Continued use of repeated doses of mannitol is therefore of doubtful value; by contrast, one or two bolus injections are useful, especially in order to obtain time for investigation and more definitive treatment (e.g., the evacuation of a hematoma), or in order to minimize the risks of a rise in intracranial pressure during a procedure such as intubation.

Views about the appropriate dosage of mannitol vary. In one study[39] mannitol was successful in reducing intracranial pressure in 27 out of 28 head injured patients, but the doses varied between 0.18 g/kg to 2.5 g/kg. Marshall and colleagues[56] have suggested that a relatively small dose of 0.25 g/kg given as a 25 percent solution at a rate of 5 g (20 cc) per minute may be as effective in the short-term as a larger dose, although the latter is more likely to produce a persistent reduction over several hours. The value of low doses has been denied by others and the most widely accepted regimen is 1 g/kg given over 10 to 15 minutes. Serum osmolality should be monitored in order to avoid levels above 320 osmoles/liter.

Mannitol may have effects other than those upon cerebral water content. It may increase cerebral blood flow independently of any change in intracranial pressure, perhaps by a rheological mechanism or perhaps by a direct vasodilatation; it can increase cardiac output; and it can also increase renal plasma flow and urine volume. Urine output should be monitored when mannitol is being given and fluid replacement adjusted accordingly.

Diuretics

Acetazolamide inhibits carbonic anhydrase and reduces the rate of CSF formation, perhaps by impeding sodium transport in the choroid plexuses. Reduction in intracranial pressure might result from the lowered CSF volume or because the lower rate of CSF formation encourages clearance of edema into the ventricles (p. 61). The diuresis produced by acetazolamide is probably not of major importance for effects upon intracranial pressure, but stronger diuretics such as frusemide, which will dehydrate a patient, can be used for this purpose. At present it is not clear whether their beneficial effects depend solely upon increasing plasma osmolality by dehydration or whether they have direct actions upon transport mechanisms in the brain.

Steroids

The response to steroids of many patients with brain tumors is often so dramatic that no one doubts their effectiveness in this situation. By contrast, the value of steroids in head injury remains uncertain in spite of studies both in patients and in animals with experimental injuries.

It has been believed that the beneficial effects of steroids in a patient with a brain tumor are due to an effect upon the blood-brain barrier and a reduction in perifocal edema. Yet improvement may take place without any change in intracranial pressure and without any effect upon edema (as detected by CT scan). The

241

basis for the beneficial effect of steroids after head injury can only be speculative at present. Steroids seem most likely to be effective when there is edema in association with a defective blood-brain barrier, and the incidence of both edema (as opposed to brain swelling or raised intracranial pressure) and blood-brain barrier dysfunction is unknown in the clinical situation. Steroids may also stabilize cellular membranes and so prevent the harmful effects of lysozome rupture and free radical action. The beneficial effects of steroids in experimental studies are greatest when they are given before the lesion is produced, but are not usually evident until 24 hours after trauma and do not appear to depend upon the level of dosage.[89] Pretreatment with steroids has been reported to reduce the complication rate among patients undergoing the controlled trauma of cortical resection for epilepsy,[76] but this is impossible in head injured patients. Gurdjian and Webster,[31] Sano and colleagues,[81] Sporachio,[84] and French[21] described clinical benefit in response to steroid therapy in uncontrolled series of head injured patients. Subsequent experience was, however, less impressive.[32] A controlled study was undertaken by Ransohoff[75] in severely head injured patients, employing 1 to 5 mg methylprednisolone every 6 hours, commencing within 24 hours of admission. Survival was doubled in the steroid treated group, but the difference was not significant and no benefit was seen in patients with subdural hematomas. Other controlled studies[37,55] also failed to show any beneficial effects from steriods. In contrast are the results of two controlled studies carried out in Germany, which employed much higher doses of steroids than previously: an initial bolus of 48 mg of dexamethasone followed by 8 mg every 2 hours in one study[26] and two injections of 100 mg dexamethasone followed by 4 mg four times a day in the other.[16] In both studies survival was higher among patients treated with the high-dose steroids when compared with those receiving conventional doses or no steroids, but in at least one study there was considerable disability among the extra survivors in the steroid treated group. More recent studies, however, have not shown any clear benefit,[13] and there is no firm evidence that high-dose steroids should be given to severely head injured patients.

Hyperventilation

Hyperventilation can reduce intracranial blood volume both by active vasoconstriction and perhaps also by an effect upon central venous pressure. It may also reduce CSF formation. The use of ventilation and hyperventilation in head injured patients has been discussed previously (p. 225).

Hypothermia

The ability of hypothermia to protect the brain when oxygen delivery is decreased or absent is well established. The magnitude of protection is related to the extent of the decrease in temperature: at 28°C the cerebral circulation can be interrupted for at least 8 minutes; at 15°C the brain of an infant can tolerate as much as an hour of circulatory arrest. Cold decreases the rates of biochemical reactions; decreasing body temperature is accompanied by increasing cerebral metabolic depression, and it is likely that the protective effects of hypothermia are related to the depression of cerebral metabolism.

Hypothermia increases survival after an experimental head injury of moderate severity,[79] but early clinical studies did not give encouraging results. Some patients appeared to improve as temperature was reduced, but relapsed when rewarmed and often died. Hypothermia was also associated with systemic complications such as pneumonia and gastrointestinal bleeding. Because of these problems, hypothermia fell out of vogue in the management of head injury. However, James and associates[39] have recently reported that hypothermia (27–36°C), induced by placing a patient between blankets and using ice bags, reduced intracranial pressure by an average of 50 percent in 6 out of 15 head injured patients. The maximum effect could take several hours to detect. Hypothermia alone is not recommended as a treatment for head injury, but it may be of value in combination with other agents that depress metabolism, such as barbiturates.

Hyperbaric Oxygen

Like hypothermia, hyperbaric oxygen has had its vogue in the treatment of brain damage. Also, as with hypothermia, a patient's intracranial pressure may fall during treatment, and his condition appear to improve temporarily, but permanent benefit does not seem to ensue. After treatment is discontinued there may be a rebound increase in intracranial pressure.[67] Moreover, the effect of hyperbaric oxygen depends upon the cerebrovascular response to hypocapnia being intact, and hyperventilation may be equally effective and simpler.[65]

Barbiturates

Barbiturates and many other anesthetics depress cerebral metabolism (probably by stabilizing electrically active membranes and decreasing the work of the brain). It seems certain that they can protect experimental animals against some of the metabolic, structural, and functional effects of a variety of experimental ischemic insults. This applies whether the drugs are given before or shortly after the induction of ischemia. Many aspects of their use are, however, at present uncertain: their precise mode of action; the appropriate time, duration, and dosage of administration; and whether they have additive effects with other measures, such as hypothermia. The maximum depression of cerebral metabolism occurs with a relatively low dose of barbiturates, yet some reports indicate that large doses are necessary in order to demonstrate a protective effect in the experimental animal. Also, if the protective effects of barbiturates were due only to the energy-sparing effects of the depression in electrical activity that they produce, then when the degree of ischemia is sufficient to abolish electrical activity they should be ineffective. This does not seem to be so, and they may even have beneficial effects when cerebral ischemia has been severe enough to deplete all the brain's energy reserves. In these circumstances their benefits may lie in controlling the destructive processes that are initiated once the circulation is reestablished. At the cellular level these actions may include a decrease in lipid peroxidation (p. 51) and a reduction of lysosomal activity. Barbiturates may also increase blood flow to an area of damaged brain, either because the reduction in the metabolic demands in the normal parts of the brain results in the redistribution of blood flow to the damaged area or because overall perfusion is improved as a result of the reduction in the intracranial pressure that can be achieved when they are given.

In clinical studies Shapiro and colleagues[83] have reported that some patients with raised intracranial pressure that had been unresponsive to other treatments showed reduced pressure when pentobarbitone was given. Subsequently, Marshall, Smith, and Shapiro[58] treated 25 patients whose intracranial pressures were greater than 40 mm Hg for at least 15 minutes, despite treatment with steroids, hyperventilation, mannitol, and CSF drainage. Pentobarbitone (3–5 mg/kg) reduced intracranial pressure in 19 patients. After the initial loading dose, pentobarbitone was continued at the rate of 1 mg/kg/hour, yielding a blood level of 2.5 to 4 mg percent and being associated with an EEG frequency of 2 to 5 Hz. The rate of administration was also controlled in order to adjust cerebral perfusion pressure to between 60 and 70 mm Hg. Proportionally similar doses of barbiturates have been given to 20 head injured children who were either flaccid or who had abnormal motor responses and intracranial pressure levels above 20 mm Hg. Fifteen made moderate or good recoveries. The use of these dosages of barbiturates results in depression of respiration, so that all patients require controlled ventilation, and in many cases systemic hypotension is also a problem. The question whether barbiturates can improve the outcome of severely head injured patients cannot at present be satisfactorily answered, and the proponents of this therapy are proceeding to randomized controlled trials.[64] In the meantime, we would advise against their use in ordinary clinical practice, outside of such trials.

Influence of Medical Treatments upon Outcome

The efficacy of the measures discussed above in lowering elevated ICP and, in occasional patients, in halting or reverting an impending tentorial compression, does not seem to be followed consistently by improved outcome.

Indeed, reviewing mortality over recent decades, Langfitt[50] concluded that there had been little improvement in spite of the application of several measures designed to control the secondary events that threaten life after injury. Three explanations are possible. One is that therapy is ineffective. Another is that more efficient resuscitation and transportation enable more hopelessly injured patients to reach special centers, where they soon die; this maintains a high mortality rate, even though other patients are doing better than previously. The third is that methods of assessment vary so much from place to place, or from time to time, that like is not compared with like, and the value of effective treatment is thereby obscured.

The last is the most readily dealt with, by the use of standardized systems for assessing initial severities, subsequent progress, and ultimate outcome. This has already been done for over 1000 patients prospectively collected as part of a collaborative study based on Glasgow, Netherlands, and Los Angeles.[42] Although methods of clinical assessment were rigorously controlled in this study, no attempt was made to standardize treatment, but the therapies used were recorded. There were marked differences between the three countries in the frequency with which some treatments were used (Table 5). Some methods of therapy were more often used in the more severely injured patients, but even when these factors, the age of the patient, and the presence or absence of hematoma were allowed for, statistical analysis showed that there was no difference in outcome when steroids were administered. Tracheostomy, intubation, controlled or triggered ventilation, use of osmotics, or removal of the bone flap (after evacuation of an IC hematoma) was each associated with a *higher* mortality than occurred in patients of similar severity and age who were not so treated. This effect was independent of the presence of a major chest injury, although this was the reason for some patients

244

Table 5. Frequency of treatments and outcome in head injured patients who were in coma for 6 hours at different centers

	Glasgow n=507	Los Angeles n=224	Netherlands n=302
Steroids	24%	99%	34%
Tracheostomy	10%	66%	15%
Intubation/			
tracheostomy-3D	38%	70%	61%
Assisted ventilation	18%	62%	28%
Bone flap removed (% of			
craniotomies)	28%	93%	92%
Osmotics	86%	78%	69%
Dead or Vegetative (6 months after			
injury)	49%	54%	50%

(Data from Jennett et al.[42])

having tracheostomy and ventilation; it was also the same irrespective of the stage after injury at which the patient was admitted to the neurosurgical or neurological unit. Moreover, we could find no evidence that series of patients treated with each of these therapies had better outcomes than was predicted on the basis of data from patients not so treated (p. 327).

The uniformity of the outcomes for series of patients well matched for severity, but treated by different techniques, does not prove that these various methods may not be effective for some patients in some circumstances. It does, however, suggest that methods that can be applied in the experimental laboratory, where it is possible to control intracranial events over a matter of hours, may not be easy to translate into successful clinical use as a routine matter over days and weeks. Provided that patients receive a high standard of basic care, which concentrates upon the avoidance of complications, outcome seems predominantly determined by age and severity of brain damage. A parallel study in medical coma has come to similar conclusions.[5] Reports of series of patients, who have been managed "intensively" or "aggressively" and who have apparently better outcomes than those in the Data Bank,[6,8,57,60] have not achieved as close a match as is required for the evidence of efficacy to be completely convincing. Differences in the time when severity of injury is assessed, the age distribution, the proportion of patients with a hematoma, and the size of the sample can all make significant changes in the estimated mortality (p. 336).

There is a need for studies in order to determine the most effective combination of methods of treatment already in general use; those recently introduced in a few centers, such as barbiturates; and those that may be considered in the future. These last include such compounds as the alkalizing agent THAM;[1] dimethylsulfoxide (DMSO), which has diuretic, vasodilatatory, and anti-inflammatory properties; and the inhibitors or antagonists of catecholamines, prostaglandins, and other substances that may be involved in the biochemical process whereby brain damage is aggravated. It is unrealistic to expect that the effect of any of these will be such a dramatic change that there will not be a need for rigorously conducted studies to detect any benefit they confer. Due consideration must be given to how

245

soon after injury intensive treatment begins, as there is good evidence that adverse secondary events begin to operate within a few hours. It may be that the good results reported already are partly derived from the prompt application of conventional active measures rather than the introduction of certain specific additional treatments.

Pharmacological Treatment for Persisting Disability

Gerstenbrand suggested that some of the disorders in the "apallic syndrome" might be due to a deficiency in dopaminergic activity and might therefore be improved by administration of L-dopa.[25] Several workers have reported low CSF levels of HVA, a dopamine metabolite, and increased 5HlAA (a serotonin metabolite) in such patients. Some, but not all, patients with abnormal motor responses and loss of contact (and awareness), but with normal arousal (sleep/wake cycles), are clearly more responsive when taking L-dopa. The presence of dopaminergic neurons and synapses, which are structurally intact but whose function is impaired, is probably essential for a response to take place. Marked improvement appears to occur only in the first month or two of injury, and then may merely anticipate what would have occurred naturally.

PRIORITIES IN MANAGEMENT OF MULTIPLE INJURIES

Multiple injuries, of which one is a head injury, present problems in initial assessment and early management (Fig. 7). The demands of the cranial and extracranial injuries may conflict, and unless wise decisions about priorities are made by surgeons of appropriate seniority, tragedies can result. The effect that other injuries may have on initial impressions about the severity of brain damage has already been discussed (p. 97). Once initial resuscitation is completed the diagnostic scene must be reviewed, and established or suspected injuries listed. Some may require early urgent measures (including investigations under anesthesia, e.g., CT scan), but from the head injury viewpoint only those that are immediately life-threatening should be dealt with immediately. It is important during the first 24 hours after injury, when the intracranial conditions may undergo so much change, that those concerned with monitoring brain dysfunction should not be deprived of the opportunity to maintain careful clinical observation—as would be the case if the patient were under anesthesia for a long period for definitive nonurgent surgery for extracranial injuries.

But anesthesia and operative procedures may also directly aggravate brain damage, unless due care is taken to avoid the use of anesthetic agents that cause cerebral vasodilatation, and that may therefore raise intracranial pressure; and to avoid hypotension and hypoxia, which may threaten brain oxygenation. The need for early intervention for extracranial conditions that are not life-threatening, but in which the ultimate result may be affected by undue delay, must be balanced with the risk of further brain damage. It is of little benefit to have a good cosmetic result for facial fractures, or functional restoration of tendons and nerves, if the patient is thereby made a worse cerebral cripple than he need be.

The first priority is undoubtedly to secure the injured person's grip on life, but management evolves progressively, with resuscitation, assessment, diagnosis, and treatment being interdependent. Moreover, the clinical picture will often change considerably during the course of resuscitation, with new and helpful signs

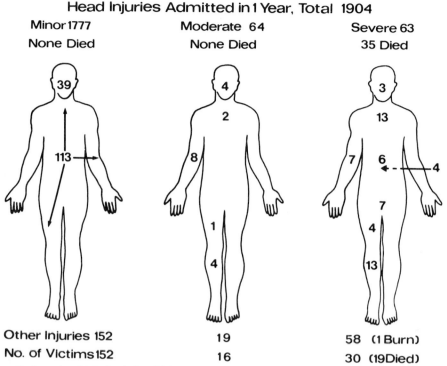

Figure 7. Associated injuries in head injured patients admitted to the Birmingham Accident Hospital. (Redrawn from London[54])

emerging like rocks from the sea as the tide of shock or acute respiratory embarrassment recedes.[54] Nevertheless it is useful to consider what action may be needed immediately, what is urgent, what must be expedited, and what can be deferred.

AN OUTLINE OF THE EARLY MANAGEMENT OF HEAD INJURY

I. **Normal consciousness. No focal signs**
    X-ray skull
    Suture any scalp laceration
    Treat other injuries
    Consider need for admission

II. **Impaired consciousness or focal signs**
    Assess brain function—establish a baseline on the coma scale and assess pupils, focal signs, and eye movements
    Actively seek to exclude associated injuries
    X-ray skull
    Consider possible influence of alcohol and other drugs on the patient's state
    Consider whether definitive neuroradiological investigation is required immediately or should be deferred until evidence of lack of improvement or of deterioration
    Evacuate unilateral lesion with shift of midline

Consider whether continuous monitoring should be limited to clinical recording or should include measurement of intracranial pressure or respiratory pattern or other parameters

Consider whether any immediate drug treatment is required (e.g., anticonvulsants, antibiotics, or steroids)

III. **Early management of unconscious patient with possible multiple injuries**

Immediate resuscitation (within minutes)

Airway—clear by positioning and suction, and insert whatever mechanical airway can be tolerated

Breathing—administer oxygen-enriched mixture if spontaneous respiration present; otherwise give artificial ventilation

Circulation—restore normotension; temporary head-down may be accepted, although it will increase intracranial venous congestion and so raise intracranial pressure; insert large bore i.v. cannula

Urgent assessment and action (within minutes or first hours)

Assess—consciousness; visceral injuries; spinal injuries; major limb injuries

Arrange—x-rays of spine; chest; abdomen; skull

Action

Pneumo/hemothorax with mediastinal shift; flail chest—drain; (?) ventilate

Spinal injury—collar; back board or halter traction; immobilize limb injuries in splints

Ruptured spleen/liver—diagnostic paracentesis; (?) laparotomy

Suspected early intracranial hematoma—CT scan or operate

Appraise—need for monitoring of intravascular (systemic/pulmonary/central venous) and intracranial pressures

Administer—prophylaxis against tetanus and other infections; (?)drugs acting on damaged brain; (?) anticonvulsants

Expedite in first 24 hours

Skeletal traction to reduce and immobilize a cervical spine injury

Operation for

Intracranial hematoma

Compound depressed fracture of skull

Gut/bladder perforation into peritoneum

Continued hemorrhage from crushed kidney

Compound limb fracture

Closed limb fracture needing internal fixation to facilitate in management (e.g., with vascular injury)

Primary suture of tendons/nerves

Primary suture of face and other lacerations

Defer for up to 1 to 2 weeks

Internal fixation of limb and spinal fractures

Faciomaxillary wiring

Repair of CSF leak

REFERENCES

1. AKIOKA, T., OTA, K., MATSUMOTO, K., ET AL.: "The effects of THAM on acute intracranial hypertension. An experimental and clinical study." In Beks, Bosch and Brock (eds.): *Intracranial Pressure, III.* Springer Verlag, Berlin, 1976, pp. 219–223.

2. ALLISON, S. P.: *Metabolic aspects of intensive care.* Br. J. Anaesth. 49:689–696, 1977.

3. APUZZO, M. L. J., WEISS, M. H., PETERSONS, V., ET AL.: *Effect of positive end expiratory pressure ventilation on intracranial pressure in man.* J. Neurosurg. 46:227–238, 1977.

4. ATTAR, S., BOYD, D., LAYNE, E., ET AL.: *Alterations in coagulation and fibrinolytic mechanisms in acute trauma.* J. Trauma 9:939, 1969.

5. BATES, D., CARONNA, J. J., CARTLIDGE, N. E. F., ET AL.: *A prospective study of nontraumatic coma: methods and results in 310 patients.* Ann. Neurol. 2:211–220, 1977.

6. BECKER, D. P., MILLER, J. D., WARD, J. D., ET AL.: *The outcome from severe head injury with early diagnosis and intensive management.* J. Neurosurg. 47:491–502, 1977.

7. BRANSTON, N. M., SYMON, L., CROCKARD, H. A., ET AL.: "Dependence of the cortical evoked response on the local tissue blood flow in baboons and its sensitivity to arterial PO_2." In Harper, Jennett, Miller, et al. (eds.): *Blood Flow and Metabolism in the Brain.* Churchill Livingstone, Edinburgh, 1975, pp. 14.22–14.26.

8. BRUCE, D. A., GENNARELLI, T. A., AND LANGFITT, T. W.: *Recovery from coma due to head injury.* Crit. Care Med. 6:254–269, 1978.

9. CAVENESS, W. F., AND LISS, H. R.: *Incidence of post-traumatic epilepsy.* Epilepsia 2:123–129, 1961.

10. CHRISTENSEN, M. S.: *Prolonged artificial hyperventilation in cerebral apoplexy.* Acta Anaesth. Scand. Suppl. 62, 1976.

11. COHEN, P. J., REIVICH, M., AND GREENBHOM, L. J.: "Electroencephalographic changes induced by 100% oxygen breathing at 3 atmospheres in man." In Brown, and Cox (eds.): *Proceedings of the 3rd International Congress on Hyperbaric Medicine.* National Academy of Sciences, Washington, D.C., 1966.

12. COLD, G. E., JENSEN, F. T., AND MALMROS, R.: *The effects of $PaCO_2$ reduction on regional cerebral blood flow in the acute phase of brain injury.* Acta Anaesth. Scand. 21:359–367, 1977.

13. COOPER, P. R., MOODY, S., CLARK, W. K., ET AL.: *Dexamethasone and severe head injury: a prospective double-blind study.* J. Neurosurg. 51:307–316, 1979.

14. DOMONKOS, J., AND HUSZAK, I.: *Effect of hydrogen ion concentration on the carbohydrate metabolism of brain tissue.* J. Neurochem. 4:238, 1959.

15. EALES, G., AND SEVITT, S.: *Coagulation and fibrinolysis in injured patients.* J. Clin. Pathol. 17:1–13, 1969.

16. FAUPEL, G., REULEN, H. J., MULLER, D., ET AL.: "Double blind study on the effects of dexamethasone on severe closed head injury." In Pappius, and Feindel (eds.): *Dynamics of Brain Oedema.* Springer Verlag, New York, 1976, pp. 337–343.

17. FEIG, P. U., AND McCURDY, D. K.: *The hypertonic state.* N. Engl. J. Med. 297: 1449, 1977.

18. FISHMAN, A. P.: *Pulmonary oedema: a new dimension.* Circulation 46:390–408, 1972.

19. FLEISCHER, A. S., RUDMAN, D. R., PAYNE, N. S., ET AL.: *Hypothalamic hypothyroidism and hypogonadism in prolonged traumatic coma.* J. Neurosurg. 49:650–657, 1978.

20. FORREST, J. B.: *The effect of hyperventilation on pulmonary surface activity.* Br. J. Anaesth. 44:313–320, 1972.

21. FRENCH, L. A.: *The use of steroids in the treatment of cerebral oedema.* Bull. N.Y. Assoc. Med. 42:301–311, 1966.

22. FREY, C., HUELKE, D. F., AND GIKAS, P. W.: *Resuscitation and survival in motor vehicle accidents.* J. Trauma 9:292, 1969.

23. FROST, E. A. M.: *Respiratory problems associated with head trauma.* Neurosurgery 1:300–305, 1977.

24. FROST, E. A. M., AND GILDENBERG, P. L.: *Effects of positive end expiratory pressure in intracranial pressure and compliance in brain injured patients.* J. Neurosurg. 47:195–200, 1977.

25. GERSTENBRAND, F.: *Das traumatische apallische syndrom.* Wien. Springer Verlag, New York, 1967.

26. GOBIET, W., BOCK, W. J., LEISEGANG, J., ET AL.: "Treatment of acute cerebral oedema with high dose dexamethasone." In Beks, Bosch, and Brock (eds.): *Intracranial Pressure, III.* Springer Verlag, Berlin, 1976, pp. 231–235.

27. GORDON, E.: *Controlled respiration in the management of patients with traumatic brain injuries.* Acta Anaesth. Scand. 15:193–208, 1971.

28. GORDON, E.: "Management of acute head injuries by controlled ventilation." In Rias, Llaurado, Nalda, et al. (eds.): *Recent Progress in Anaesthesiology and Resuscitation*. Exerpta Medica, Amsterdam, 1975, pp. 784–789.

29. GORDON, E., AND ROSSANDA, M.: *Further studies on cerebrospinal acid-base states in patients with brain lesions*. Acta Anaesth. Scand. 14:97, 1970.

30. GRUBER, V. F., AND RITTMAN, W. W.: *Hypovolaemic shock—therapy of hypervolaemia and respiratory insufficiency*. Triangle 13:91, 1979.

31. GURDJIAN, E. S., AND WEBSTER, J. E.: *Head Injuries—Mechanism, Diagnosis and Management*. Little, Brown and Co., Boston, 1958.

32. GUTTERMAN, P., AND SHENKIN, I. M.: *Prognostic features in recovery from traumatic decerebration*. J. Neurosurg. 32:330–335, 1970.

33. HAIDER, W., LACKNER, F., SCHLICK, W., ET AL.: *Metabolic changes in the course of severe acute brain damage*. Eur. J. Intensive Care Med. 1:19, 1975.

34. HENDRICK, E. B., AND HARRIS, L.: *Post-traumatic epilepsy in children*. J. Trauma 8:547, 1968.

35. HOFF, J., NISHIMURA, N., AND PITTS, L. H.: "A quantitative method of neurogenic pulmonary oedema in cats." In McLaurin (ed.): *Head Injuries*. Grune & Stratton, New York, 1975, pp. 141–145.

36. HOFFMAN, E.: *Mortality and morbidity following road accidents*. Ann. R. Coll. Surg. Engl. 58:233, 1976.

37. HOYT, H. J., GOLDSTEIN, T. P., REIGEL, D. H., ET AL.: *Clinical evaluation of water-soluble steroids in the treatment of cerebral oedema of traumatic origin. A double blind study*. Clin. Pharmacol. Ther. 13:141, 1972.

38. ILLINGWORTH, G., AND JENNETT, B.: *The shocked head injury*. Lancet ii:511–514, 1965.

39. JAMES, H. E., LANGFITT, T. W., KUMAR, V. S., ET AL.: *Treatment of intracranial hypertension. Analysis of 105 consecutive continuous recordings of intracranial pressure*. Acta Neurochir. 36:189–200, 1977.

40. JENNETT, B.: *Early traumatic epilepsy*. Arch. Neurol. 30:394–398, 1974.

41. JENNETT, B., AND CARLIN, J.: *Preventable mortality and morbidity after head injury*. Injury 10:31–39, 1979.

42. JENNETT, B., TEASDALE, G., FRY, J., ET AL.: *Treatment for severe head injury*. J. Neurol. Neurosurg. Psychiatry 43:289–295, 1980.

43. KATSUDURA, K., YAMADA, R., AND SUGIMOTO, T.: *Respiratory insufficiency in patients with severe head injury*. Surgery 73:191–199, 1973.

44. KELMAN, G. R.: *Interpretation of CVP measurements*. Anaesthesia 28:209, 1971.

45. KING, L. R., MCLAURIN, R. L., LEWIS, H. P., ET AL.: *Plasma cortisol levels after head injury*. Ann. Surg. 172:975–989, 1970.

46. KNOWLES, H. C., JR., AND KING, L. R.: "Personal communications. Cited by McLaurin and King." In Vinken, and Bruyn (eds.): *Handbook of Clinical Neurology 24*. North Holland Publishing Co., Amsterdam, 1973.

47. KRENN, J., STEINBEREITHNER, K., SPORN, P., ET AL.: "The value of routine respiratory treatment in severe brain trauma." In *Advances in Neurosurgery*. Vol. 3. Springer Verlag, Berlin.

48. KULNER, A., ROQUEFEUIL, B., VIGVIE, E., ET AL.: "Artificial ventilation in cerebral oedema—cerebral analysis of manometric and gasometric conditions." In Schurmann, Brock, Reulen, et al. (eds.): *Advances in Neurosurgery*. Springer Verlag, Berlin. 1973, pp. 178–190.

49. LANCET: Editorial—*Preventing secondary brain damage after head injury*. Lancet ii:1189–1190, 1978.

50. LANGFITT, T. W.: *Measuring the outcome from head injuries*. J. Neurosurg. 48:673–678, 1978.

51. LAWLER, P. G. P., AND NUNN, J. F.: *Intermittent mandatory ventilation. A discussion and a description of necessary modifications to the Brompton Manley ventilator*. Anaesthesia 32:138–147, 1977.

52. LINDHOLM, C. E., AND GRENVIK, A.: "Flexible fibreoptic bronchoscopy and intubation in intensive care." In Ledingham (ed.): *Recent Advances in Intensive Therapy*. Churchill Livingstone, Edinburgh, 1977, pp. 47–66.

53. LINDHOLM, C. E., OLLMAN, B., SNYDER, J., ET AL.: *Flexible fibreoptic bronchoscopy in critical care medicine*. Crit. Care Med. 2:250, 1979.

250

54. LONDON, P. S.: "The management of persons with multiple injuries." In Robb, and Smith (eds.): *Accident Surgery*. Butterworths, London, 1964, pp. 95–184.

55. LONG, D. M., AND MAXWELL, R. E.: "Steroids in the treatment of head injury." In Vinken, and Bruyn (eds.): *Handbook of Clinical Neurology 24*. North Holland Publishing Co., Amsterdam, 1976, pp. 627–635.

56. MARSHALL, L. F., SMITH, R. W., RAUSCHER, L. A., ET AL.: *Mannitol dose requirements in brain injured patients*. J. Neurosurg. 48:169–172, 1978.

57. MARSHALL, L. F., SMITH, R. W., AND SHAPIRO, H. M.: *The outcome with aggressive treatment in severe head injuries. I. The significance of intracranial pressure monitoring*. J. Neurosurg. 50:20–25, 1979.

58. MARSHALL, L. F., SMITH, R. W., AND SHAPIRO, H. M.: *The outcome with aggressive treatment in severe head injuries. II. Acute and chronic barbiturate administration in the management of head injury*. J. Neurosurg. 50:26–30, 1979.

59. MCKAY, G. M.: *Some features of traffic accidents*. Br. Med. J. 4:799, 1969.

60. MCLAURIN, R. L., AND KING, L. R.: "Metabolic effects of head injury." In Vinken, and Bruyn (eds.): *Handbook of Clinical Neurology 24*. North Holland Publishing Co., Amsterdam, 1976, pp. 109–131.

61. MICHENFELDER, J. D., AND SUNDT, T. M., JR.: *The effect of $PaCO_2$ on the metabolism of ischaemic brain in squirrel monkeys*. Anaesthesiology 38:445, 1973.

62. MILLER, J. D.: "Effects of long term controlled ventilation in intracranial hypertension." In Lundberg, Ponten, and Brock (eds.): *Intracranial Pressure, II*. Springer Verlag, Berlin, 1975, pp. 467–469.

63. MILLER, J. D.: *The search for optimal management of head injury*. Med. Coll. Virginia Q. 13:97–106, 1977.

64. MILLER, J. D.: *Barbiturates and raised intracranial pressure*. Ann. Neurol. 6:189–193, 1979.

65. MILLER, J. D., AND LEDINGHAM, I. MCA.: *Reduction of increased intracranial pressure*. Arch. Neurol. 24:210–216, 1971.

66. MILLER, J. D., SWEET, R. C., NARAYAN, R., ET AL.: *Early insults to the injured brain*. J. A. M. A. 240:439–442, 1978.

67. MOGAMI, H., HAYAKAWA, T., KANAS, N., ET AL.: *Clinical application of hyperbaric oxygenation in the treatment of acute cerebral damage*. J. Neurosurg. 31:636–643, 1969.

68. MOSS, E., GIBSON, J. S., AND MCDOWALL, D. G.: *The effects of nitrous oxide, althesin and thiopentone on ICP during chest physiotherapy in patients with severe head injury*. Proceedings of the 4th ICP Symposium, 1979.

69. MOSS, G., STAUNTON, C., AND STEIN, A.: *Cerebral aetiology of the "shock lung syndrome."* J. Trauma 12:885–890, 1972.

70. OBRZUT, A., JARZYNA, A., SKRZYDLEWSKI, Z., ET AL.: *Thrombo-elastographical evaluation of the coagulation system of the blood and fibrinolysis in craniocerebral injuries*. Minerva Neurochir. 11:42, 1967.

71. PAPO, I., AND CARUSELLI, G.: "Intracranial pressure monitoring in intensive care patients suffering from acute head injury." In Beks, Bosch, and Brock (eds.): *Intracranial Pressure, III*. Springer Verlag, Berlin, 1976, pp. 110–113.

72. PITTS, L. H., SEVERINGHAUS, J. W., MITCHELL, R. A., ET AL.: "The role of increased intracranial pressure in the production of neurogenic pulmonary oedema." In Lundberg, Ponten, and Brock (eds.): *Intracranial Pressure, II*. Springer Verlag, Berlin, 1975, pp. 319–323.

73. PLUM, F., POSNER, J. B., AND SMITH, W. W.: *Effect of hyperbaric-hyperoxic hyperventilation on blood brain and cerebrospinal fluid*. Am. J. Physiol. 215:1240, 1968.

74. PRICE, D. J., AND SLEIGH, J. D.: *Control of infection due to Klebsiella aerogenes in a neurosurgical unit by withdrawal of all antibiotics*. Lancet ii:1213–1215, 1970.

75. RANSOHOFF, J.: "The effects of steroids on brain oedema in man." In Reulen, and Schurmann (eds.): *Steroids and Brain Oedema*. Springer Verlag, Berlin, 1972.

76. RASMUSSEN, T., AND GULATI, D. R.: *Cortisone in the treatment of post-operative cerebral oedema*. J. Neurosurg. 19:535–544, 1962.

77. RICHARD, K. E., ELSNER, A., AND FIELDER, V.: "The behaviour of intraventricular pressure under discontinuous long term controlled ventilation in cases of severe brain lesions." In Lund-

251

berg, Ponten, and Brock (eds.): *Intracranial Pressure, II.* Springer Verlag, Berlin, 1975, pp. 485–489.

78. ROSE, J., VALTONEN, S., AND JENNETT, B.: *Avoidable factors contributing to death after head injury.* Br. Med. J. 2:615–618, 1977.

79. ROSOMOFF, H. L., SHULMAN, K., AND RAYNOR, R.: *Experimental brain injury and delayed hypothermia.* Surg. Gynecol. Obstet. 116:27–32, 1960.

80. ROSSANDA, M., SELENATI, A., VILLA, L., ET AL.: *Role of automatic ventilation in treatment of severe head injuries.* J. Neurosurg. Sci. 17:265–270, 1973.

81. SANO, K., HATANAKA, H., KAMANO, S., ET AL.: *Steroids and the blood brain barrier with special reference to the treatment of brain oedema.* Neurol. Med. Chir. 5:21–43, 1963.

82. SCOTTISH HEAD INJURY MANAGEMENT STUDY: *Head injuries in Scottish hospitals.* Lancet ii:696–698, 1977.

83. SHAPIRO, H. M., WYTE, S. R., AND LOESER, J.: *Barbiturate-augmented hypothermia for reduction of persistent intracranial hypertension.* J. Neurosurg. 40:90–100, 1979.

84. SPORACHIO, R. R., LIN, T. H., AND COOK, A. W.: *Multiple prednisolone sodium succinate in acute craniocerebral trauma.* Surg. Gynecol. Obstet. 121:513–516, 1965.

85. STAUB, N. C.: *Pulmonary oedema.* Physiol. Rev. 54:678–811, 1974.

86. STEINBOK, P., AND THOMPSON, G. B.: *Metabolic disturbance after head injury. Abnormalities of sodium and water balance with special reference to the effects of alcohol intoxication.* Neurosurgery 3:9–15, 1978.

87. SWAN, H. J. C., GANZ, W., FORESTER, J., ET AL.: *Catheterisation of the heart in man with the use of a flow directed balloon-tipped catheter.* N. Engl. J. Med. 283:447, 1970.

88. THEODORE, J., AND ROBIN, E. D.: *Pathogenesis of neurogenic pulmonary oedema.* Lancet ii:749–751, 1975.

89. THORNHEIM, P. A., AND McLAURIN, R. L.: *Effect of dexamethasone on cerebral oedema from cranial impact in the cat.* J. Neurosurg. 48:220–227, 1978.

90. TRINKLE, J. K., RICHARDSON, J. D., FRANZ, J. L., ET AL.: *Management of flail chest without mechanical ventilation.* Ann. Thorac. Surg. 19:355, 1975.

91. VANDER ARK, G. D.: *Comments on respiratory problems associated with head trauma.* Neurosurgery 1:305, 1977.

92. VAN DER SANDE, J. J., VELTKAMP, J. J., BOEKHOUT-MUSSERT, R. J., ET AL.: *Head injury and coagulation disorders.* J. Neurosurg. 49:357–365, 1978.

93. VECHT, C. J., SIBINGA, C. T. S., AND MINDERHOUD, J. M.: *Disseminated intravascular coagulation and head injury.* J. Neurol. Neurosurg. Psychiatry 38:567–571, 1975.

94. YATES, D. W.: *Airway patency in fatal accidents.* Br. Med. J. 2:1249–1251, 1977.

95. YEN, J. K., RHODES, G. R., BOURKE, R. S., ET AL.: *Delayed impairment of arterial blood oxygenation in patients with severe head injury: preliminary report.* Surg. Neurol. 9:323–327, 1978.

96. YOUNG, B., RAPP, R. P., PERRIER, D., ET AL.: *Early post-traumatic epilepsy prophylaxis.* Surg. Neurol. 4:339–342, 1975.

CHAPTER 10

Recovery After Head Injury

Recovery of function after acute brain damage is a remarkable phenomenon, the mechanism of which is almost wholly obscure. There is much controversy about the kind of recovery to be expected under various circumstances, and about how to distinguish recovery that is spontaneous from that which is related to specific therapeutic interventions. Clarification of this complex problem calls for analysis of several separate issues:

1. Describing the *process of recovery*, its rate and sequence, by measuring changes in the patient's state, on a time scale appropriate to the interval after injury—initially day-to-day, then over weeks or months.

2. Assessing the *outcome*, once this has become relatively stable. This requires definition of the nature of the mental and physical disabilities and of the social consequences of different combinations of these disabilities.

3. *Predicting* the ultimate degree of disability after severe injury, to facilitate management decisions.

4. Identifying those factors that can *influence recovery*, favorably or unfavorably, and that can be controlled or manipulated.

5. Understanding the *biological substrate of recovery*, in order to devise ways and means of affecting it favorably.

This chapter will deal with this last topic, the early stages of recovery from coma, the postconcussional syndrome, and the principles of prediction. Subsequent chapters will be concerned with persisting neurophysical (Chapter 11) and mental disabilities (Chapter 12); with the assessment of ultimate outcome (Chapter 13); and with the prediction of recovery after severe injury (Chapter 14).

STRUCTURAL SUBSTRATE OF RECOVERY AND OF SEQUELAE

The lack of a good animal model for reproducing the clinical or pathological features of the acute stage of human head injuries has already been discussed (p. 20). The experiments of Ommaya (p. 22) have indicated some of the transitory changes in the intracranial milieu associated with a blow to the head. These include the mechanical movement of the brain and alterations both in intracranial pressure and in cerebral blood flow; these all have secondary effects on the electrical and metabolic activity of the brain. However, even these hard-won data shed only a dim light on the mechanism of concussion—if by this is meant the temporary suppression of activity in large areas of the brain following a blunt impact. It is even more difficult to study the process of recovery at the functional or structural level. Achieving the prolonged survival of badly brain damaged animals is difficult, both in practical terms and because there may be ethical objections. Moreover, large numbers of animals would be required if recovering brain was to be examined at varying intervals after injury.

This makes it all the more important to undertake systematic clinical observations during recovery from brain damage. Standardized methods are required that will measure changes in performance over time, so that recovery curves can be constructed for various different functions. The time scale of recovery, as revealed by such curves, may indicate a greater likelihood of one mechanism of recovery than of another. Moreover, it may be possible to judge the effect of therapeutic interventions if these produce changes in these curves, careful study of which might provide a basis for distinguishing between spontaneous recovery and the results of therapy—which is so important in assessing the role of specific methods of rehabilitation.

The rapid recovery of consciousness in a matter of minutes after apparently complete suspension of brain function as a result of a blow to the head invites comparison with the aftermath of an epileptic fit or of (nontraumatic) subarachnoid hemorrhage. It is reasonable to assume that such a rapidly reversible process has a biochemical (or electrochemical) basis. The functional interference may be primarily at a metabolic level (e.g., interference with cerebral oxygenation by a vascular mechanism such as spasm, vessel distortion, or alteration in perfusion pressure), or it may be the result of flux in transmitters or their inhibitors caused by neuronal discharges (or the withdrawal of tonic influence). It is still uncertain whether one part of the brain is crucial to the phenomenon of sudden temporary unconsciousness, but the weight of evidence is in favor of primary dysfunction over an extensive area of the brain rather than of a focal lesion in the brain stem—which was previously believed to underlie many of the features associated with "concussion."

When the delay before improvement starts is measured in hours or days, it seems likely that this improvement represents the return of activity to a neuronal system that had remained structurally intact but was functionally disordered. However, in either structural or functional disorders, the key to resolution may simply be the disappearance of whatever factor originally triggered that development. To what extent head injury may result in a disruption of synaptic contact and whether the restoration of such contacts contributes to recovery are matters of speculation.

The role of mechanical factors in causing continuation of neurological dysfunction and the value of relieving mechanical distortion of neural structures as an aid to recovery are controversial. When a surgeon removes an intracranial hematoma there is often an immediate improvement in the patient's condition, particularly in his level of consciousness and in those neurological signs that are attributable to brain stem distortion (pupil dilatation, unilateral decerebrate rigidity of the limbs). In the less critically affected patients, however, the removal of an intradural hematoma may have little immediate effect on the function of hemiplegic limbs. Particularly when this operation is done several days after injury, the slow improvement that occurs over the succeeding weeks may be no more than a continuation of the process of natural recovery already began before operation. Neither the rate of recovery nor the ultimate degree of function achieved may have been materially influenced by the surgical intervention. With a well-compensated hematoma for which surgery is not deemed necessary, recovery of function may occur long before the resolution of the mechanical lesion, as shown on serial CT scans.

The other common cause of focal brain damage is a depressed fracture of the skull vault. When this is associated with neurological focal signs, these seldom resolve immediately after elevation of the fracture, and it is presumed that they are due to damage sustained at the time of impact. However, there are occasional instances of rapid restoration of function when a depressed fracture is elevated, which suggests that dysfunction can occasionally be due to deformation either of neural structures, or more likely of vessels.

Recovery of function that occurs over months or years after brain damage depends on quite different mechanisms, the natures of which are ill-understood. It is widely held that regeneration in the mammalian central nervous system does not occur to any extent. Although recent animal experiments indicate that axonal sprouting and restoration of synapses can occur in certain areas, it is doubtful whether this can result in normal function.[12,15] Claims for improvement of fixed deficits weeks or months after stroke, related to surgical or chemical interventions designed to improve local cerebral blood supply, suggest that there can be functionally inactive areas of brain that will revive in response to manipulation of factors that affect local cerebral oxygenation. There is no information about how often such a circumstance occurs after brain damage that is primarily ischemic (e.g., stroke), let alone after head injury (which is often complicated by ischemic damage).

In these circumstances it seems likely that most late recovery (say, after a month) is due to the functional use of alternative or redundant neural pathways. The greater potential of children for recovery is usually ascribed to a greater plasticity of the nervous system; but this is not necessarily the explanation, because children also have a greater capacity for learning, and much of recovery may be a learning process. The less good recovery of older patients is probably related in part to reduced neuronal reserve and to the more limited availability of alternative structural pathways; but there is also a reduced capacity to learn and perhaps a less responsive vascular system.

Residual disabilities are much more frequent than newly developing complications. Epilepsy is the only common complication that develops after a time; late pathological events, such as obstructive hydrocephalus and caroticocavernous fistula, are relatively rare and make a trivial contribution to the sum of disability in a population of head injured survivors. Residual organic sequelae after head injury depend largely on the net effect of impact and secondary brain damage. However, there is little knowledge about the clinicopathological correlations at this stage. Autopsy data are largely confined to early deaths, with some data from patients who have remained in hospital for months or years with major degrees of irreversible brain damage. The nature and extent of the lesion in less severely affected survivors is largely unknown, except for occasional opportunistic observations on the brains of patients who have made a reasonable recovery before dying of other causes. However, in such circumstances there is seldom good clinical data about either the original injury or the sequelae in the intervening period; clinicopathological correlations cannot therefore be established.

Psychologists, armed with tests designed to distinguish between lesions in different parts of the brain, naturally wish to classify patients as having damage in various locations and to seek confirmation from clinical features, such as the site of a skull fracture, of an intracranial hematoma, or of neurological signs. Unfortunately, deductions based on such evidence are often misleading; for example, the fracture in a third of cases is contralateral to the site of the major brain damage, and this is seldom the *only* site of damage. It is reasonable to assume that patients who survive for years have widespread, if less severe, brain damage similar to that which characterizes injuries that are fatal in the first few weeks after injury. If that is so, then attempts by clinicians and psychologists to localize the site of damage responsible for persisting sequelae are bound to be frustrated, except for the identification of the most gross lesions. Analysis of the complex syndromes of disability on a symptomatic basis may, however, be invaluable in planning therapy, although treatment should not be too confidently based on the supposed anatomical site of the lesion.

In survivors after stroke, however, it may be more valid to draw deductions about the site of the pathology, because the lesions are much more discrete and are usually not accompanied by the "background noise" of widespread brain damage—unless the patient already suffers from diffuse cerebral arteriosclerosis.

Much effort has been expended in recent years on the study of sequelae after stroke, and it is natural that parallels should be drawn with head injury. Apart from the more focal nature of the lesion in stroke, however, there are other differences. Head injured patients are younger and are usually otherwise healthy; even when disabled they mostly have a normal life expectation. The older stroke victims not only have a lower survival rate in the acute stage (if severely enough affected to be in coma), but even after an initial period of recovery they may suffer another stroke or develop cardiac or renal decompensation. The mental disabilities that are so prominent a feature of head injured patients are less often seen in stroke victims, whose disability tends to be predominantly neurophysical. There are also differences in the social circumstances of these two groups of patients. Head injured patients, often on the threshold of their career and either still dependent on parents or relatively newly married, present different problems from those of the mature person with an established marriage, and children already grown up.

RECOVERY FROM COMA

The patient who has been in coma for several days begins to emerge from this state by opening the eyes at times—evidence that the mechanisms concerned with wakefulness are recovering. The next step, in patients who are not to remain vegetative and are not completely aphasic, is that words are uttered, at first occasional and random, or commands are obeyed; or both these functions may return together. In some patients there is a period of noisy, disinhibited behavior: cursing, attempts to get out of bed, perhaps aggressive attitudes to those around. The patient is almost always amnesic for all events during this period of disturbed behavior, which is sometimes termed "cerebral irritation" or more appropriately, "traumatic delirium." The intensity and duration of this phase of recovery varies considerably. Whether these variations reflect damage to different areas of the brain, are a function of the pretraumatic personality traits of the patient, or are related to environmental factors is unclear. Certainly bifrontal injury is frequently followed by a prolonged period of confusion, even though such patients often begin to speak within a day or so of injury. Some factors appear to aggravate this state, in particular confinement to bed, which is often necessary because of extracranial injuries; the restraints that may then be necessary tend to make matters worse. Physiological factors about which the patient is unable to communicate rationally may add to his frustration: a full bladder, thirst, or pain from associated injuries. Sedative drugs are sometimes given in an attempt to control disturbed behavior, but they may merely add to the patient's confused state of mind.

Dealing with this state is never easy, but anticipation of those factors mentioned that may be aggravating the situation may reduce agitation. Sedation should be restricted to night time, when it is justified, if only for the sake of other patients. Limiting restraint, avoiding unnecessary periods in bed, having the patient in a ward rather than a side room (where some degree of sensory deprivation can add to the patient's confusion), encouraging frequent short visits from relatives—these may all reduce disturbed behavior. Although this kind of behavior is more readily tolerated in an acute mental unit, only if it seems to be continuing for more than a few days is it appropriate to arrange temporary transfer to a psychiatric ward. It is necessary to emphasize to the staff of such a ward that this is a temporary state and to ensure that the patient's natural recovery is not impeded by heavy sedation. Families will need reassurance at this stage because, having ceased to worry about the survival of the patient, they may now begin to fear for his sanity. In fact most patients who are disturbed in this active kind of way make a reasonable recovery—it takes a well coordinated brain, structurally speaking, to produce such elaborately disorganized behavior.

In the next phase the patient is quiet and his conduct may seem unremarkable, but direct enquiry reveals that he is still confused about temporal, spatial, and even personal orientation; he will be amnesic subsequently for this period of semiautomatic behavior. However, casual observers often regard patients in this stage as having already recovered and may even discharge them from hospital. Such patients may be able to make statements to legal authorities and the police, which they may subsequently deny, because they are amnesic for the encounter. Investigations suggest that the end of post-traumatic amnesia, as assessed later in recovery, corresponds closely with the return of complete orientation, as assessed at the time. They also indicate that the end of PTA marks a crucial stage in the recovery process and that it is paralleled by the restoration of other mental skills. Moreover, the duration of PTA is closely related to the ultimate degree of recovery and to the likelihood of certain sequelae. It appears to be a reliable guide to the severity of diffuse brain damage (p. 89), which has been reflected in the acute stage by the depth and duration of coma.

Once the patient is out of PTA, he may begin to display other, more subtle, abnormalities of behavior, but these may be more in the way of changes in aspects of his personality that are obvious only to those who have known him before the injury. In general, apathy is more common than overactivity at this stage, and this may prove a hindrance for the rehabilitation staff. Relatives are now relieved to find improvement and may be hopeful that the rapid changes recently seen will continue, and that the unusual behavior patterns will give way to the patient's former self. At this stage recovery may be accelerated by return home to a familiar environment. But the family should be warned that the patient may not be wholly responsible, and that erratic behavior is still to be expected; the patient may be intolerant of his children and subject to outbursts of violence and impulsive behavior that are unlike his old self. Close relatives must also be prepared for

257

the inevitable slowing up in the rate of recovery and led to expect some persisting changes in personality, in motivation, and in speed of performance, particularly of motor tasks involving complicated sequences of events. A family is less likely to develop anxieties and tensions if they have been properly prepared for this altered behavior by early counseling.

POSTCONCUSSIONAL SYMPTOMS AND SYNDROME

Many patients after mild head injury complain for a time of headache and dizziness, and sometimes also of poor concentration and memory, fatigue, and irritability. This constellation of subjective complaints is remarkably consistent from one patient to the next, but there is great variation in the degree and duration of these complaints, and in the extent to which they prove disabling. Because some patients remain off work for long periods with symptoms of this kind after trivial head injury, there has long been a view that psychological factors rather than organic damage to craniocervical structures predominate in their causation. This view has been robustly promoted by Miller, in particular in his lectures on "accident neurosis."[14] However, most recent evidence supports the concept that these symptoms have an organic basis, but that they usually subside rapidly; only in a few patients do symptoms persist and secondary depression or anxiety develop.

This topic was extensively reviewed by several authors at a conference in 1969 on the Late Effects of Head Injury. The account that follows will mostly refer to this and to data published since then. At that meeting Teuber drew attention to one likely reason for the discrepant results, and consequently divergent views, of different observers, namely, the varying populations that they had studied.[20] Up to that time there had been no prospective studies on large series of head injured patients, including those who had no persisting complaints. Some series, such as those of Miller,[14] were drawn largely from medicolegal practice; they were naturally weighted with patients who had residual complaints long after injury, as well as with the confusing influence of impending litigation. Another variation is the time after injury when assessment is made. Lewin has pointed out that when a patient with a fractured femur complains of pain in his leg and limps during the first few weeks on his feet, this is not designated as a complication, nor as a post-traumatic syndrome.[11] Similarly, after head injury there is a period during which headaches, dizziness, and some reduction in mental capacity should be regarded as part of the normal recovery process. The time scale that should be regarded as natural for the resolution of these symptoms after injuries of varying severity is not, however, clearly defined. The development of a syndrome due to secondary influences, whether traumatic or motivated by considerations of gain from litigation, should be suspected only when symptoms appear disproportionate in degree or duration to the severity of injury, or when complaints appear anew after a period of satisfactory recovery.

The view that there is an organic basis for these symptoms rests on two main strands of evidence. One is the revised concept of concussion that has developed as a result of new insights into the neuropathological substrate of head trauma and of careful studies of neuro-otological and psychological function after mild injuries. The other kind of evidence comes from questioning series of patients, including those who do *not* have residual complaints, about symptoms that they suffered in the early stages after head injuries.

258

The term "postconcussional syndrome" was coined at a time when part of the definition of concussion was that there was no organic damage, only transitory functional disorder. This implied that persisting symptoms had to be explained on psychological factors. Pathologists have now been able to demonstrate lesions in patients who have died after recovering from mild injury. It is now accepted that even brief concussion usually entails some structural damage to the brain.

Neuro-otological examinations of patients who show no abnormal signs on routine clinical examination have revealed a high incidence of vestibular dysfunction and of asymmetrical, high-frequency hearing loss (p. 278). This would provide an explanation for the dizziness and hyperacusis which are common complaints.

Psychological tests that involve measuring the processing of information (e.g., paced auditory serial addition, PASAT) have shown a very high incidence of abnormality within a day or so of injury, even in patients whose PTA was less than 1 hour.[6] Half these mildly injured patients performed normally on this test after 2 weeks, but 10 percent were still abnormal at 35 days, and these patients had postconcussional symptoms; these tended to subside *pari passu* with the restoration of normal performance on this psychological test. This would explain the loss of concentration of which so many patients complain.

In a more recent investigation[23] the same observers found impairment on tasks involving vigilance and recent memory a year or more after mild concussion when testing was carried out under conditions of mild hypoxia (by simulating conditions at high altitude); matched controls who had not been concussed showed significantly less impairment at high altitude, compared with performance under normal conditions.

Direct evidence of a relationship between organic damage and postconcussional symptoms has appeared in several recent reports. In one series of 145 patients examined 4 to 5 weeks after injury,[16] patients who were still complaining of multiple postconcussional symptoms more often had a PTA exceeding 15 minutes; and they more often had had, when examined 24 hours after injury, either headache, diplopia, anosmia, or other CNS signs. Kay[10] compared three groups of patients: those who had recovered except for one symptom at 3 to 6 months; those who had more than one postconcussional symptom at that time; and those suffering manifest residual brain damage (Table 1). The postconcussional group more often had disorders of smell, vision, or hearing, or had had an

Table 1. Symptoms after discharge from neurosurgical ward

	None or One Symptom (=Recovered) n=268	Post-Concussional Symptoms n=94	Residual Brain Damage n=61
Conscious level on admission*	1.5	1.6	3.0
Duration of PTA*	2.2	2.4	3.9
Skull fracture	21%	21%	59%
Intracranial hematoma	5%	12%	41%
Disordered smell, hearing, vision	11%	32%	45%

*1–5 scale, higher is worse.
(Prepared from data in Kay, Kerr, and Lassman[10])

259

intracranial hematoma, than had the recovered group; these organic features were even more frequent in the patients with residual brain damage. Many of the brain damaged patients in this series had headache and dizziness at follow-up, and this is at variance with the fact that many severely injured patients deny ever having suffered from these symptoms. At the other end of the severity scale, most patients who suffer a mild injury do complain of some symptoms, at least briefly. Even after injury on the football field, 60 percent of concussed players complained of headache and 54 percent of dizziness, for a time.[3]

The duration of symptoms and the extent of the disability caused by (or attributed to) them are the features that distinguish postconcussional neurosis from the normal postconcussional syndrome. On the other hand, Cook has commented on how brief was the period of disability after concussion when this had been suffered on the rugby football field.[3] Only 17 percent of footballers lost time from work, and 80 percent of these were off work for less than a week. Only 14 percent continued with symptoms for more than 2 days. In another study[4] the same author showed that patients who were claiming compensation more often had symptoms (including headache) than those not seeking legal redress; the latter also had a shorter PTA and longer periods off work (Table 2).

In a group of patients with residual complaints seen by a psychiatrist,[13] headache and dizziness were again prominent, with memory disorders and depression also common. This series excluded patients with pending litigation, but 17 of the 27 cases had already had claims settled and were still complaining. Although no patient had a skull fracture, nor PTA exceeding an hour, five of them remained unemployed and six had suffered reduction in occupational status. Several of these patients had stable pretraumatic personality, which had not protected them against the development of marked postconcussional symptoms. On the other hand, many observers have commented on the frequent association of premorbid personality traits with the development of persisting post-traumatic symptoms. It may be that this determines the reaction to the injury and its subsequent symptoms; in particular, previous traits may predispose to depression, which Cartlidge[2] found a frequent feature in those who developed symptoms after an initial period of recovery.

The most complete prospective study of head injuries has been that recently reported by Cartlidge.[2] Admissions to a neurosurgical unit (372 patients) were assessed on discharge, at 6 months, 1 year, and 2 years; 40 percent had PTA of less than 1 hour, 20 percent 1 to 12 hours, and the rest for longer periods. More than a third of patients had headache on discharge, but less than a fifth had headaches when seen at a year; by contrast almost as many patients had dizziness at a year as had complained of this symptom on discharge (Table 3).

Of those who complained of headache and dizziness at the time of discharge

Table 2. Postconcussional patients

	Compensation Claim	No Claim
Some symptoms	96%	85%
Headache	85%	70%
Mean loss of work	88 days	24 days
PTA >5 minutes	37%	65%

(From Cook, with permission[4])

Table 3. NSU head injury discharges (n=372)

	On Discharge	6 months	1 year	2 years
Headache	36%	27%	18%	24%
Dizziness	19%	22%	14%	18%

(From Cartlidge, with permission[2])

from hospital, 59 percent were free of these symptoms when seen 6 months later. By contrast almost half of the patients who were complaining of these symptoms 6 months after injury had acquired them since discharge from hospital, having been symptom-free in the early post-traumatic period. Those with evolving symptoms of headaches and dizziness more often had depression and intended to seek compensation (Table 4). Dizziness in the earlier stages was often accompanied by positional nystagmus, which became less common as the interval from injury increased. Nystagmus was seldom found in patients with acquired dizziness. The frequency with which symptoms were found was not too dissimilar from that found in Barr and Ralston's report[1] from a peripheral hospital, or that of Steadman and Graham[18] from a city hospital (Table 5). These are lower than the incidence reported sooner after injury (Table 6). Rutherford[16] found 51 percent of 145 concussed patients complaining of at least one symptom 4 to 6 weeks after injury, and two thirds of them had more than one symptom.

The exact mechanism of persisting symptom production is unclear.[19] The dizziness so often complained of can readily be related to labyrinthine concussion, and hyperacusis to damage to the hearing mechanisms.[21] Indeed, these patients have complaints identical with those who have had no trauma but have positional vertigo. Loss of concentration and memory may be a reflection of defective information processing, as revealed by the PASAT test. The patient who returns too soon to work may find that he cannot cope, particularly with jobs that require simultaneous attention to several separate factors. Finding that he cannot manage, he is liable to develop fatigue, tension, and depression; a vicious cycle is then initiated, which aggravates both the mental symptoms and the headache.

The headache is the most difficult to explain. There are many possible causes for persisting headache after head injury, including pain in scalp scars, neuralgia of occipital or supraorbital nerves, precipitation of migraine in predisposed subjects,[5,7] and occasionally serious intracranial complications, such as hydrocephalus or chronic subdural hematoma. In the majority of patients, however, the

Table 4. Frequency of certain features in two groups of patients 6 months after discharge from neurosurgical ward (n=372)

	In Patients With	
	Subsiding Symptoms	Acquired Symptoms
Positional nystagmus	45%	5%
Depression	12%	39%
Compensation	24%	51%

(From Cartlidge, with permission[2])

Table 5. Persistence of postconcussional symptoms years after injury

	Cartlidge[2] 306 2 yr	Barr & Ralston[1] 306 c.4 yr	Steadman & Graham[18] 400 5 yr
Headache	24%	35%	12%
Dizziness	18%	25%	

headache has the characteristics associated with tension headache in patients who have not suffered trauma. That is to say the pain has no specific time pattern during the day, is often described as a tight band around the head, and there is frequent involvement of the neck and occipital region; it is resistant to analgesics. Indeed, there are some who believe that a major factor in post-traumatic headache is associated soft tissue trauma to the neck, or aggravation of pre-existing cervical spondylosis.[8] It must be remembered that most patients who have a bang on the head, even without alteration in consciousness, develop some headache, and that some subarachnoid bleeding is an almost invariable complication of moderate and severe injury. In a study of recovered (symptom-free) patients, those with post-concussional symptoms and those with brain damage, headache was most frequently found in the group with postconcussional symptoms; but a fifth of the recovered patients had also had headache.[10]

This condition is more readily prevented than treated, and there may be a clue to this in the relative immunity that severe injury appears so often to confer. Such a patient never knew the unpleasantness of the early headache and meningism caused by subarachnoid hemorrhage. His first memory was to awake free of headache, surrounded by people pleased to welcome him back to consciousness. His family are relieved that he has recovered from coma and may regard every sign of improvement as a triumph; meanwhile they expect (and demand) little of the patient. The victim of mild injury enjoys no such care and consideration, although his remembered experience may be more upsetting and haunting than anything in the memory of the severely injured patient. He wakes in strange surroundings, with a bad headache, bewildered by what has happened to him. And within days he may find that he is expected to resume normal life, with the facile reassurance that nothing serious has happened to him.

It has been suggested that admission to hospital, followed by reassurance and graded resumption of activity, will reduce the incidence of symptoms.[22] A contrary view is that admission to hospital can itself act as additional psychological trauma and may convince the patient that something serious has happened. Certainly overnight admission to an accident or general surgical ward, followed by summary dismissal next morning, is unlikely to be beneficial in this respect, whatever its merits in safeguarding against serious intracranial complications.

Table 6. Postconcussional symptoms at various intervals after injury

	Cook[4] at any time	Rutherford[16] 4–6 wk	Cartlidge[2] 6 mo	Merskey[13] Years
Headache	60%	25%	27%	93%
Dizziness	54%	15%	22%	89%
Mental	—	8–9%	—	70–80%

The prolonged reduction in PASAT that Gronwall and Wrightson found after even mild injuries led them to explore two alternative approaches to rehabilitation.[6] One was to treat all patients after mild concussion for a period of 2 to 3 weeks. The other was to arrange follow-up at 1 month and to take into treatment only those with persisting symptoms. Against the latter, seemingly more economic, policy they warned that patients who had already begun to develop disabling symptoms were more difficult to restore to normal than those who were treated from the beginning. On the other hand, they recognized that many patients without treatment would in fact recover satisfactorily. In a subsequent study of patients who had been sent home from the accident department within a few hours of injury, they found that, although 80 percent of patients with less than 12 hours of PTA returned to work in less than a week, more than half had adverse symptoms for 2 to 3 weeks. Slowness and fatigue were common, and many felt useless in the evening and went early to bed, even though they were back at work.[23]

Our conclusion is that the damage done by, and the symptoms subsequently suffered after, mild head injuries are frequently underestimated. Several factors contribute to this. One is that many of the hospital doctors who deal with mildly injured patients are unfamiliar with recent work in this field, and in any event are not used to dealing with the largely subjective complaints that are the feature of these patients' persisting disability. On the other hand, those who are accustomed to dealing with severe head injuries are apt to view the mildly concussed patient as fortunate to have escaped serious brain damage—a comparison of little significance to the patient. There seems little doubt that these patients' symptoms may become intensified and prolonged largely because their doctors do not pay due attention to the disability that they cause and therefore do not give the support and protection that is needed during the few weeks following concussion. What is needed is to explain to the patient and his family that, although he has fortunately escaped serious brain damage, it will take a few weeks before he is completely right, and that he should expect some headache and dizziness for a time, and perhaps some temporary limitation of mental capacity. It should be pointed out that the patient should not too soon resume stressful work, particularly that requiring mental concentration. He should be seen again, so that the doctor can assess progress, decide if symptomatic drugs are needed, and offer further advice about the resumption of various normal activities.

PROGNOSIS AFTER HEAD INJURY

What is appropriate management for the individual head injured patient depends on what probabilities are put on the likelihood of complications after milder injuries, or of recovery after the more severe. Until recently it was regarded as very difficult to predict events after head injury, and many management policies were based on the almost total uncertainty of what would happen. Three examples can be given. *Intracranial hematoma* is known to occur in a small proportion of mildly injured patients, but in them a serious situation can develop relatively rapidly. In the hope of increasing the likelihood that, if this complication should develop, early diagnosis will be made and more timely treatment instituted, thousands of fully conscious patients come into hospital every year for observation after recent head injury, many of them probably unnecessarily. With *late traumatic epilepsy,* another uncommon but much less dangerous complication, un-

263

certainty about the risks leads to underuse of prophylactic anticonvulsants, and so to many patients needlessly having fits (p. 287). The reason that drugs are not more widely used is that surgeons are unsure about the risk of epilepsy associated with different types of head injury. A third area is in the management of *severe head injuries,* for which several elaborate and expensive methods of treatment are available. Some of these patients make a good recovery, but even after extensive therapeutic endeavors many still die, and some survivors remain permanently and severely brain damaged. Uncertainty in the early stages about the potential for recovery obliges doctors to continue with intensive therapy, even when they suspect that irreversible brain damage has already occurred, and to treat, with unnecessarily elaborate (and sometimes hazardous) methods, patients who would recover with "ordinary" care.

In each of these three instances important clinical decisions depend on the clinician's estimate of what is likely to occur with or without certain interventions—whether they be admitting to hospital, giving anticonvulsants, or providing intensive therapy. These represent special instances of the principle of triage in the delivery of medical care, a concept originally applied in military surgery in which surgeons with restricted medical resources had to anticipate dealing with large numbers of casualties. In such circumstances necessity demands a decision about which patients are in need of urgent treatment, as distinct from those not badly enough injured to need it, or those too seriously affected to benefit from it. The parallel between this and the selection of critically ill civilian patients for intensive care is obvious. But it is not always realized that a not dissimilar principle applies to the admission of mildly injured patients to hospital, and to the administration of anticonvulsants, or indeed to the use of a special investigation such as CT scanning. Nor is it only a matter of restricted resources; most interventions have other costs, in the form of additional risks or side-effects, or the inconvenience of travelling to special facilities. These costs have to be balanced against the expected benefits. In each of these instances, rational decision-making should depend on balancing the costs and benefits expected from alternative lines of action. The balancing of the trade-off between these, as applied to individual patients, is one of the most important functions of any doctor. This complex business of decision-making is influenced by cultural and socioeconomic factors, as well as by the personalities of the physician, of the family, and also of the patient if he is sentient and sane.

But the expectation of what will happen, biologically rather than socially, in a variety of clinical situations, is one of the most weighty factors that the doctor has to balance in his mind when reaching decisions about appropriate action. What are the chances, the odds, the probability, that this particular patient will develop a hematoma, or will have late epilepsy, or will recover to a certain degree from a severe injury? Estimates of this kind have traditionally depended on the experience of the individual doctor, but it is now increasingly realized that predictions can be much more effectively calculated by probability statistics. By this means an individual clinician can have at his disposal a "past experience" of similar cases that far exceeds what he could hope to gain in the longest professional lifetime. Moreover this data can be made available to him in a much more reliable form than one man's memory could ever provide.

Making a prognosis about a patient is as old as medicine itself. Indeed, it constituted the main activity of physicians (as distinct from surgeons) until the therapeutic possibilities of the last 50 years changed the scene. Because so many methods of treatment are now available, it is easy to forget the importance of prognosis. It has always been vital information for the patient and his family to have, no matter whether or not the course of the condition could be influenced by treatment. Nowadays prognosis is also essential if doctors are to be able to judge the extent to which various methods of management do in fact influence the natural history, so as to be in a position to make wise decisions about what to do for individual patients.

Until recently prognosis was largely informal and usually nonstatistical—depending on no more than the identification of factors that were more often associated with a given future event than were others. It was known that patients with a skull fracture were more likely to develop an intracranial hematoma, that gunshot wounds were more often followed by epilepsy than closed injuries, and that patients in coma soon after injury more often died than those who were not. But how *much* more likely does each of these prognostic factors make a given outcome? And what is the effect of several factors combined, each of which alone is known to predispose to a particular event? These questions can be answered only by the analysis of large series of patients and by the use of formal statistical methods. This approach may also make it possible to reach more accurate predictions about individual patients. It is easy to overlook the limited value, in practical terms, of knowing that 80 percent of patients with a given characteristic will follow a certain course, if there are no clues as to whether the patient under treatment is one of the 80 percent who will, or of the 20 percent who won't, behave in this particular way.

Practicalities of Prognosis

There are practicalities in making a formal estimate of the probability of various events occurring to an individual patient. It is first necessary to declare what events are to be predicted. These may be complications, such as the occurrence of a hematoma or of epilepsy, which either happen or do not, or they may be a set of states of health (or degrees of recovery) after severe injury. In either case it is essential to define the events to be predicted. These alternative outcomes must be a set of mutually exclusive classes. Events have time courses, and these must be taken account of when outcomes are specified. These are of particular importance when predicting events that may be far in the future, such as the development of late epilepsy, or the ultimate degree of recovery after severe injury; the occurrence of an acute intracranial hematoma or the question of survival is a more immediate prediction.

The next step, having defined outcomes to be predicted, is to identify predictive criteria. This entails the accumulation of a large number of patients with information about their early state and also about their outcomes. Information about this early state has to be collected according to standardized methods, which can be used reliably by the various clinicians who wish to use the predictive system. The establishment of "data banks" of clinical cases is of value not only for making predictions about individual patients, but also for comparing the outcomes in different series of patients. These may be successive patients in a single center; or patients in different hospitals, different cities, or different countries; or patients matched in formal trials of a specific form of therapy.

Having assembled an adequate data bank, it is possible to identify features in the early stages after injury that influence outcome. These will enable estimates to be made of the distribution of outcomes in groups of patients, e.g., that X percent of patients with feature Y will develop epilepsy. But the interactions between different features can also be explored—both how often they occur together (their dependence) and what their combined effect is on outcome. From this will emerge combinations of predictive criteria, which can be made available to the clinician in various forms. There will likely be some combinations of features that seem always to be associated with given outcomes, and these will include most of those features already "known" by doctors. However, experience indicates that relatively few patients have features that make the outcome obvious. A more generally useful approach is to develop tables that indicate the relationship of outcome to various combinations of factors. This will make it feasible in some instances to quote a probability for an individual patient reaching one or more specified outcomes, and, for series, to estimate the proportional distribution of outcomes. This approach will be discussed in more detail in the chapters that deal with calculating the risk of late epilepsy (p. 283) and predicting outcome after severe head injury (Chapter 14).

REHABILITATION

Surgeons concerned with the management of head injuries in the acute stage are apt to overlook the need for a planned program of rehabilitation. Unless they make a practice of routine follow-up visits and, when they do see a patient, allow time to discover from him and from his family the true range of his mental and physical disabilities, surgeons can easily underestimate the extent of the difficulties encountered by head injured patients after they leave the surgical ward. The bias of rehabilitationists is different; they are apt not to realize the capacity for spontaneous recovery, and so may claim more credit for specific techniques of remedial therapy than is sometimes justified. No doubt this derives from their experience with patients who have residual disabilities months after injury, when they are first seen by rehabilitation staff.

Discussions about rehabilitation are sometimes confused by the different interpretations put on the term by different practitioners. Sometimes rehabilitation seems to be synonymous with the whole treatment of the patient, or the treatment of the patient as a whole. This leads to slogans such as "rehabilitation begins at the road-side"; and at a later stage to the term "long-term rehabilitation," which in effect means the long-term care of the patient with a static condition of disability. Nor should the assessment or diagnosis of disability be confused with its treatment. The discussion that follows is concerned with formal rehabilitation, which makes use of those trained professionally in physical, speech, and occupational therapy. It may involve also the participation of social workers, psychologists, and psychiatrists. It is advantageous for this to begin while the patient is still in the acute surgical ward, even though the main site for such activity will usually be in the rehabilitation center in which the patient stays at a later stage or which he visits from home. It is vital to ensure that continuity of care is maintained when the patient leaves the acute surgical unit, and to make sure that sensible and sympathetic advice is given to the patient's family soon after injury, and also to the patient once he is able to understand the situation.

Objectives

By suitable intervention the hope is that recovery may be accelerated and the degree of persisting disability reduced. Four separate approaches are possible:
1. Restoring old skills (for damaged parts)
2. Teaching new skills (for unaffected parts)
3. Retrieving lost ground
4. Influencing attitudes of the patient, family, and therapeutic team

Perhaps the most important is to influence the attitudes of the patient and family regarding the predicament resulting from brain damage. In the early stages after severe brain damage, relatives will matter more than the patient, because he will be a relatively passive partner. The family needs to be prepared for the kind of difficulties likely to occur, and to be given realistic short-term objectives and some hint of the ultimate degree of recovery that is expected. Later on it may be necessary to retrieve lost ground, both in terms of attitude and of secondary adverse or negative reactions on the part of patient and relatives. Once this has been done, the question is what balance to aim for between restoring old skills and learning new skills that depend on the functioning of undamaged parts of the brain. Once it is clear, for example, that one hand will recover little function, it is important to concentrate on maximizing the use of the other side. Similarly, nonverbal modes of communication may have to be developed if dysphasia is severe and persistent.

In the first month the main objectives are to prevent complications, particularly to prevent contractures of the limbs; to predict outcome; and to prepare the family for the likely time course and degree of recovery.

In the next 3 to 6 months every effort should be made to promote recovery by specific graded activities. In the late stage, after 6 months, when neurological recovery has largely been completed, the need is to analyze the patient's disability and capability, and to encourage the patient to adapt physically, to accept mentally, and to adjust socially.

Assessing Effectiveness

Until recently there were no generally agreed upon methods for monitoring the process of recovery, or the degree of recovery finally reached. This partly accounts for the lack of good evidence as to the effectiveness of specific rehabilitation procedures on disability caused by brain damage. Another difficulty is to quantify the amount and type of treatment given, on account of the degree of overlap between what is done by different kinds of therapists, and of the tendency for substitution therapy to be given by nonprofessionals if formal rehabilitation is not available or is incomplete. Is walking of the patient by nurses on the ward to be regarded as physical therapy? Is devoted attention by an educated mother to her son's recovery of the ability to communicate by verbal, visual, and auditory modes equivalent to speech therapy? Is the attempt of father or employer to interest the brain damaged young man in regaining old skills of hobbies or work a form of occupational therapy? If skilled therapists are available, how much of what they achieve should be attributed to methods with a theoretical background, as compared to those developed empirically from working with previous cases? In any event, how much does rehabilitation owe to the general psychological effect of those around the patient taking an interest, offering encouragement, setting goals—rather than to the use of particular physiologically based patterns of activities? Considering that the mental components of disability tend to predominate after brain damage, it would be surprising if the creation of an environment that was stimulating, understanding, and well structured was not found to be important. To admit this is not to dismiss or to diminish the importance of the separate contributions of different therapists; but there is a need to attempt to distinguish the contribution of the various specific methods of therapy, in order to discover the most effective way to plan a rehabilitation program and the emphasis to lay on its different components.

Questions of the same kind should be asked about rehabilitation as are routinely posed when drug treatment is under review. These include consideration of which patients to treat, when to treat, with what intensity (e.g., dosage), and when to stop. What are the desired effects, and are there adverse reactions? Is there evidence of a placebo effect, and can patients become dependent on therapy (if not actually addicted)?

One of the most important factors in rehabilitation is that there should be some continuity of care, once the postprimary stage is reached. Specific problems such as communication difficulties, spasticity, ataxia, or perceptual disorders require analysis by therapists experienced in the assessment of these deficits; there must be diagnosis before treatment. Once treatment begins, progress should be monitored in order to determine when a plateau is reached; this may indicate a need to change the method of treatment or that therapy should now be discontinued. Therapy should be biased towards the pragmatic and the practical: less on what muscle movements can be performed in the artificial setting of the therapy room and more on what would be possible and necessary at home. At the earliest opportunity those aspects of therapy that can be carried out by family members should be taught to them. They will often be able and willing to provide much more intensive and continuous therapy than is practical or economic within the formal setting of a hosptial; and it may greatly benefit the patient to be at home, and to be free of the need for repeated journeys to a rehabilitation center.

REFERENCES

1. BARR, J. B., AND RALSTON, G. J.: *Head injuries in a peripheral hospital. A five year survey.* Lancet ii:519–522, 1964.

2. CARTLIDGE, N. E. F.: *Post-concussional syndrome.* Scot. Med. J. 23:103, 1977.

3. COOK, J. B.: "The effects of minor head injuries sustained in sport and the post-concussional syndrome." In Walker, A. E., Caveness, W. F., and Critchley, M. (eds.): *Late Effects of Head Injury.* Charles C Thomas, Springfield, 1969, pp. 408–413.

4. COOK, J. B.: *The post-concussional syndrome and factors influencing recovery after minor head injury admitted to hospital.* Scand. J. Rehabil. Med. 4:27–30, 1972.

5. FRIEDMAN, A. P.: "The so-called post-traumatic headache." In Walker, A. E., Caveness, W. F., and Critchley, M. (eds.): *Late Effects of Head Injury.* Charles C Thomas, Springfield, 1969, pp. 55–71.

6. GRONWALL, D., AND WRIGHTSON, P.: *Delayed recovery of intellectual function after minor head injury.* Lancet ii:605–609, 1974.

7. GUTHKELCH, A. N.: *Benign post-traumatic encephalopathy in young people and its relation to migraine.* Neurosurgery 1:101–105, 1977.

8. JACOBSON, S. A.: "Mechanisms of the sequelae of minor craniocervical trauma." In Walker, A. E., Caveness, W. F., and Critchley, M., (eds.): *Late Effects of Head Injury.* Charles C Thomas, Springfield, 1969, pp. 35–45.

9. JENNETT, B.: "Late effects of head injuries." In Critchley, M., O'Leary, J., and Jennett, B. (eds.): *Scientific Foundations of Neurology.* F. A. Davis, Philadelphia, 1972, pp. 441–451.

10. KAY, D. W. K., KERR, T. A., AND LASSMAN, L. P.: *Brain trauma and post-concussional syndrome.* Lancet ii:1052–1055, 1971.

11. LEWIN, W.: *Rehabilitation needs of the brain injured patient.* Proc. R. Soc. Med. 63:28–32, 1970.

12. MATTHEWS, D. A., COTMAN, C., AND LYNCH, G.: *An electron microscopic study of lesion-induced synaptogenesis in the dentate gyrus of the adult rat. 1. Magnitude and time course of degeneration.* Brain Res. 115:1–21, 1976.

13. MERSKEY, H., AND WOODFORD, J. M.: *Psychiatric sequelae of minor head injury.* Brain 95:521–528, 1972.

14. MILLER, H.: *Accident neurosis.* Br. Med. J. 1:919–925, 1961.

15. RAISMAN, G.: *Neuronal plasticity in the septal nuclei of the adult rat.* Brain Res. 14:25–48, 1969.

16. RUTHERFORD, W. H., MERRETT, J. D., AND McDONALD, J. R.: *Sequelae of concussion caused by minor head injury.* Lancet i:1–4, 1977.

17. SHETTER, A. G., AND DEMAKA, J. J.: "The pathophysiology of concussion: review." In Thompson, R. A., and Green, J. R. (eds.): *Advances in Neurology.* vol. 22. Raven Press, 1979, pp. 5–15.

18. STEADMAN, J. G., AND GRAHAM, J. G.: *Head injuries: an analysis and follow-up study.* Proc. R. Soc. Med. 63:23–28, 1970.

19. Taylor, A. R.: *Post-concussional sequelae.* Br. Med. J. 3:67–71, 1967.

20. TEUBER, H. L.: "Neglected aspects of the post-traumatic syndrome." In Walker, A. E., Caveness, W. F., and Critchley, M. (eds.): *Late Effects of Head Injury.* Charles C Thomas, Springfield, 1969, pp. 13–34.

21. TOGLIA, J. U.: "Dizziness after whiplash injury of the neck and closed head injury." In Walker, A. E., Caveness, W. F., and Critchley, M. (eds.): *Late Effects of Head Injury.* Charles C Thomas, Springfield, 1969, pp. 72–83.

22. TUBBS, O. N., AND POTTER, J. M.: *Early post-concussional headache.* Lancet ii:128–129, 1970.

23. WRIGHTSON, P.: Personal communication, 1978.

CHAPTER 11

Neurophysical Sequelae

Most reports on physical deficits are based on series of patients who have persisting complaints. Those that are the result of an attempt to follow-up a whole group of injured patients seldom include a searching neurological examination. How often minor deficits are found, particularly after the less severe injuries, depends on how carefully they are sought. For these various reasons the true frequency of various kinds of deficits after injuries of differing severity is not known.

Many patients have temporary deficits that resolve during the first few months after injury. Focal signs of damage to the cerebral hemisphere were found soon after injury in 20 percent of a large series of patients with compound depressed fracture,[8] but only half of these had residual deficits 6 months after injury. Many more patients with acute intracranial hematoma had hemiparesis soon after injury (61%), but 6 months later only half of them still had a deficit. Cranial nerve dysfunction can frequently be found in the early weeks after less severe injuries, and this often resolves; most common are disorders of the middle and inner ear mechanisms, of ocular movements, and of accommodation.

Persisting physical deficits were more common after severe injuries. Over 300 patients with injuries severe enough to have caused unconsciousness or post-traumatic amnesia of a week or more were reviewed 20 years later by Roberts.[15] He found three main patterns of neurological disability in those who regained consciousness. *Hemiparesis* was the main disability in 40 percent, although it was slight in the majority of these. Some 20 percent had a *brain stem syndrome* with asymmetrical cerebellar and pyramidal signs; more of these patients had a history of early post-traumatic deterioration than did patients with other types of persisting disability, and this was interpreted as indicating the development of secondary brain stem damage from raised ICP and shift. In 5 percent the state was described as *athetoid pseudobulbar,* a combination of bilateral pyramidal and extrapyramidal signs. About 25 percent of this series had no neurological deficit; the others had abnormalities outside this classification.

The frequency of occurrence of neurophysical disabilities 6 months after injury was examined in 150 survivors in Glasgow who regained consciousness following severe head injury (Data Bank series). The commonest findings were disorders related to dysfunction in the cerebral hemispheres and in the cranial nerves (Table 1). The brain stem and pseudobulbar syndromes described by Roberts were sel-

Table 1. Neurophysical sequelae at 6 months after injury

	All Cases n=150	After Intracranial Hematoma n=77	No Intracranial Hematoma n=73
Any cerebral hemisphere dysfunction	65%	62%	67%
Cranial nerve palsy			
All cases	37%	38%	36%
As only sign	13%	10%	15%
Ataxia	9%	4%	14%

(From Jennett, Snoek, Bond, et al.[9])

dom encountered, but his finding that a quarter of the patients had no neurological abnormalities was confirmed.[9]

CEREBRAL HEMISPHERES

Pathological evidence indicates that the brunt of the impact damage from blunt injury falls on the cerebral cortex (contusions) and on the subcortical white matter (shearing lesions). Secondary ischemic damage, which is common in fatal cases and must presumably also affect some survivors, most often affects the cortex and the basal ganglia (p. 35). In many patients who remain disabled, there has also been an intradural hematoma, which has caused secondary focal brain damage in the cerebral hemisphere, particularly in the temporal lobe. In 935 cases of severe head injury in the Data Bank study there was clinical evidence during the acute stage of cerebral hemisphere damage in 89 percent; a third of these (28% of all cases) had early evidence of *bilateral* hemisphere damage.

In the 150 Glasgow survivors after severe injury, 49 percent had hemiparesis and 29 percent dysphasia, while 21 percent had both (Table 2). Hemianopia occurred in only 5 percent of patients, and then usually in association with other signs of hemisphere damage. About half of the 150 patients had had an intracranial hematoma removed. Hemiparesis was more common in patients *without* intracranial hematoma, and this was still so when the small number of patients with depressed fracture was removed from the series without hematoma. Epilepsy was, however, very uncommon in diffuse injuries without depressed fracture or hematoma (3 percent had late fits); more than 90 percent of patients with epilepsy had had either a depressed fracture or a hematoma. That is what would have been expected from other studies that we have made on traumatic epilepsy (p. 281). Epilepsy in this series of severe injuries was associated with persisting signs of hemisphere damage in 59 percent of cases; only 6 percent of the whole series had epilepsy as the sole sign of hemisphere damage.

CRANIAL NERVE DEFICITS

The frequency of occurrence of these has been reported in several large series of head injuries, but it is difficult to know how head injury was defined for such purposes. In any event, the overall incidence is not of great significance in practical management—of more importance is to know the potential for recovery and the likely disability that these deficits incur, because in few (if any) circumstances

Table 2. Sequelae of cerebral hemisphere damage at 6 months after injury

	All Cases $n=150$	After Intracranial Hematoma $n=77$	No initial Hematoma $n=73$
Hemiparesis			
All cases	49%	56%	62%
As only hemisphere sign	24%	14%	34%
Dysphasia			
All cases	29%	32%	26%
As only sign	7%	10%	4%
Hemiparesis + dysphasia	21%	17%	26%
Hemianopia			
All cases	5%	5%	5%
As only sign	1%	1%	1%
Epilepsy			
All cases	17%	25%	8%
As only sign	8%	12%	1%

(From Jennett, Snoek, Bond, et al.[9])

is therapeutic intervention possible. Recognition of these lesions in the early stages will minimize the confusion that can occur from the misinterpretation of disorders of pupil reactions, eye movements, or facial movements—which may be wrongly ascribed to central dysfunction. In the later stages it is important to consider what contribution cranial nerve palsies make to overall disability.

In the 150 patients assessed 6 months after severe injury, cranial nerve palsies were found in 32 percent and in 14 percent of the series these were the only persisting signs. They were somewhat more common in patients who had had an intracranial hematoma. The most common to be affected was the optic nerve, some of these palsies being due to severe craniofacial injuries. Deafness and disorders of external ocular muscles were both more common than anosmia. Some patients with basal skull fractures had more than one cranial nerve involved. Exhaustive accounts of individual cranial nerve palsies after trauma are contained in the *Handbook of Neurology;* the brief account that follows is largely based on chapters in that text.

Anosmia

Loss of sense of smell is reported by about 7 percent of patients admitted to hospital with a head injury, and the first is the only cranial nerve to be commonly affected after milder injuries. About half of the patients with anosmia have had less than an hour's PTA; but the incidence is much higher (20%) in patients who have been unconscious than in those who have not. Detection depends on the patient's response, and therefore it is only survivors who can complain or who are questioned or tested, and any evidence emerges from them. Among the milder injuries, occipital blows are often reported. In such cases there is often no fracture, and the assumption is that contrecoup damage has occurred, probably to the olfactory filaments transversing the cribriform plate. But most patients with anosmia have been unconscious and have a fracture, and this fracture is most often frontal. About 50 percent of the patients with CSF rhinorrhea from anterior fossa fracture have anosmia, and in those who have had surgical repair the incidence of anosmia is about 80 percent.

Many patients recover and most do so within 3 months; again this depends on how carefully evidence of anosmia is sought in the early stages. When PTA exceeds 24 hours, anosmia is usually permanent. When recovery occurs it is usually complete, although some patients have distorted sensation (parosmia), and some remain unable to detect certain smells (olfactory scotomata). Occasionally recovery is reported after years, and Sumner[19] suggests that a central lesion may then be the explanation. He also suggests such a lesion (e.g., contusion on the under surface of the frontal lobe) as the probable cause for the loss of both smell and taste that is occasionally reported after relatively mild concussion, and also after episodes of generalized cerebral hypoxia, such as cardiac arrest.

Patients vary in the extent to which they complain of loss of taste when they are anosmic. The sight of food becomes important in such circumstances, no doubt because gustatory memory is involved. While the subtleties of flavor cannot be tasted, trigeminal taste will persist and can be shown by the ability to detect salt, vinegar, and sugar. Specific loss of trigeminal taste can occur with facial nerve lesions associated with petrous fractures, and occasionally with specific trigeminal damage.

The significance of anosmia for the patient is readily overlooked, particularly if he has recovered well in other respects from an injury that initially threatened his life. But anosmia can rightly form a basis for compensation, not only for the loss of many of the pleasures of life, but for interference with occupation (e.g., in cooks, food handlers, and wine and tea tasters), and for loss of ability to detect dangerous smells (e.g., of escaping gases or of burning). Formal testing then becomes important, and the most reliable recognized test odors are coffee, tar, oil of lemon, and almond (benzaldehyde). Ammonia is useful in detecting sham anosmia, as the lacrimation cannot be hidden by the patient who claims to sense nothing when sniffing the bottle.

Visual Pathways

These may be affected anywhere from the retina to the calcarine cortex. Penetrating injuries, caused by missile fragments or by pointed instruments, may affect any part of the system and are the only frequent cause of lesions to the optic radiation. Blunt injuries most often affect the intracanalicular part of the optic nerve; the chiasm is involved much less frequently (by a factor of 5 to 25 times less). The frequency of lesions of the occipital cortex is hard to determine because cortical blindness is often transitory and probably goes undetected in many cases.

Optic nerve lesions are usually in the canal, where it is difficult to show a fracture; but there may be an associated orbital or anterior fossa fracture. Autopsy has shown hemorrhagic, ischemic, and shearing lesions.[5] Almost any type of field defect can be found, when the lesion is incomplete. Most often there is complete monocular blindness of immediate onset (with an unreacting pupil); and this can occur after injuries that are quite mild in terms of general brain damage, especially in children. Recovery is rare and the disc usually becomes pale within 3 to 4 weeks. Lesions anterior to this may affect the retinal vessels, which are either thread-like and thin, or congested as in central vein thrombosis. Chiasmal lesions cause bitemporal hemianopia, probably owing to ischemia of the vulnerable central part of the chiasm; like nerve lesions, these are usually present immediately after injury and neither progress nor improve, but delayed lesions do occasionally occur.

Lesions of the calcarine cortex are not uncommon, but unless evidence is actively sought, temporary hemianopia or cortical blindness may be overlooked. In both adults and children, such blindness is often delayed for hours or days after injury and may then only last for half an hour, though more often it lasts for several hours and sometimes days. It is seldom followed by persisting hemianopia. This fact, together with the delay in onset and the temporary nature of the disorder, raises doubts about whether this symptom is a reflection of impact damage. It would be more readily explained by hypoxia or ischemia, though whether on the basis of focal spasm in response to injury, or to a form of migraine precipitated by the injury, is speculative. When the condition is marked, there may be aphasia and agnosia from involvement of the adjacent brain, and these rather than hemianopia probably account for persisting reading difficulties when they occur.

Disorders of the Oculomotor Nerves and Connections

In the acute stage after injury, abnormal eye movements are common and are usually a temporary phenomenon.[16,22] Patients examined in the first few minutes after mild concussion may show nystagmus and/or skew deviation, which disappear within minutes. Patients who are in coma for hours or days may have partially dysconjugate roving or reflex (vestibulo-ocular) eye movements, which return to normal as consciousness is regained. The assumption is that such disorders reflect dysfunction in the brain stem, but do not indicate structural lesions that lead to sequelae. When disorders of conjugate gaze are discovered in fully conscious patients who have recently had a head injury, the diagnosis of multiple sclerosis should always be considered (the episode perhaps precipitated by trauma); this is said to be the only common cause of bilateral internuclear paralysis after mild injury.

Diplopia is a common complaint after recovery from the acute stage of head injury and there are many causes. Often the problem lies in the orbit and this symptom need not indicate intracranial damage, nor even involvement of nerves. It does not need much dislocation of the globe or mechanical restriction of movement to produce ocular imbalance, and this can result from orbital fractures, blood, edema, or the escape of air or CSF into the orbit. The ocular muscles or the nerve branches to them may be involved by these factors also. In some cases no definite lesion, mechanical or neurological, can be found; such cases frequently respond to orthoptic treatment.

Third nerve palsy is not uncommon, either as a result of impact injury or (more often) of tentorial herniation. Impact lesions are most often in the superior orbital fissure; but they can be at the apex of the orbit when the optic nerve is also involved, or in the wall of the cavernous sinus when the fourth, fifth, and sixth nerves are also affected. Recovery is the rule, but upward movement may remain restricted.

Sixth nerve palsy is usually associated with fracture of the petrous temporal or sphenoid bones. But it may also occur subsequent to lumbar puncture or because of phenytoin intoxication—either of which may be associated with head injury. Recovery is again usual.

Seventh and Eighth Cranial Nerves

These are frequently damaged together by petrous fractures, which are of two kinds: the more common and less serious longitudinal, and the transverse (Fig. 1). These have distinct clinical features that usually make it possible to know which type of fracture has occurred, even if radiology is negative, which it often is with the longitudinal type (Table 3). However, mixed fractures and syndromes do occur. Moreover, facial palsy is sometimes seen without evidence of a petrous fracture, since it is occasionally caused by lacerations that have damaged fibers (or the trunk) in their extracranial course. Bilateral inner ear concussion can also happen without fracture.

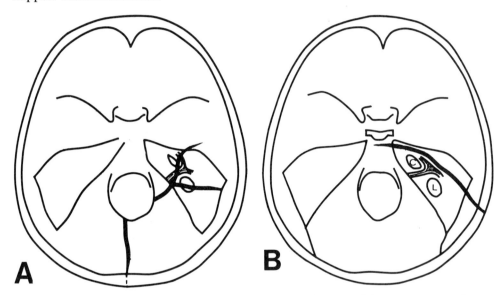

Figure 1. Usual course of transverse (**A**) and longitudinal (**B**) fractures of the petrous temporal.

Facial Palsy[12,13]

When associated with transverse fracture, the paralysis is usually immediate and complete, while with longitudinal it may be delayed, usually by 2 to 3 days. Delayed palsy is usually followed by recovery over a period of 6 to 8 weeks. Sometimes a partial weakness is immediately apparent and then becomes complete later. The site of the lesion can be deduced from the involvement of the lachrymal and salivary secretion, and the involvement of taste in the anterior two thirds of the tongue; return of taste usually occurs before recovery of facial power and is a useful sign of impending recovery. Electrical tests can be difficult to interpret, and there is not yet an ideal battery of such tests on which to base prognosis. Steroid treatment given to all petrous fractures as soon as they are admitted to hospital will reduce the incidence of delayed facial palsy.[12] Although otologists frequently recommend surgical decompression, the view of most neu-

Table 3. Fractures of the petrous temporal bone

	Transverse	Longitudinal
Frequency	10–20% of fracture	80–90% of petrous fracture
Impact	Fronto-occipital—severe	Temporoparietal—often milder
Spread from	Foramen magnum	Temporal squama vault (ipsilateral)—¼ from contralateral side via sphenobasilar suture
Drum/meatus	Hemotympanum	Bloody otorrhea (in c. 50%); CSF otorrhea (c. 5%)
Battle's sign	−	+ (usually with otorrhagia)
Labyrinth damage	+ (lateral type)	−
Ossicle damage	−	+ (incus dislocated)
Inner ear damage	+ (medial type)	−
Facial palsy	30–50%	10–25%

rosurgeons is that, since most delayed palsies recover (at least partially) and most immediate lesions remain permanent whatever is done, operative intervention is seldom justified.

Eighth Nerve Dysfunction

Lesions can occur in several locations in the cochleovestibular system, often in more than one place at a time (Table 4). Damage may be central (brain stem nuclei and pathways), in the nerves in the internal auditory meatus, in the end-organs (labyrinth, utricle, or organ of Corti), or in the ossicular chain. *Vestibular dysfunction* may be manifest in vertigo or ataxia, or both. Nystagmus may be evident on testing; it can be spontaneous or may be seen only after suddenly changing the position of the head. It may be observed directly, but electronystagmography allows nystagmus to be recorded with the eyes closed; this increases the sensitivity of the test, because fixation can suppress nystagmus in some circumstances. Drugs and reduced alertness will also affect the response. Even after quite mild injuries, without petrous fracture, many patients can be shown, by using these tests, to have vestibular dysfunction, even when there is no nystagmus on routine clinical examination (including positional change). These abnormalities can persist for a year or more. This is one piece of evidence that supports the organic basis for some aspects of the postconcussional syndrome (p. 258). The symptoms

Table 4. Frequency of eighth nerve dysfunction after head injury

	All Closed Head Injuries	With Skull Fracture	With Temporal Fracture
Vestibular Function			
Dizziness	58%	58%	87%
Nystagmus	27%	36%	42%
Calorics abnormal	60%	—	—
Audiological Function			
Hearing loss	52%	—	—
Neurosensory hearing loss	60%	—	—

(From Toglia and Katinsky,[21] with permission.)

277

caused by vestibular dysfunction usually subside within a few weeks, although vertigo on change of position can persist. When vestibular symptoms occur with a petrous fracture, the damage is usually in the end-organ, but almost a third of cases without a fracture are thought to have a central lesion (in the brain stem nuclei).

Audiological tests show an abnormality in more than half the patients tested in a number of large series, although the kind of patients admitted to examination is not clearly defined (Table 5). *Hearing loss* is commonly sensorineural, often bilateral, and associated with transverse petrous fractures. It affects the high frequency range and is similar to that caused by exposure to high intensity noise. The lesion is most often in the organ of Corti, which is believed to be damaged by concussion. Conductive deafness is common with longitudinal fractures; it may be temporary if caused by blood in the middle ear system, but permanent impairment may be due to disruption of the ossicular chain, the one type of hearing loss that may respond to surgical treatment. *Tinnitus* is a common complaint, which frequently occurs after mild injuries and is then unassociated with hearing loss or vestibular dysfunction. When it is accompanied by bilateral sensorineural deafness, the tinnitus is usually unvarying in intensity and can be shown to correspond to sound in the range 3000 to 6000 Hz, either as a pure tone (ringing) or filtered white noise (hissing). Tinnitus with unilateral conductive deafness is of more variable intensity and is usually described as roaring.

Table 5. Audiometry in 100 cases of head injury

Neurosensory Hearing Loss	
Bilateral symmetrical	36
Bilateral asymmetrical	10
Unilateral	21
Conductive Deafness	3
Mixed	1
Normal	29

(From Toglia and Katinsky,[21] with permission.)

Last Four Cranial Nerves[6]

Traumatic lesions in this region are usually extracranial in location and are largely confined to gunshot wounds.[6] Occasionally a severe pontobulbar syndrome may affect the nerves also, but distinction between the central and peripheral components of the resulting "bulbar" syndrome is often difficult.

DELAYED COMPLICATIONS

Head injury is so common that it is inevitable that some patients who develop one or other of a wide variety of neurological conditions will be found to have previously sustained an injury. Sometimes when there is a valid causal relationship (e.g., epilepsy or meningitis), the association with injury may not be recognized by the clinician. He may not be told about the head injury, because the patient sees no connection between it and his present complaint; or the clinician may dismiss the head injury as unrelated to the present condition either because the injury was relatively mild or because it happened long ago. However, epilepsy declares itself more than 4 years after injury in 25 percent of cases, while meningitis caused by basal skull fracture may occur 10 years or more after injury. The time lapse since injury is therefore no reason for excluding trauma as a cause of these conditions. Moreover, both of these complications can follow an injury that was associated with a relatively brief period of unconsciousness and that might be considered in retrospect to have been relatively mild.

More common than overlooking a connection with trauma are unjustified attempts to invoke trauma as a cause, or at least as having precipitated an illness that is almost certainly unrelated to injury. A legal claim may be made for damages against those held responsible for head injury, and doctors will then be asked to testify to the probable strength of the connection.

Vascular Conditions

The patient admitted with a head injury is sometimes found to have a recently ruptured aneurysm or an intracerebral hemorrhage in a site that is typical of a primary vascular accident rather than trauma. It will usually be found in such circumstances that the patient sustained his head injury because he fell owing to the immediate effect of spontaneous intracranial hemorrhage, although this may be difficult to establish beyond doubt. While aneurysmal rupture may be associated with circumstances that lead to a surge in blood pressure, there is no evidence that head injury can precipitate the rupture of a congenital aneurysm or can trigger intracerebral hemorrhage associated with hypertension or atherosclerosis.

Occasionally a patient with what appears to be a spontaneous intracerebral hemorrhage gives a history of a head injury some days or weeks previously. The question then arises as to whether this is an instance of *spatopoplexie* as described by Bollinger (p. 157). There is no rule by which to judge the connection between two events of this kind, both of which are relatively common. Even at autopsy after a fatal hemorrhage it may be impossible to do more than form an opinion on the balance of probabilities. But common sense requires that not too long an interval between injury and the symptoms of hemorrhage should elapse; if there is some continuity of symptoms recorded during this period, the association may be easier to sustain.

Very occasionally *aneurysms* form on the carotid artery, in the region of the base of the skull related to a fracture. Less often aneurysms occur on the meningeal or scalp vessels; these are probably false aneurysms. Should these be revealed by angiography, then an association with trauma is reasonable.

Carotid thrombosis occasionally occurs a few days after head injury and is presumably related to associated trauma in the neck. There is no evidence that an ischemic stroke months or years after a head injury, which is found to be due to carotid occlusion in the neck, can be causally related to the preceding trauma. When this complication occurs soon after injury, usually in a young patient without atheroma, hemiplegia develops before (and sometimes without) any marked alteration in consciousness. If edema and shift develop following infarction of the temporal lobe, then the clinical picture of deepening coma and dilated pupil may develop and will be clinically indistinguishable from an intracranial hematoma. CT scanning and angiography will indicate the true nature of the pathology.

Caroticocavernous fistula is a rare sequel of trauma. A fracture is relatively seldom found and the injury it follows has often been mild. About a quarter of patients have no history of trauma at all, and this raises the possibility that a predisposing condition, such as an intracavernous aneurysm of the carotid artery, may be a factor even in some of the traumatic cases. When the lesion follows penetration of the orbital region by sharp instruments or by missiles, there is no reason to doubt that the fistula is solely traumatic in origin. With trauma as obvious as this, symptoms begin within 24 hours in about a third of cases, in a quarter of the rest in the first week, and in the next two months in a fifth. As time passes it is reasonable to raise doubts as to the connection with trauma, especially if this has been mild.

The consistent feature is a subjective bruit, which can usually be heard by an observer with a stethoscope; it may be stopped (or markedly reduced) by carotid compression. Proptosis is usual and may be pulsatile; a degree of edema and chemosis commonly develops—although sometimes only after some weeks of delay. Limited ocular movements may be mechanical or due to involvement of the nerves of the muscles; the sixth is the commonest to be recognizably involved—but there may be complete external ophthalmoplegia. Vision is affected in about half the patients and a quarter may become blind. Occasionally the trigeminal nerve is involved.

Spontaneous resolution occurs in some cases, but how often is uncertain; nor is there any means of predicting which cases will resolve. In some patients the bruit stops abruptly after carotid angiography, although whether this is due to the contrast medium or to the carotid compression employed at the end of this procedure is uncertain. Even when the bruit ceases, the orbital swelling, proptosis, and chemosis sometimes continue, as may occur after surgical obliteration of the fistula. An orbital decompression may then be required.

There are numerous ingenious techniques for achieving occlusion of the fistula. Internal carotid ligation in the neck is reported to be successful in about two thirds of cases when the common carotid is tied, and in three quarters when the internal carotid is occluded. Unless due care is taken to monitor the effects on the cerebral circulation, this operation carries a certain morbidity and mortality associated with cerebral ischemia. A higher rate of success attends "trapping," when the internal carotid is clipped both intracranially and in the neck; if the ophthalmic artery can be included in the internal trapping, the results are significantly better. Various methods of embolizing the fistula, with or without carotid ligation, have been evolved in recent years—some based on intracranial approaches, others on "posting" emboli up the carotid, which has been exposed in the neck. No one surgeon can report a large series of cases, but Stern[17] has reviewed the various reports thoroughly and concludes that experience is still insufficient for any one technique to be firmly recommended as clearly better than the alternatives.

Post-traumatic Hydrocephalus

The availability of CT scanning is making known the frequency and extent of ventricular dilatation after various kinds of head injury, and the time course of the natural history of this condition. Information at present available is patchy and views about the clinical importance of post-traumatic hydrocephalus are therefore controversial. It is, however, clear that three kinds occur: that caused by wasting of white matter after severe injury (ex vacuo); that caused by impairment of circulation of the CSF owing to adhesions in the pathways, probably secondary to bleeding (obstructive); and communicating hydrocephalus (normal pressure). Obstructive hydrocephalus is rare, but will declare its presence by the development of symptoms of raised intracranial pressure, which will be relieved by a shunting operation. The real problem is to distinguish between the other two forms of hydrocephalus. A firm diagnosis of normal pressure hydrocephalus is likely to be made only when a patient who has already recovered to a considerable degree from injury develops new symptoms (mental impairment and disorder of gait); diagnosis depends on these characteristic clinical features and on evidence of retarded CSF circulation. As when this condition occurs spontaneously, only a proportion of patients respond favorably to shunting, and there are no criteria to identify with certainty which patients these are. In a large study of hydrocephalus of all kinds after head injury, only a quarter of those diagnosed as having normal pressure hydrocephalus responded well to shunting.[26]

Intracranial Tumors

Isolated reports are made of meningiomas developing in relation to injuries of scalp and skull, and of gliomas in patients with previous injuries. A systematic long-term study at the Mayo Clinic disclosed no increased risk of either type of tumor over many "patient years" of follow-up after head injury.[11]

Late Traumatic Epilepsy

This is by far the most frequent of delayed complications, yet it occurs in only about 5 percent of all patients admitted to hospital after nonmissile head injury. After some types of injury the risk is much higher than this, particularly when there has been an intracranial hematoma or a compound depressed fracture with certain other features, or when an early fit has occurred (in the first week after injury).

In the study of 150 *severe* injuries[9] followed for more than a year after injury, 15 percent had epilepsy; this would certainly have been higher had the follow-up been longer. The incidence was twice as great in those with severe disability; 20 of 22 severely disabled patients with epilepsy had either an intracranial hematoma or a depressed fracture. This confirms the findings of our previous traumatic epilepsy study,[8] which was based on different patients.

The significance of epilepsy as a disabling symptom depends on whether there are other disabling features, and it was the only physical disability in almost half the patients in whom it occurred after severe injury. It also depends on the extent to which it interferes with the life-style of the particular patient. Young men on the threshold of their careers may have their future options appreciably limited by the occurrence of epilepsy, even by the threat of its developing. Many patients will regard the restriction on car driving that epilepsy entails as one of the most disabling aspects of this complication, even those who are not vocational drivers.

Time of Onset

The case for recognizing fits in the first week as a distinct category (early epilepsy) has been made already (p. 236). What proportion of patients are regarded as having begun within the first year depends on whether or not these early fits are regarded as the beginning of traumatic epilepsy or not. It depends also on how long the patients are followed, because a small number of additional

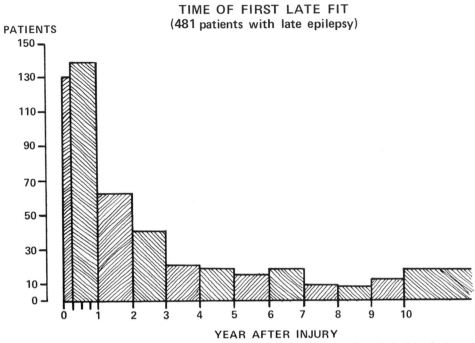

Figure 2. Time of first late fit in 481 nonmissile injuries. The first 3-month period of the first year is separated. In this series 56 percent had their first *late* fit in the first year. If fits occurring in the first year only were included, the first year figure would be 76 percent.

cases develop even after 4 years, and these will dilute the first year fraction. In Jennett's study[8] of 481 patients with late epilepsy beginning within 4 years of injury (Fig. 2), 56 percent had their first *late* fit in the first year (27 percent within 3 months of injury); of those developing epilepsy within the first 5 years after a missile injury, 73 percent had their first fit within a year of injury.

Type of Fit

About 40 percent of patients have at least some fits with focal features, but focal motor attacks (limited to twitching of the face or a limb), which are common in the first week after injury, are seldom encountered. Over 70 percent of patients have attacks in which they become unconscious. In a fifth of patients, the seizures are of temporal lobe type, and when these attacks begin they may not always be immediately recognized as being epileptic in origin. Petit mal has not been encountered as a form of post-traumatic epilepsy.

Persistence of Fits

Whether or not fits will persist once the first late seizure has occurred is an important question. Prior to our study there were several references to post-traumatic epilepsy, mostly after missile injuries, having died out after a time; this led to the concept that seizures were perhaps a manifestation of a certain stage in the healing process. In 1962 we proposed that *remission* of epilepsy was a safer term than cessation, and that 2 years without fits might be a reasonable (if arbitrary) definition of remission.[7] This definition was used also by Caveness,[1] who pointed out that clinicians frequently recommend discontinuation of anticonvulsant drugs in adults after 2 years without fits, and that 2 years without fits is the rule for granting a driving license in many of the United States (it is 3 years without any daytime fits in the U.K.). In a series of combat victims from Korea, 56 percent were still having fits 4 years later and 47 percent at 8 years;[1,3] there was no difference between missile and nonmissile injuries. Of patients who had three or more fits in the first year, two thirds still had frequent fits 8 years after injury.

In Jennett's study of nonmissile injuries,[8] 75 percent of patients continued to have epilepsy for years after the onset. And, as Caveness found, even a remission of 2 or more years was frequently followed by reappearance of fits. Temporal lobe epilepsy was more often persistent, as was epilepsy that had been delayed in onset for more than 2 years after injury. There was no clear association between other features and the likelihood of persistence of remission. It must be concluded that once a patient suffers even one late fit, there is a high probability that he will continue to have epilepsy, although this may be well controlled by anticonvulsants. Even if there is a remission of 2 years, there remains a significant probability that further fits will occur.

Prediction of Fits

Because this complication occurs relatively seldom among head injuries as a whole, but can occur in patients who are otherwise well recovered, and may not develop until years after injury, there is a premium on the doctor's ability to predict the likelihood of its occurrence. On this will depend decisions about prophylactic anticonvulsants, about how the patient should be advised for his future, and about what guidance to give to lawyers concerned with claiming compensation for the patient.

A review of current practice of board-certified neurosurgeons (early in 1972) in regard to pharmacological prophylaxis for post-traumatic epilepsy revealed a wide diversity of opinion about the indications for medication; 40 percent did not use drugs routinely, most of them because of uncertainty about the indications, or because the risk was considered too low to justify treatment.[14] It was estimated that as many as 100,000 Americans yearly might be suffering convulsions because they were not receiving therapy. Statistical studies over the past decade have established the levels of risk associated with different kinds of injury, and uncertainty about this can no longer be a valid excuse for not giving prophylactic anticonvulsants.

The major study has been by Jennett, whose detailed findings have been collected in a monograph.[8] Various separate findings from this study have been confirmed by different observers in other countries, and there seems little reason to doubt his conclusions, which were based on a study of over 800 patients with traumatic epilepsy following nonmissile head injury. The absolute incidence reported will vary according to the duration of follow-up; although more than half of those who develop late epilepsy have their first fit within a year of injury, in 25 percent of Jennett's cases the onset was delayed for 4 years or more. On the basis of a minimum follow-up of 4 years, he estimated that 5 percent of patients admitted to hospital develop late epilepsy. The majority of such patients continue to

283

Table 6. Main factors increasing incidence of late epilepsy

No early epilepsy	29/868	3%	P<0.001
Early epilepsy	59/238	25%	
No hematoma	27/854	3%	P<0.001
Hematoma	45/128	35%	
No depressed fracture	27/832	3%	P<0.001
Depressed fracture	76/447	17%	

(From Jennett,[8] with permission.)

suffer from fits for years, and most have attacks that render them unconscious—although there are often focal features at the beginning of a fit.

Three factors increase the risk of late epilepsy significantly (Table 6). In patients with neither a depressed fracture nor an acute intracranial hematoma the risk of epilepsy is low, whether or not there has been prolonged unconsciouness (PTA > 24 hr), unless there has been an early fit (Table 7). The influence of early epilepsy is therefore most powerful in these patients, whose risk of late epilepsy would otherwise be low. Early epilepsy increases the risk of late epilepsy as much after trivial as after serious injuries, and whether early epilepsy was confined to a single fit, repeated fits, or consisted of status. Children are somewhat less liable to develop late epilepsy after an early fit, but the risk of late epilepsy is still significantly greater if there has been a seizure during the first week (Table 8).

In patients with depressed fracture, the risk of late epilepsy varies greatly according to four features: whether the dura is torn, there are focal signs, the PTA exceeds 24 hours, or there has been early epilepsy. On the other hand, the site of fracture, whether the bone fragments are removed or replaced, or indeed whether the fracture is elevated or not, makes little difference to whether or not late epilepsy develops. Varying combinations of the four influential factors are associated with a range of risks of late epilepsy between 3 percent and 70 percent (Fig. 3). High risk combinations occur relatively seldom, and, using the predictive criteria evolved, it is possible to recognize that some 40 percent of patients with depressed fracture have a risk of epilepsy of less than 5 percent (Fig. 4).

Table 7. Late epilepsy after injuries without depressed fracture or intracranial hematoma

	All Cases	PTA < 24 hr	PTA > 24 hr
All cases	2%	1%	4%*
No early epilepsy	1%	1%	1.5%
After early epilepsy	26%	22%	30%

*Confirmed from Glasgow Data Bank, 2/63 = 3%.
(From Jennett,[8] with permission.)

Table 8. Incidence of late epilepsy at different ages

| | Jennett[8] | | Stowsand[18] |
	> 16 years	< 16 years	< 15 years
No early epilepsy	21/638　3%	8/230　4%	8/230　4%
After early epilepsy	39/120　33%	20/118　17%	8/40　20%
	P<0.001	P<0.001	P<0.001

It is natural that the EEG record should be looked to for clues to the likelihood that epilepsy will develop. Patients who have suffered more severe brain damage more often have EEG abnormalities and are more prone to develop epilepsy. These EEG abnormalities become less marked as time from injury increases, but they do so less quickly in patients who develop late epilepsy (Table 9). However, this difference becomes significant only a year or more after injury, and it is therefore not a useful predictive criterion. Moreover, most serious brain damage that is associated with EEG abnormalities is obvious clinically (depressed fracture, intracranial hematoma, prolonged PTA, or focal signs); the EEG is therefore not providing additional data. Furthermore, some 20 percent of patients who subsequently develop late epilepsy have a normal EEG in the early stages after injury. Although this is a significantly greater proportion than obtains in patients who remain free of epilepsy, it does mean that a normal EEG cannot be regarded as reassuring. Our conclusion that the EEG is not helpful in predicting late epi-

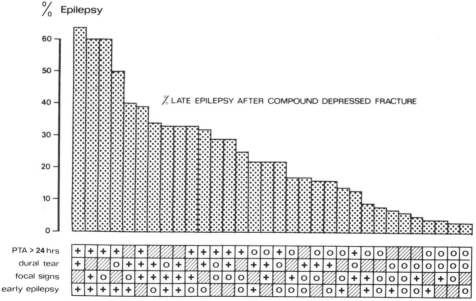

Figure 3. Proportion of patients developing late epilepsy after compound depressed fracture (at least 1 year follow-up). Different groups of patients are shown, according to four features, with the calculations based on knowledge of three of these four features (as information is often missing about one of them). (From Jennett,[8] with permission.)

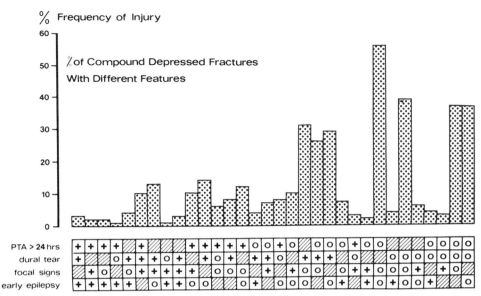

Figure 4. Frequency of occurrence of various combinations of epileptogenic features in 1000 depressed fractures. Same ordering (from left to right) as in Figure 3; most cases are on the right, where the risk of epilepsy is least. (From Jennett,[8] with permission.)

lepsy is in accord with other contemporary views,[4,20,25] and this appears, therefore, to be a consensus in the present state of knowledge.

Late Epilepsy after Missile Injuries

This is much more common than epilepsy after nonmissile injury and has shown remarkable consistency during successive wars over the last 50 years (Table 10). Improved early care of these open injuries, with a greatly reduced subsequent infection rate, has not made any difference in the incidence of late epilepsy. Presumably this is because epilepsy is related to the amount of brain damage; thus the epilepsy rate is higher when the dura is torn, when PTA is prolonged, and when there is damage to more than one lobe of the brain or a track deep enough to reach the ventricle.[3]

Table 9. Frequency of abnormal EEG records at varying intervals after injury

Time Since Injury	No Late Epilepsy	Late Epilepsy	p
< 4 mo	76%	83%	NS
4–12 mo	59%	67%	NS
1–2 yr	64%	71%	NS
> 2 yr	46%	73%	<0.001

(From Jennett,[8] with permission.)

Table 10. Epilepsy after missile injuries in four wars[2,3]

	World War I	World War II		Korea	Vietnam
	Ascroft (n=316)	Walker (n=295)	Russell (n=820)	Caveness (n=211)	Caveness (n=802)
All cases	35%	34%	—	35%	33%
Dura torn	41%	—	43%	42%	43%

Prophylactic Anticonvulsant Therapy

High risk patients can now be recognized with confidence by the end of the first week, many of them within 1 or 2 days of injury. What level of risk justifies anticonvulsants will be a matter of opinion; we consider that 20 percent is certainly an indication for drugs. How long they should be continued is also a matter for discussion. The residual risk after an interval has passed without epilepsy having occurred can be calculated;[10] this is the best guide to when discontinuation should be considered. If no individual calculation is made, then 2 years would seem a reasonable time for initial treatment. Checks on blood levels should be done regularly to ensure compliance with whatever regimen has been prescribed.

A new approach to prophylaxis was proposed and tested by Young and associates.[23] This entailed the establishment of adequate blood levels of phenytoin as soon after injury as possible, certainly in the first 24 hours. An intravenous loading dose (11 mg/kg body weight) was followed by intramuscular injections sufficient to maintain 10 to 20 μg/ml blood level. Oral dosage was substituted as soon as was practical, and an attempt made to maintain this for 1 year. However, it was found that only a third of patients were still taking medication a month after injury, and half of these had inadequate blood levels. In spite of this there was a lower than expected number of patients who developed epilepsy during the first year after injury. This suggested that the effect of treatment had been at least partly due to preventing the development of an epileptic focus, rather than suppression of epileptic activity. More studies with larger numbers of patients will be needed to confirm this preliminary report. Such treatment may also reduce the incidence of early epilepsy, but it can never be wholly successful, because many of the fits occur in the first hour or so after injury.

REFERENCES

1. CAVENESS, W. F.: *Onset and cessation of fits following craniocerebral trauma.* J. Neurosurg. 20:570–583, 1963.

2. CAVENESS, W. F., MEIROWSKY, A. M., RISH, B. L., ET AL.: *The nature of post-traumatic epilepsy.* J. Neurosurg. 50:545–553, 1979.

3. CAVENESS, W. F., WALKER, A. E., AND ASCROFT, P. B.: *Incidence of post-traumatic epilepsy in Korean veterans as compared with those from World War I and World War II.* J. Neurosurg. 19:122–129, 1962.

4. COURJON, J. A.: "Post-traumatic epilepsy in electroclinical practice." In Walker, A. E., Caveness, W. F., and Critchley, M. (eds.): *Late Effects of Head Injury.* Charles C Thomas, Springfield, 1969, pp. 215–227.

5. CROMPTON, M. R.: *Visual lesions in closed head injury.* Brain 93:785–792, 1970.

6. FISHBONE, H.: "Irreversible injury of the last four cranial nerves (Collet-Sicard syndrome)." In Vinken, P. J., and Bruyn, G. W. (eds.): *Handbook of Clinical Neurology.* vol. 24. North Holland Publishing Co., 1976, pp. 179–181.

7. JENNETT, B.: *Epilepsy after Blunt Head Injuries*. ed. 1. Heinemann, London, 1962.

8. JENNETT, B.: *Epilepsy after Non-Missile Head Injuries*. ed. 2. Heinemann, London, 1975.

9. JENNETT, B., SNOEK, J., BOND, M. R., AND BROOKS, N.: *Disability after severe head injury: Observations on the use of the Glasgow Outcome Scale*. J. Neurol. Neurosurg. Psychiat. 44:285–293, 1981.

10. JENNETT, B., TEATHER, D., AND BENNIE, S.: *Epilepsy after head injury. Residual risk after varying fit-free intervals since injury*. Lancet ii:652–653, 1973.

11. KURLAND, L.: "Head injuries at the Mayo Clinic." In Rose, C. F. (ed.): *Clinical Neuro-Epidemiology*. Pitman, London, 1980.

12. POTTER, J. M., AND BRAAKMAN, R.: "Injury to the facial nerve." In Vinken, P.J., and Bruyn, G. W. (eds.): *Handbook of Clinical Neurology*. vol. 24. North Holland Publishing Co., Amsterdam, 1976, pp. 105–117.

13. PUVANENDRAN, K., VITHARANA, M., AND WONG, P. K.: *Delayed facial palsy after head injury*. J. Neurol. Neurosurg. Psychiatry 40:342–350, 1977.

14. RAPPORT, R. L., AND PENRY, J. K.: *A survey of attitudes toward the pharmacologic prophylaxis of post-traumatic epilepsy*. J. Neurosurg. 38:159–166, 1973.

15. ROBERTS, A. H.: *Long-term prognosis of severe accidental head injury*. Proc. R. Soc. Med. 69:137–140, 1976.

16. ROBERTS, M.: "Lesions of the ocular motor nerves (III, IV and VI)." In Vinken, P. J., and Bruyn, G. W. (eds.): *Handbook of Clinical Neurology*. vol. 24. North Holland Publishing Co., Amsterdam, 1976, pp. 59–72.

17. STERN, W. E.: "Carotid cavernous fistula." In Vinken, P. J., and Bruyn, G. W. (eds.): *Handbook of Clinical Neurology*. vol. 24. North Holland Publishing Co., Amsterdam, 1976, pp. 399–439.

18. STOWSAND, D., AND BUES, E.: *Fruhanfalle unde ihre verlaufe nach hirntraumen im Kindesalter*. Z. Neurol. 198:201, 1970.

19. SUMNER, D.: "Disturbance of the senses of smell and taste after head injuries." In Vinken, P. J., and Bruyn, G. W. (eds.): *Handbook of Clinical Neurology*. vol. 24. North Holland Publishing Co., Amsterdam, 1976, pp. 1–25.

20. TERESPOLSKY, P. S.: *Post-traumatic epilepsy*. Forensic Sci. 1:147–165, 1972.

21. TOGLIA, J. U., AND KATINSKY, S.: "Neuro-otological aspects of closed head injury." In Vinken, P. J., and Bruyn, G. W. (eds.): *Handbook of Clinical Neurology*. vol. 24. North Holland Publishing Co., Amsterdam, 1976, pp. 119–140.

22. VLIET, A. G. M. VAN.: "Post-traumatic ocular imbalance." In Vinken, P. J., and Bruyn, G. W. (eds.): *Handbook of Clinical Neurology*. vol. 24. North Holland Publishing Co., Amsterdam, 1976, pp. 73–104.

23. YOUNG, B., RAPP, R., BROOKS, ET AL.: *Post-traumatic epilepsy prophylaxis*. Epilepsia, 20.

24. YOUNG, B., RAPP, R. P., PERRIER, D., ET AL.: *Early post-traumatic epilepsy prophylaxis*. Surg. Neurol. 4:339–342, 1975.

25. WALTON, J. N.: *Some observations on the value of EEG in medicolegal practice*. Med. Leg. J. 31:15, 1963.

26. ZANDER, E., AND FOROGLOU, G.: *Post-traumatic hydrocephalus*. In Vinken, P. J., and Bruyn, G. W. (eds.): *Handbook of Clinical Neurology*. vol. 24. North Holland Publishing Co., Amsterdam, 1976, pp. 231–253.

CHAPTER 12

Mental Sequelae

The most consistent consequence of a head injury is some disorder of mental functioning, either temporary or permanent. After mild injury (concussion) it has been shown that there is a measurable impairment of information processing for 2 to 3 weeks;[6] this combines with various somatic sequelae to produce the frequently encountered postconcussional syndrome, already discussed (p. 258). After more severe injury, associated with coma of some hours duration, the patient remains in a state of disordered consciousness for many hours or days, for which he is subsequently amnesic (p. 89). In patients whose PTA has exceeded 3 weeks it is almost always possible to detect impairment of performance on some test of cognitive function, even 6 months after injury, and some degree of measurable deficit is often permanent. More frequent than altered intellectual function are changes in personality; although less readily recorded or measured, these can be at least as disabling.

Many of the mental sequelae of severe injury resemble those encountered in varying degrees in patients with diffuse structural brain disorders of nontraumatic origin, such as aging or arteriosclerosis. Relatives often comment that an injury, particularly when suffered in middle age, seems to have aged the patient prematurely. It seems likely that the most frequently encountered mental sequelae are related to widespread rather than focal brain damage, which is consistent with the distribution of the initial shearing lesions and also of secondary hypoxic damage in the brain. Mental sequelae related to focal brain damage are not common, if disorders of language and of visuospatial perception are regarded as neurophysical (although the detection and monitoring of recovery of these deficits may depend on psychometric subtests). Some patients develop features associated with frontal lobe damage, and the frequency of memory disorder may be related to the tendency of the temporal lobes to be predominantly involved in many patients. However, it is unwise to overinterpret the localization of brain damage after blunt head injury, because damage is seldom confined to one lobe or even to one side of the brain (Chapter 2).

Very few patients develop symptoms akin to those suffered by psychiatric patients who have no structural brain damage (e.g., depression or psychosis); and the more severely head injured patients seldom complain of the somatic symptoms that characterize the postconcussional syndrome. It seems preferable to use the descriptive term *mental* for the deficits described in this chapter, in preference to *psychological, functional* or *psychiatric* —terms that carry interpretive implications reflecting the stance of different observers.

DEFICITS OF INTELLECTUAL (COGNITIVE) FUNCTION

The availability of large numbers of tests of IQ in general, and of subtests for different functions, has led to many reports about the range of abnormalities found after head injury. However, many of these tests depend heavily on verbal ability, which puts at a disadvantage not only patients with lesions in the left hemisphere, but also those whose capacity to manipulate language has cultural and educational limitations. Performance on IQ tests reflects what has been accumulated over a lifetime by way of intellectual habits, motivation, and cultural expectations. Test results may indicate more about these than about the psychophysiological adequacy of the brain at the time of testing. Another difficulty is to know what the functional capacity was before injury. Sometimes this may be known from the school achievements of a child prior to the accident, or for military personnel from tests undergone on entry to the service. Vocabulary allows an approximate retrospective assessment to be made because simple verbal tests tend to show little impairment after injury, perhaps because they test overlearned skills. Nonverbal tests (e.g., part of the WAIS and the Ravens Progressive Matrices) depend heavily on visuospatial ability and on motor performance; in that these test ability to reason at the time of testing, they are independent of educational and cultural influences prior to injury. On the other hand, they may be unduly affected by focal brain damage in the nondominant cerebral hemisphere, which has caused perceptual and psychomotor deficits; indeed they may be used to diagnose the presence of such neurophysical sequelae.

The balance between focal and general brain damage differs according to the kind of injury. We owe much of our knowledge about the effects of very localized brain damage to the detailed psychological follow-up and testing of military head injuries caused by missile fragments. However, all the evidence from pathological examination of brains that have sustained blunt injury indicates that damage is widespread, albeit with accentuation in certain areas.

Reitan has reported a comparison of psychological test results from patients having an intracranial tumor with those from victims of cerebrovascular accidents and with those who had suffered craniocerebral trauma.[12] The deficits found, in each of these three groups of patients, were more similar than different; patients with trauma that was judged by neurological examination to have been *unilateral* more often showed cognitive deficits that were indicative of *bilateral* pathology than did patients in the other diagnostic groups. In another series of brain damaged patients, tested many years after injury, Smith found many psychological deficits indicative of lesions in the opposite side of the brain from the primary impact.[16]

Verbal abilities are not only less severely affected in the early stages than are performance IQ tests, but they are recovered more rapidly; verbal scores have been largely recovered (if they are going to be) within 3 to 6 months, whereas performance IQ may go on improving for a year or more.[1,10] These differences in the pattern of recovery curves for various functions may account for some of the discrepancies in reports about psychological deficits after head injury, in that testing has often been carried out at widely varying intervals after injury in separate studies.

Performance tests are more severely impaired, probably because they depend on a wider range of cerebral activities and on the integration of these, than do verbal tests. They also reflect other aspects of higher mental function, such as motivation and attention, speed of performance, perseverance, and the ability to organize complex tasks over a period of time. These are in fact the kinds of deficit commonly complained of by patients and their relatives. The failure of routine IQ testing to demonstrate abnormalities in patients who are clearly not performing normally at home may be because these tests are not designed to discover these kinds of alteration in mental activity, and also because patients may perform better during the brief period and relatively abnormal situation of psychological testing than they do in real life. There may be a parallel with the effect of sleep deprivation, when subjects are found to do less well on dull, repetitive tasks requiring vigilance and sustained attention than they do on "more interesting" tasks, such as the succession of tests in an IQ battery.

Recently psychologists have begun to focus on these general aspects of mental activity and to devise appropriate means of testing them. Tests of attention and vigilance include reaction time to visual and auditory stimuli, and recognizing and checking off repeated letters or words in lists. These may be applied for varying periods (to show fatigue effects), and with the addition of various degrees of distraction of different kinds. There is evidence that the ability to screen out irrelevant information, in order to focus on the task at hand, may be one of the mental skills that patients with diffuse brain damage lose. Gronwall and Wrightson have reported that mildly concussed patients have a defect in the speed of processing information, and this is also susceptible to distraction.[6] Other tests that require the integration of many different aspects of brain function and may therefore be more appropriate when testing psychological deficits after widespread brain damage are the recognition of faces,[18] the completion of half-finished pictures, and the recognition of anomalies in sketches of various life situations.[11] These usual tests also clearly depend heavily on the integrity of the nondominant parietal lobe and may be impaired by focal damage in that location.

Another aspect of the brain's activity that it seems appropriate to try to measure is the ability to learn new tasks. This may provide a better indication of the state of the brain than the ability to reproduce previously overlearned material, or to carry out a simple task, or to solve problems one at a time in a test situation. Indeed a common complaint of patients is that while they can continue to undertake activity of a kind that was previously routine for them, and this may include work, they are unable to tackle new tasks or to learn new skills. A parallel between the effects of head injury and those of the normal aging process has already been made; it is likewise a characteristic of the elderly that they can perform well in their routine and familiar environment, but react badly to new situations (e.g., moving to a new house is often reported as having precipitated senile dementia, when it has presumably uncovered it). It might be considered that the ability to learn, after a head injury, correlates with the capacity to recover function as a whole, at least if recovery in the brain is regarded as a learning process. However, one report[13] found no correlation between the progress of patients in a rehabilitation unit and their performance on learning tasks at the beginning of treatment. Learning depends to some extent on memory, but this is a function so specifically affected after head injury, and sometimes out of proportion to other cognitive defects, that it is considered separately (p. 292).

This raises the difficult question of the interdependence of different mental

291

functions, and the extent to which one may be affected independently of others. While we have stressed the importance of dysfunction in the brain as a whole, because blunt head injury produces widespread damage, there are certain focal deficits that cognitive testing may uncover. Although these rarely occur without some deterioration of mental function as a whole, one or other of these focal deficits (such as memory) may be predominant. It may be important to recognize this, in order not to conclude that a patient has general intellectual deterioration, when many of his difficulties stem from a specific defect. Research on this matter has largely emerged from studies of missile injuries and of patients recovering from ischemic strokes, who have focal lesions without involvement of the brain as a whole. But left-sided lesions can also lead to perceptual deficits (difficulty in figure ground discrimination) and to deficits in certain motor functions, such as copying complex gestures.

Left Hemisphere Lesions

Even when patients with clinically detectable dysphasia are excluded, patients with lesions in the dominant hemisphere tend to have particular difficulty with various cognitive tests. In some of these it is clear that deficits in verbal skills are being uncovered; these are not obvious in ordinary speech, because they are evident only in the learning and retention of verbal material rather than in communication. Lishman's series of missile injuries[9] followed up many years later showed a marked correlation between left hemisphere lesions and what he termed *psychiatric disability*—a term that embraced all the features described here under *mental sequelae*.

Right Hemisphere Lesions

The visuospatial difficulties that follow these lesions may be so subtle as to require highly specialized tests in order to uncover them. They may therefore not be recognized by patients and yet be responsible for some of their difficulties. In other instances patients have clear topographical disorientation or have difficulty in recognizing faces. These deficits may in turn affect memory, in that initial registration is impaired because of the perceptual difficulty.

Frontal Lobe Syndrome

Lesions of the orbital cortex may cause personality changes, of a kind later described as defects of social restraint (p. 295), which are very marked and may be associated with hyperactivity and aggression. They may involve sexual activities and lead to criminality. Lesions of the convexity of the frontal lobe are more often associated with lack of drive and a tendency to tackle problems with a fixed strategy, because of a comparative inability to innovate or to change direction, as different tasks demand this. Milner has devised tests to detect this inability to suppress a preferred mode of response.[11]

Memory Deficits

Considering the universality of post-traumatic amnesia it is not surprising that some disorder of memorizing is a persistent complaint of many patients. Not that such a report should always be taken at its face value—it is acceptable to say that one's memory is bad, but this may prove in fact to refer to more generalized cognitive deficit or to dysphasia ("forgetting names"). When he defined post-traumatic amnesia, Russell commented that in recovery from unconsciousness the capacity to lay down on-going memory was usually the last function to return.[15] Indeed, it is one of those processes that depends on the integration of several aspects of brain function; it requires that mechanics of perception be intact and attention be adequate, so that images are clearly received. Little is known about what is needed to ensure encoding of the "memory," its persistence, and its availability for retrieval when the appropriate stimulus is applied.

A distinction should be made between recent and remote memory. It is a familiar feature of the elderly demented patient, who cannot remember from day to day or even hour to hour, that he can often vividly recall his childhood. Short- and long-term recent memory must also be recognized as different; after head injury, it is recall over the long-term that is deficient (after half an hour or so). Even patients with devastating deterioration in this form of memory may retain short-term memory and be able to repeat digits correctly; indeed, they may continue to do so if allowed to repeat the figures continuously and are not distracted. But even this short-term memory may break down if too much information is presented, and the system is overloaded. These patients are also slow at learning, although they may eventually achieve a near normal proficiency after much effort and extra time.

It is believed that short-term memory depends on neurophysiological (electrical) processes, while the finite time required for imprinting a permanent image indicates a chemical event, probably involving protein synthesis. Failure of recall may be because the "memory" was never imprinted, or has decayed, or cannot be retrieved. Sometimes cueing can release a memory that was temporarily inaccessible, suggesting that it was loss of the address to an intact imprint that was the explanation of the memory difficulty in such cases. In patients with prolonged retrograde amnesia, the usual recovery of much of the memory of events that happened prior to the injury indicates that this was a retrieval defect. By contrast there is always a permanent loss of memory for a short period immediately prior to impact, the trace of those happenings presumably never having been imprinted. This is certainly the case with post-traumatic amnesia, which remains stable and which will not yield to attempts to uncover it, such as abreaction; such techniques can, however, sometimes accelerate the return of the distant part of retrograde amnesia.

The question of how discrete memory loss can be, without there being parallel deficits in cognitive function, is a matter of dispute among psychologists. In the context of blunt head injury that causes widespread brain damage, marked memory disorder is usually associated with some impairment on standard IQ tests. Some of these tests are themselves directly affected by memory dysfunction, and some include specific memory subtests. If these are allowed for, however, there are instances of severe memory loss associated with intact routine psychometric test results; these are usually encountered after discrete lesions that affect the temporal lobes bilaterally (encephalitis or temporal lobectomy). But when the frequency of bilateral temporal lobe damage in head injury is remembered, it is to be expected that some head injured patients will have mental dysfunction consisting predominantly of problems with memory. Such patients may be considerably helped by the simple device of keeping a notebook, which will ensure that their lives are not disrupted by constant forgetting. This presupposes the preservation of sufficient drive, motivation, and insight for the patient to adopt some routine for consulting his notebook.

Until recently much of the detailed work on memory, as on other mental disorders after trauma, was based on military missile injuries. But Brooks has now begun to publish reports from series of patients with severe nonmissile head injuries, about whom there were full details of other aspects of brain damage, both in the acute and in the later stages.[23] His studies are continuing, but so far he has found that there is a good correlation between the duration of PTA and the degree of persisting memory defect in patients with more than a week's PTA. But skull fracture and focal neurological signs (including dysphasia) were not related to memory impairment, and neither was the score on standard WAIS IQ tests. He found that persisting defects, in the less severely affected, were detected only by a more searching test, such as logical memory and associate learning. Recovery of memory function (to the level of the stable deficit) occurred relatively rapidly once the patient was out of PTA, and there was seldom any significant improvement after 6 months.

Conclusions about Cognitive Tests

The objective of psychometric testing may be summarized as follows. Focal deficits may be diagnosed and disorders of integrated mental function detected and their severity assessed. This may enable advice to be given to the patient and his family and be of value also to those responsible for planning rehabilitation. Improvement may be monitored by serial testing, and this may enable a prognosis to be made and advice about the future given. It is legitimate also to recognize the opportunity that psychological testing after brain damage gives for adding to knowledge about how the brain works, and in particular how it recovers. The possibility of profitting from such data has until recently been limited by overemphasis on the features associated with focal brain damage. This tended to make psychologists less interested in the more pressing and much commoner problems of patients who suffer from the effects of diffuse brain damage, and in the light that study of these may shed on cerebral function. More innovative thinking about the kinds of tests that are appropriate is now beginning to provide a better base than was previously available for understanding this complex problem. More appropriate tests, which relate to those disorders of cognition that are complained of by patients, and are noticed by observers, are now emerging.

Psychological tests prove disappointing only to those who expect too much from them, and who are still surprised when patients who have manifest mental disability perform almost normally on standard IQ tests. It is important to remember that absence of evidence (of abnormality) is not evidence of absence.[17]

PERSONALITY CHANGE

This is the most consistent feature of mental change after blunt head injury, but there is no way to measure it. In its more subtle form this may be noticeable only to relatives or close associates, and unless they are questioned systematically, the doctor may believe that the patient has made a complete recovery.

While categorization of such a total concept as personality is difficult, it is helpful to consider three aspects of behavior when analyzing the nature of change in personality.

Drive is usually reduced and the apathy that results may be described as laziness, sloth, or simply slowness. Circumstances may, however, enable a man to carry out his work satisfactorily, particularly if this is done in a structured environment. Yet once he comes home at night and is left to his own devices and motivation, the patient may fail to follow his previous leisure pursuits, preferring to dream his evening away in an armchair. In the early stages this lack of drive may be an obstacle to successful rehabilitation, but later it may be dealt with by a near relative acting as a daily goad.

Affect most often changes in the direction of euphoria. Combined with the lack of drive this may not result in hyperactivity or hypomania, but rather in the patient's passive acceptance of his condition. This may lead him to underestimate his disabilities and to claim that he is better than he really is. That in turn may lead to a miscarriage of justice when the time comes to award damages for compensation. More florid aspects of disturbed affect are seen in patients who experience emotional lability. Inexplicable bouts of crying, or less often of laughter, may occur; patients with insight can explain that these represent the outward signs of emotion and are not mirrored by a corresponding inner feeling. In that event they are more distressing to the on-looker than to the patient. Occasionally a relative will say that a patient is better behaved or easier to live with since suffering a head injury. This will usually be when a previously aggressive individual is now quieter than he was, and this is seen as improvement.

Social restraint and judgment are qualities that individuals exercise in varying degrees, according to their personality traits and their cultural background. But when a person, who is normally well behaved socially, sensitive to the needs of others, and in control of those inner feelings of dislike and frustration that everyone experiences from time to time, becomes tactless, talkative, and hurtful, there is no doubt about the change. Such patients may be no more than a harmless nuisance to those around them, but they may be subject to outbursts of rage that are not only out of character, but frightening to the onlooker. It is sometimes questioned whether these represent episodes of temporal lobe epilepsy, but they can seldom be so explained. More often they result from some trivial frustration, which would previously never have led that particular patient to respond in this fashion. The whole picture of lack of social restraint is often referred to as "childish behavior," and indeed parts of it are reminiscent of the child not yet trained by years of social schooling by parents, relatives, and teachers.

Relationship to Previous Personality

It is useful to obtain an account from relatives about the patient's pretraumatic characteristics soon after injury, when a more unbiased version may be given than when there has been time for reflection about the consequences of injury. Even without the prospect of possible compensation, relatives are apt later to idealize the patient's previous psychosocial status, and this can make it difficult to assess the degree of change. Prior personality can best be assessed using a formal questionnaire; one of the inventories used for self-report may be modified for use by a relative, whose opinion on how the patient would have answered the various introspective questions can then be recorded.

Sometimes the personality change after injury takes the form of exaggeration of that patient's pretraumatic personality traits; or it may be a reversal of them—for example, a person previously quiet, cautious, and kind may become the opposite. It has been suggested that such patients may have been unduly dependent for their previous "model behavior" on the exercise of an undue degree of restraint, probably dependent on the frontal lobes. However, there is no consistent relationship between premorbid personality and the kind of change that follows trauma. Nor is there often a clear relationship between the type of change and the site of brain damage, although patients with frontal damage without prolonged coma sometimes show a degree of change that is more marked than would be expected from the severity of the diffuse damage.

Reactive Affective (Psychiatric) Symptoms

To suffer a head injury, even a brief concussion, is a significant experience for anyone. When the incident is mild, the patient recovers sufficiently rapidly to remember the scene of the accident, the crowd around him, the ambulance, the accident department, and admission to hospital. By contrast the more severely injured patient wakes up in hospital, often after several days or sometimes weeks of living of which his mind remains forever blank. He finds around him relatives who, unbeknown to him, have been fearing for his life, but who are now concerned for his sanity. There may be major physical problems, either related to the brain damage or to associated injuries. But insight into the situation as a whole, and its implications for the future, seldom develops for some weeks or months. For the moment, living day to day is enough. Only when he goes home is the magnitude of the effects of a severe injury on life, as it is lived as a whole, realized by the patient and his family. But at this stage improvement can usually still be recognized on a week to week scale. As this process slows down, in those whose recovery is incomplete, the probability of permanent disability is gradually realized as inevitable, and both the patient and his family enter a new phase of reaction to the situation.

Some of the more severely affected patients are so blunted or euphoric that they do not appreciate their plight. But others at this stage become not only aware but also distressed by their condition. They may react to this by frustration and anger, placing blame for much of their short-comings on either their relatives or on the doctors and therapists who are trying to help them. Others again become depressed, while some deal with the situation by denial of disability, particularly of cognitive and memory deficits, which are all too obvious to others. The relatives may likewise react with frustration, depression, or denial. However, they do not necessarily react in the same way as the injured member of the family; he may deny disability about which the relatives are aware and angry. The psychodynamics of the family can become crucial once the patient returns home, and the problem of this social reintegration is discussed under assessment of outcome. It seems possible that the mental stress and secondary mental reactions, which at present appear to be almost inevitable consequences of severe head injury, might be significantly reduced and even to some extent prevented if it became customary to offer families early psychosocial counseling to prepare their minds for the nature and the time scale of the problem that they will have to face. It has long been realized that it is the mental disability (cognitive and memory deficits and personality change) that has the most serious consequences so far as social reintegration is concerned, because this tends to evoke secondary or reactive psychiatric symptoms in the patient or his family, which then aggravate the situation.

The ability to adapt, to cope with new environmental stresses, is one of the mental capacities that head injury most consistently affects. It is never an easy matter to adjust a whole life style to a sudden and catastrophic change, such as that which commonly results from severe head injury. But after head injury this difficulty is compounded by the nature of the mental component of this change, and it is this that makes parallels with severe physical disability (such as paraplegia) so inappropriate. Another factor in determining the psychological reaction to injury is the pretraumatic psychosocial status of the patient. Head injured patients are far from being a random sample of the population; many have evidence of previous antisocial behavior and of disturbed family life. In some areas alcoholism is frequent among the head injured, and children with severe head injuries include many from disturbed or deprived homes. The youth of the patient is another factor that influences reaction to injury; the average age of survivors after severe head injury is under 30, and many are in their late teens or early 20s. The problems of adolescence, or of early married life, are compounded with those of brain damage. This particularly affects relationships with parents. But relationships with peer groups and the consequences of the injury for the future, for the completion of education and for career prospects, are also important.

Cognitive and memory deficits are closely related to the extent (and to a lesser degree, to the location) of brain damage;[8,12,16] no such association can be discerned between brain damage and the mental response to the injury. Indeed, there may be marked discrepancy between the degree of measurable disability and the reaction to it, this being most marked when the normal postconcussional symptoms are prolonged and exaggerated into an accident neurosis (p. 258). But after severe head injury, the response appears to depend more on the pretraumatic endowments and characteristics of the patient and his social setting, both within the family and outside it, and on the insight and motivation that are preserved. The social consequences of a combination of mental and physical disability are crucial also, and are discussed later with assessment of outcome (p. 306). What is certain is that patients in the upper socioeconomic groups show a greater capacity to cope with the mental consequence of brain damage, even though they may suffer more from awareness of the loss of mental powers that were previously their pride. Similarly, their families have more resources of adaptation and more options open to them.

Precipitation of Presenile Dementia or of Psychosis

Because boxers' brains have some of the characteristics of Alzheimer's disease, it has been claimed that one head injury may precipitate this condition. It seems more likely that in such circumstances the process was already active prior to injury, but that it was still compensated clinically; the additional brain damage caused by trauma then reduces the reserve on which compensation depended.

There are a small number of cases of schizophrenia that appear to have been precipitated by head injury. This is more likely to be on a psychodynamic basis than by reason of the site or degree of brain damage. Similarly, depressive illness after head injury is usually reactive and related to the mental or physical disability that is persisting.

A certain number of cases of normal pressure hydrocephalus are related to preceding trauma. This and other forms of post-traumatic hydrocephalus are discussed elsewhere (p. 280).

FREQUENCY DISTRIBUTION OF MENTAL SEQUELAE AFTER SEVERE HEAD INJURY

It is difficult to know what the true frequency of various mental sequelae is, for two reasons. One is that most reports previously published have been of series collected by psychiatrists or psychologists and comprised patients referred because they had residual problems in the mental sphere. The other is that data about the initial severity of injury are either not available to those concerned with assessing late sequelae, or the means whereby they are assessed differ greatly between one series and another. Inevitably, therefore, there are widely varying estimates of the frequency and significance of these sequelae.

The scale of occurrence of such sequelae has been analyzed in some detail for a series of 150 patients from Glasgow who had been severely injured (6 hours in coma).[7] Two thirds of these patients had personality changes and two thirds had one or more measurable cognitive deficits. Significant personality changes were found in more than 60 percent, even in patients who had no cognitive deficit and in those who had no physical deficit. On the other hand, patients who had no personality change seldom had significant physical or cognitive deficits. The most common measurable mental deficit was memory impairment, both verbal and nonverbal. Performance IQ was also frequently impaired, representing deficits in the completion within a time limit of complex visuospatial tasks. Memory and performance skills depend on the integration of functions that are widely represented in the brain and are therefore predominantly affected after diffuse brain damage. Verbal and constructional skills, which are presumed to be organized more focally, are less often affected.

PROGRESSIVE DEMENTIA: CUMULATIVE BRAIN DAMAGE

Systematic studies of boxers in Britain have established that some of those who fought hundreds of fights, before there were proper medical controls, developed a stereotyped syndrome.[14] This was progressive and continued to worsen long after fighting had finished, and these men often ended their lives in mental hospitals. Memory impairment was the prominent feature, but there was also severe generalized intellectual loss. Many of the victims had rage reactions, some of which might have been in the form of temporal lobe epilepsy. Physical features consisted of ataxia, spasticity, rigidity, and tremor. The brains of a number of ex-boxers have been exhaustively studied pathologically by Corsellis and his colleagues.[4] Some of the findings appear to be unique to this condition, but some features resemble Alzheimer's disease (pp. 12 and 39).

There are other sports that carry a risk of repeated concussion, such as horse-riding, American football, and rugby football (p. 12). The order of magnitude of the number of injuries is quite different, however, from that formerly sustained by boxers, and the pathological substrate is almost certainly different. However, concern is now being expressed about the possible cumulative effects of several episodes of head injury, some of which may be more severe than those usually occurring in the boxing ring. Neurologists have reported four professional jockeys in one hospital who became disabled by temporal lobe epilepsy and persisting mental impairment after repeated riding accidents.[5] These accidents had sometimes been followed by PTA lasting hours or days, and one jockey had fractured his skull on no less than 10 occasions. It is not suggested that these men have the same syndrome as boxers, but they do provide further evidence that the effects of a series of only moderate injuries may be cumulative; the cumulative effects of more minor concussion have been commented on by others (p. 12).

REFERENCES

1. BOND, M. R., AND BROOKS, D. N.: *Understanding the process of recovery as a basis for the investigation of rehabilitation for the brain injured.* Scand. J. Rehab. Med. 8:127–133, 1976.
2. BROOKS, D. N.: *Recognition memory and head injury.* J. Neurol. Neurosurg. Psychiatry 37:794–801, 1974.
3. BROOKS, D. N.: *Long and short term memory in head injured patients.* Cortex 11:329–340, 1975.
4. CORSELLIS, J. A. N., BRUTON, C. J., AND FREEMAN-BROWNE, D.: *The aftermath of boxing.* Psychol. Med. 3:270–303, 1973.
5. FOSTER, J. B., LEIGUARDA, R., AND TILLEY, P. J. B.: *Brain damage in national hunt jockeys.* Lancet i:981–987, 1976.
6. GRONWALL, D., AND WRIGHTSON, P.: *Delayed recovery of intellectual function after minor head injury.* Lancet ii:605–609, 1974.
7. JENNETT, B., SNOEK, J. BOND, M., ET AL.: *Disability after severe head injury* (in press).
8. LEVIN, H. S., GROSSMAN, R. G., ROSE, J. E., ET AL.: *Long term neuropsychological outcome of closed head injury* (in press).
9. LISHMAN, W. A.: *The psychiatric sequelae of head injury: a review.* Psychol. Med. 3:304–318, 1973.
10. MANDELBERG, I. A., AND BROOKS, D. N.: *Cognitive recovery after severe head injury. 1. Serial testing on the Wechsler Adult Intelligence Scale.* J. Neurol. Neurosurg. Psychiatry 38:1121–1126, 1975.
11. MILNER, B.: "Residual intellectual and memory deficits after head injury." In Walker, A. E., Caveness, W. F., and Critchley, M. (eds.): *The Late Effects of Head Injury.* Charles C Thomas, Springfield, 1969, pp. 84–97.
12. REITAN, R. M.: "Psychological testing after craniocerebral injury." In Youmans, J. R. (ed,): *Neurological Surgery.* vol. 2. W. B. Saunders, Philadelphia, 1973, pp. 1040–1048.
13. RICHARDSON, A.: "Rehabilitation following central nervous system lesions." In Youmans, J. R. (ed.): *Neurological Surgery.* vol. 3. W. B. Saunders, Philadelphia, 1973, pp. 2010–2024.
14. ROBERTS, A. H.: *Brain Damage in Boxers.* Pitman Medical Publishing Co., London, 1969.
15. RUSSELL, W. R.: *Cerebral involvement in head injury. A study based on the examination of 200 cases.* Brain 55:549–603, 1932.
16. SMITH, E.: *Influence of site of impact on cognitive impairment persisting long after severe closed head injury.* J. Neurol. Neurosurg. Psychiatry 37:719–726, 1974.
17. TEUBER, H. L.: "Neglected aspects of the post-traumatic syndrome." In Walker, A. E., Caveness, W. F., and Critchley, M. (eds.): *The Late Effects of Head Injury.* Charles C Thomas, Springfield, 1969, pp. 13–34.
18. WARRING, E., AND JAMES, M.: *An experimental investigation of facial recognition in patients with unilateral cerebral lesions.* Cortex 3:317, 1967.

CHAPTER 13

Assessment of Outcome

The outcome of serious illness is a matter of concern for the patient and his family, for therapeutic teams involved, and for society as a whole. The patient and his family are concerned with the quality of survival, and means are needed to measure this. Therapeutic teams dealing with the critically ill need to know what success their efforts achieve, in order to assess the comparative efficacy of alternative methods and to devise prognostic criteria, and also for their own satisfaction and the maintenance of morale. The concern of society derives from the need to meet the expense of early treatment and of subsequent support for the disabled survivors; in any cost-benefit equation the main component of benefit must be the outcome of the illness.

In spite of these humanitarian, scientific, and economic requirements, the characterization of the initial diagnosis and severity of serious illness attracts much more attention than does the description and classification of outcome in survivors. Head injury is no exception, although the need for accurate assessment is all the more pressing in the case of survival after brain damage, because persisting mental and physical deficits have a marked effect on the quality of life. When survival is achieved after acute failure of other bodily systems, the patient is usually sound in mind. Although functional reserve in one system may be diminished, he can usually accommodate to this situation; moreover, survival with these conditions is often for only a limited period, because there is progressive disease. Survival with brain damage caused by injury is often prolonged and is usually associated with mental impairment, which may seriously interfere with the capacity to cope with disability.[5]

Not only does this make the assessment of disability after brain damage of particular importance, but it makes it peculiarly difficult. The patient himself may lack insight, and the main burden of the disability in terms of distress and suffering may fall on his family or friends. Variations in the terms used to describe the state after brain damage reflect the bias of observers, some of whom tend to take an optimistic view, while others assume a pessimistic stance. Optimistic assessment tends to result from a superficial examination, with undue emphasis on the physical recovery rather than on the mental handicap. Those who were concerned with the expenditure of extraordinary treatment efforts in the acute stage, when the patient was in life-threatening coma, are particularly apt to overestimate the degree of recovery, because of the contrast between the patient's overall state now as compared with then. On the other hand, too pessimistic a view may be expressed by clinicians who list every detectable deficit disclosed by neurological examination, regardless of whether it contributes significantly to disability. Members of the family may view the patient's premorbid state in an overly generous light and may then ascribe to the effects of injury what may prove to have been unsatisfactory psychosocial adjustment to life long before the accident; to this extent they may overstate the disability. Either undue optimism or pessimism is inimical to realistic appraisal and may be a hindrance to better understanding of the needs of individual patients, as well as to the acquisition of knowledge about the effects of management methods that were used either in the acute stage or in the rehabilitation period.

The assessment of outcome after any serious illness should comprise three steps, according to those who have made a special study of this problem. First, the indicators of outcome have to be identified, namely, the functions that treatment or management should aim to restore. Then scales must be devised by which to measure the degree to which these have been achieved. The interaction of these two will then describe a state of health, or an overall outcome.[7]

INDICATORS OF OUTCOME

1. *Removal of threat to life* is the obvious objective of management in the acute phase, and mortality rates provide a ready measure of achievement of this aim. Apart from the crucial issue of the quality of survival, however, the fact of death itself may sometimes be a less straightforward index of outcome from an episode of brain damage *per se* than it first appears to be. Death caused by brain damage may be delayed, while early death that appears to be the result of brain damage may be due to other factors.

2. *Relief of symptoms* is perhaps of less obvious importance, at least as a primary objective, because the brain damaged patient in the early stages is not suffering in the usual sense of the word. Even in the later stages, lack of insight may limit the distress of the patient, although some are only too keenly aware of their plight.

3. *Reduction of dependency* is relatively easily measured in administrative terms, in that discharge from the intensive care unit, from the acute surgical ward, and from hospital itself, each represents a progressive stage in recovery. Although duration of stay in each stage provides a measure of the rate of recovery, this may be deceptive, in that it can depend more on local policies and on the level of family support than on biological recovery. Return to home is often regarded as a satisfactory end result (recently espoused with enthusiasm by geriatricians and psychiatrists); but this again may indicate more about the family than about the state of the patient, because exceptional family efforts may make it possible for some very dependent patients to go home.

4. *Social reintegration* should always be the aim of medical treatment, in as much as this means restoring the patient to his previous activities. However, this is more difficult to measure than it might appear to be, and too often recourse is taken to using "return to work" as an index of recovery. This often proves to be less than satisfactory, particularly for patients who did not previously "work" (e.g., housewives and the unemployed). Failure to return to work may reflect a decision to retire early or, in times of high unemployment, the local economic situation. Moreoever, the range of occupations is so diverse that the interaction

between a particular disability and that patient's job can produce all kinds of anomalies—minimal disablement may be a bar to some work, while serious disability may be compatible with return to other kinds of employment. A broader view of social reintegration than return to work is required and should take account of social relationships and leisure activities.

OUTCOME SCALES

A number of exclusive categories are required if outcome is to be compared between one patient and another, or between different series of patients. Those already used in reports of head injuries over the past 10 years show a wide variety of terms. These include recovery, restitution, and reintegration (on the optimistic side); and sequelae, deficit, invalid, dementia, and apallic (on the pessimistic side). Qualifying terms include prolonged, persisting, and permanent (of coma or invalidism); and severe, serious, partial, and slight (of disability).

A number of scales have been devised for stroke assessment,[23] but these tend to be biased towards subdivisions of severe disability (Table 1). The same is true for some recently introduced specifically for head injuries,[19,22,24,26] and also for one widely used in assessing patients with cancer.[16] Relative degrees of dependence are of considerable significance for the elderly, who make up the bulk of stroke patients; but for the head injured survivor, whose average age is under 30 years, we maintain that any degree of dependence merits classification as severe disability. The scales depicted in Table 1 are only the simplest of the many that have been devised; many methods for assessing stroke patients consist of a complex analysis of various aspects of daily living, each of which may be scored by the degree of independence (or assistance needed). Others score muscle power limb by limb or joint by joint.

Table 1. Classification of disability (conscious survivors)[13]

Head Injury and Nontraumatic Coma		Stroke		Head Injury		Cancer
Glasgow Scale Jennett & Bond		Rankin[23] (1957)	Adams[1] (1963)	Najenson[22] (1974)	Stover & Zeiger[26] (1976)	Karnofsky[16] (1951)
(1975)[11] 3 point	1978[13] 6 point					
Severe Disability	5 4	4 3	3 2	2	2 3 4 5	2 3 4 5 6
Moderate Disability	3 2	2	1	3 4	6	7 8
Good Recovery	1 0	1		5	7 8	10

Glasgow Outcome Scale

A more appropriate approach for brain damaged survivors is a scale based on the overall social capability (or dependence) of the patient, which will take account of the combined effect of specific mental and neurological deficits, but without listing these as part of the definition. This was the purpose of the Glasgow Outcome Scale, which was devised for brain damage in general,[11] because it was required for studies both of head injury[14] and of nontraumatic coma.[2] Its successful use in collaborative international investigations has established that it can be reliably and readily used by different observers. When 150 Glasgow survivors after severe head injury were classified independently by a neurologist and by a neurosurgeon, there was over 90 percent agreement, both for assessments at 6 months and at 12 months after injury.[13] Four categories of survival are recognized:

1. Vegetative State. This condition of nonsentient survival was defined by Jennett and Plum,[12] and has been described on page 85, where its differentiation from other states that are characterized by reduced responsiveness associated with wakefulness is fully discussed. These other states are associated with awareness, while it is part of the definition of the vegetative state that there is no evidence of psychologically meaningful activity, as judged behaviorally, because the cerebral cortex is out of action. After head injury this state is most often the result of severe diffuse shearing white matter damage (p. 26). But it may also result from secondary neocortical necrosis, caused by cardiac arrest. It is possible that in some cases the combination of moderately severe impact damage, with the effects of secondary raised intracranial pressure and subsequent brain stem distortion, together with widespread hypoxic brain damage owing to cerebral perfusion failure, may produce this state, without there having been a single incident serious enough to produce profound and general neocortical necrosis, such as is associated with cardiac arrest. After nontraumatic coma (particularly after stroke), patients may be recognized as vegetative within a day or so of the ictus, because the eyes are open.[19] After head injury, however, it is usually a week or so before the eyes open; this period of coma is considered to be the result of the inactivation of the ascending reticular system by the impact injury to the subcortical white matter. How soon a patient can be considered to be in a persistent vegetative state is discussed later (p. 311).

The case for preferring "vegetative state" to other terms, such as "permanent coma," "apallic syndrome," or "persisting dementia," has been argued elsewhere.[12] We believe that the criteria for the definition of this state should be strict, and that patients who show any evidence of meaningful responsiveness, who obey even simple commands or who utter even single words occasionally, should be assigned to a higher category of recovery—severely disabled. The use of the term "partial apallic syndrome" by some authors seems likely only to promote confusion and to reduce the usefulness of a classification of outcome that includes such a category.[15]

2. Severe Disability (conscious but dependent). Patients in this category are dependent on some other person for some activities during every 24 hours. The worst affected are severely disabled physically, often with spastic paralysis of three or four limbs, sometimes with dysarthria and dysphasia as well; marked dysphasia, which limits communication, is the major handicap in some. Marked physical deficits such as these are always associated with severely restricted mental activity; however, there are some patients who have little or no persisting neurological disability but who are so severely affected mentally that they require permanent supervision, usually in a mental hospital. Such patients do not all have severe organic dementia; some have become so disinhibited, irresponsible, and even psychopathic following their head injury that they are quite incapable of conducting their day-to-day life. The least affected of those in the category of severe disability are patients who are communicative and sensible, though usually with marked impairment of cognitive and memory function on testing, who are dependent for only certain activities on others—perhaps dressing, feeding, or cooking their meals. Such a person could not be left to fend for himself, even for a weekend. He is not independent and must therefore be regarded as severely disabled on our classification. Many severely disabled patients are permanently institutionalized, but this should not be part of the definition, because occasionally even totally dependent patients are able to be at home.

3. Moderate Disability (independent but disabled). These patients look after themselves, can travel by public transport, and some are capable of work. This may be of a sheltered kind, but certain disabilities are compatible with return to the patient's own occupation. For example, a patient with severe dysphasia may be able to carry out complex nonverbal tasks—one such man who was a shepherd could readily control his dogs by whistling. A patient with a blind eye would be in this category, or one who had bilateral deafness, because these are also compatible with economic independence in certain kinds of work. Sometimes indulgent employers allow a man to resume work, although in truth he is being "carried" by his colleagues and is functioning nowhere near his previous level. For this and other reasons we do not believe that return to work in itself should be central to classifying ultimate disability. Most patients in the category of moderately disabled have either memory deficits or personality changes, varying degrees of hemiparesis, dysphasia or ataxia, post-traumatic epilepsy, or major cranial nerve deficits. Notice that the degree of independence required to reach this category is of a higher degree than that commonly described, particularly by geriatricians, as "independent for ADL" (see p. 314). Patients able to attend to their personal needs in their own room, but to do no more than this, would be judged severely disabled on the Glasgow scale.

4. Good Recovery. This need not imply the restoration of all normal functions; there may be persisting sequelae such as bilateral anosmia, or mild impairment on some psychological tests. But the patient is able to participate in normal social life and could return to work (although he may not have done so). Just as some moderately disabled patients do work, quite a number of those with good recovery do not—the possible reasons for which are many.

Number of Categories

According to the purpose for which a classification is devised, it may require more or fewer categories than those described above (Table 2). When seeking statistical relationships between early features and outcome, it is necessary to avoid having too many, and we have frequently made use of a reduced number, usually by merging dead and vegetative patients at one end of the scale, and moderate disabilities and good recoveries at the other. However, when it is wished to analyze the rate and degree of recovery, or to recognize improvement within

Table 2. Variations on the Glasgow Outcome Scale[13]

Extended Scale	Original Scale	Contracted Scales			
Dead	Dead	Dead	Dead or Vegetative	Dead or Vegetative	Dead
Vegetative	Vegetative	Dependent			
Degree of Disability: 5	Severely Disabled		Severely Disabled		
4					Survivors
3	Moderately Disabled			Conscious	
2		Independent	Independent		
1	Good Recovery				
0					
Total Categories 8	5	3		2	

one large category, it is helpful to subdivide the upper three categories into a better and a worse grade for each, as has been suggested recently by Smith.[25]

Component Disabilities in Different Outcome Categories

In only a quarter of 150 Glasgow head injury survivors previously described (p. 271) was the physical disability more prominent than the mental; in more than half the mental component of the disability was judged to be more important (Table 3). There was a similar preponderance of mental disability in each of the three categories of conscious survivors. In a more detailed study of a series of 56 patients from a larger series, Bond[4] has explored other aspects of the relationship between social handicaps and aspects of the mental and physical sequelae (Table 4). He likewise showed that mental disability contributed more significantly to overall social handicap.

When physical, cognitive, and personality deficits were classified each into three grades of severity in 61 patients for which full information was available,

Table 3. Component disabilities in different outcome categories[13]

Balance of Disability	Good Recovery n=55	Moderate Disability n=60	Severe Disability n=30	Total n=145
Mental worse	56%	48%	63%	54%
Physical worse	27%	30%	23%	28%
Equal	17%	22%	13%	18%
Mental ≥ Physical	73%	70%	76%	72%

Table 4. Correlations between different handicaps[4]

Social Handicap	vs Physical Handicap	vs Mental Handicap
Social handicap as a whole	<0.001	<0.001
Work capacity	<0.02	<0.01
Leisure	NS*	<0.001
Family cohesion	NS	<0.001
Sexual activity	NS	NS

*NS = not significant

the relation of these deficits to the different outcome categories could be analyzed (Table 5). Deficits in patients who had made a good recovery were mostly mild changes in personality. In those with moderate disability, personality change and physical disability were recorded in about equal proportions. More detailed analysis of the neurophysical sequelae showed that in the good recoveries these were most commonly mild hemiparesis, cranial nerve palsies, or infrequent epilepsy. In the moderately disabled, hemiparesis was again prominent and was sometimes severe; and dysphasia was much more frequent than in the good recoveries. Cranial nerve palsies were more common and sometimes severe, and ataxia was not uncommon. In both these upper grades of recovery, personality changes were common, but these were more frequent and more severe in the moderately disabled than in the good recoveries. There was no marked difference between measurable aspects of disability in the moderate and the severely disabled, largely owing to the small number of severely disabled patients in whom formal cognitive testing was feasible. This emphasizes the value of making an overall clinical judgment, rather than depending on a detailed analysis and basing a calculation of overall disability by adding the individual disabilities thus revealed. Indeed, the conclusion reached at the end of this detailed investigation was that although it was of interest to discover the nature of the component disabilities that resulted in the patient being allocated to a given outcome category, allocation to that

Table 5. Relationship of degree of deficit to outcome category[13]

Degree of Deficit (3 = severe)		Good Recovery n=29	Moderate Disability n=23	Severe Disability n=9
Physical	1	26	8	1
	2	3	15	6
	3	0	0	2
Personality	1	16	2	0
	2	13	17	1
	3	0	4	8
Cognitive	1	28	17	0
	2	1	4	2
	3	0	2	7
Total	1	29	12	0
Disability	2	0	10	1
	3	0	1	8

category did not require such a detailed analysis. In fact, it could be reliably done on the basis of a brief outpatient interview by use of a structured questionnaire.

WHEN TO ASSESS OUTCOME

It is surprising how seldom reports on outcome make specific reference to how long after injury the assessment was made. Most deaths occur in the first week, but the process of recovery in survivors may continue for months, and, indeed, it is often asserted that substantial recovery may occur even after years. What interval is chosen for assessment depends to some extent on how detailed a categorization is required. Division into deaths and survivors can reasonably be made at the time of discharge from intensive care, although there will be a few late deaths among those who are vegetative or severely disabled. But any attempt to record the ultimate degree of disability at this stage would really be a prediction, not an assessment; confusion arises unless this distinction is made. As time passes prognosis becomes more confident, but it should still always be made clear whether the expected or the actual state is being described, and if the latter, at what interval after injury assessment of actual outcome was made.

It is important to know the shape of recovery curves in order to judge the extent to which alternative therapies are altering them; in order to make practical decisions about rehabilitation (in particular how long various techniques should be continued); and in order to be able to make plans for the future of patients who seem likely to remain disabled.

Anecdotes about unexpected late recoveries many months or years after severe head injury lead some clinicians to encourage patients' relatives and therapists to look forward to continued recovery over a long period of time, when this may in fact be unrealistic. What is required for practical purposes is to determine an interval after injury by which time most of the recovery will have occurred in most of the patients. What is meant by most of the recovery will depend on how accurate a scale of measurement is used to judge outcome.

In the Data Bank study there were more than 500 survivors 3 months after injury, and their recovery has been analyzed, at 6 months and 12 months (Table 6; Fig. 1). By the end of the year there were more good recoveries and fewer severely disabled patients; this was not only due to improvement in those with severe disability, but because some of these had died during the period of follow-up. Of those who made a good or moderate recovery by 12 months, two thirds had already reached this level within 3 months of injury and 90 percent had done so by 6 months (Table 7). In the 150 patients from Glasgow, who were studied in more detail, it was confirmed that 10 percent of patients who were severe or moderate at 6 months moved up to become moderate or good, respectively, by 1 year. Only 5 percent of 82 patients followed for more than 18 months showed improvement after 12 months sufficient to change outcome category.

This is not to deny that recovery may continue after 6 months in many patients in whom the improvement is not sufficient to justify a change of category on the three-point scale we have used. Indeed, when the six-point outcome scale was applied to the subset of 150 survivors in Glasgow, we found that 20 percent changed by one category between 6 and 12 months; and in half of these this meant that they moved into a different category on the three-point scale (Fig. 2).

There is other evidence to support the view that most recovery occurs in most patients within the first 6 months. The recovery curves based on severe injuries

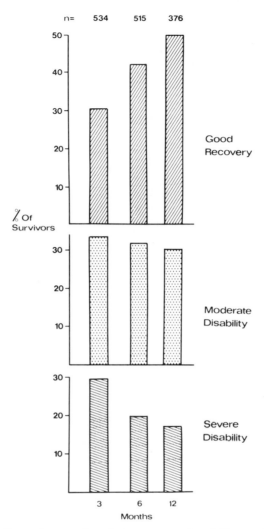

Figure 1. Distribution of conscious survivors between categories of Glasgow Outcome Scale at 3, 6, and 12 months after injury.

Table 6. Survivors after severe head injury

| | | Survivors at | |
Outcome	3 months n=534	6 months n=515	12 months n=376
Vegetative state	7%	5%	3%
Severe disability	29%	19%	16%
Moderate disability	33%	34%	31%
Good recovery	31%	42%	50%
Moderate/Good	64%	76%	81%

309

Table 7. Attainment of final outcome category[13]

Outcome 1 year after injury	n	Already in this category by	
		3 mo.	6 mo.
Moderate disability	118	62%	92%
Good recovery	236	69%	90%

followed for 20 years by Roberts[24] show that almost all who made good recoveries had done so by 6 months. A recent carefully conducted study of recovery after stroke by Brocklehurst[6] also showed little further restoration of various physical capacities between 6 months and 1 year (Table 8).

We maintain, therefore, that 6 months after injury is an appropriate time to

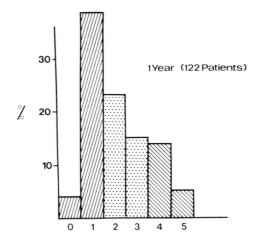

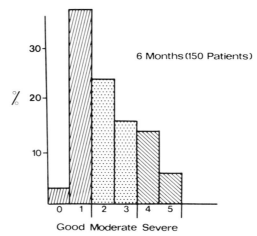

Figure 2. Distribution on 6-point scale for conscious survivors at 6 and 12 months.

310

Table 8. Functional state of 94 stroke survivors

	Improvement by 6 months (%)	Improvement by 1 year (%)
Power	21	22
Mobility	54	61
Independence	48	49
ADL*	44	47
Walking pattern	42	44

*ADL = activities of daily living
(From Brocklehurst, J.,[6] with permission)

assess outcome and is not too long to maintain contact with the majority of patients; this is the basis of our statistical studies into predictive criteria (p. 320).

COURSE OF THE VEGETATIVE STATE

Since the vegetative state was defined by Jennett and Plum in 1972[12] the term has come into general use, and although individual clinicians encounter relatively few such patients, there are now at least three large series of patients with data about their course. These are the Japanese epidemiological study,[8] the cases from the Anglo-American collaborative project on nontraumatic coma,[2] and the head injury Data Bank cases.[14] Two questions that can be discussed with reference to these three series are: How soon after an episode of acute brain damage can the vegetative state be recognized? What is the subsequent course of the patients diagnosed as vegetative (in particular, do these patients ever regain consciousness or independence)? The answers that are given to these questions depend critically on how rigorously the vegetative state is defined.

We have always emphasized that this term should be confined to patients who show no psychologically meaningful response, as well as having the characteristic physical features of sleep/wake rhythms with periods of eye opening, and also abnormal motor responses in all four limbs. However, there are authors who appear to include in their reports patients who say occasional words; and some European authors have even used the term "partially apallic," to add to the confusion. In the first few weeks after an episode of brain damage, when this has been caused by head trauma, it can sometimes be difficult to be certain whether a patient is in fact vegetative or should be classified as (very) severely disabled. Indeed, when assessment was made 1 month after head injury in 94 patients who were considered to be in one or other of these states, we assigned only 59 percent confidently as vegetative; 7 percent of these, as compared with 13 percent of those about whom we were doubtful, eventually became independent, although disabled. Such improvement was always obvious within 3 months of injury, and no patient diagnosed as vegetative 3 months after injury gained independence; consciousness was regained in 10 percent of patients who were regarded at 3 months as vegetative, but all these patients remained totally dependent. These findings indicate that in many cases the vegetative state can be recognized with confidence 1 month after injury, but that when there is doubt, the possibility of recovery to moderate disability may be entertained at this early stage. About a

311

third of these doubtful cases will have died by 3 months, and in those still vegetative the possibility of regaining an independent existence can then be virtually excluded.

The pattern of recovery after nontraumatic coma is somewhat different, perhaps because there is no concussive element, but possibly also because of the older age of most of the patients. In many instances the vegetative state was recognized within a week of the ictus, and in a proportion of these it was suspected on the first day after the episode of brain damage.[19] This was because the eyes began to open sooner after nontraumatic brain damage than after head injury. Of patients diagnosed as vegetative after nontraumatic coma, 56 percent had their eyes open in the 4 to 7-day epoch, compared with 26 percent after head injury. It seems likely that the nontraumatic patients who became vegetative without a long preceding period of coma had sustained a focal lesion, usually in the brain stem. After head injury the vegetative state is a sequel of diffuse white matter lesion, or of widespread hypoxic brain damage in the cortex and elsewhere, or of severe brain stem distortion from a supratentorial mass lesion. The first two of these lesions, and in most cases the third, have a period of deep coma before the eyes begin to open and the vegetative state can be recognized. When the vegetative state was diagnosed at 1 month after a nontraumatic coma-producing episode of brain damage, the chances of regaining independence were virtually nil.[19] The early death rate was also higher in the nontraumatic cases, probably because the patients were older and often suffering from systemic disease.

How long young head injured patients who are in the vegetative state (at 3 months) may survive is of some importance. This is of particular concern to lawyers when calculating appropriate personal damage claims following accidents, and who have to consider the possibility of many years of dependent existence. The average age of head injured patients in the Data Bank study who survived in this state was 27 years; their normal expectation of life would therefore be some 45 years. There is as yet no evidence as to whether such patients could survive for this long, because the kind of intensive care that has made the early rescue of these badly brain damaged patients possible began to be widely used only about 20 years ago. The longest head injured vegetative survivor known to us died 18 years after sustaining his injury in 1959. A review of over 100 vegetative patients in Japan revealed that two thirds were still alive 3 years later.[8] This was an etiologically mixed group of patients, which included some with developmental and degenerative disorders—although about a third were a result of trauma and a third of an episode of hypoxic brain damage.

How long these patients *can* live and how long they *do* live may be different. It will be pointed out later that a consensus is emerging that survival in the vegetative state is worse than death (p. 314). It follows from this that in the event of complications developing, such as respiratory tract infections, many doctors would regard it as good medical practice not to intervene actively by giving antibiotics, if the family is in agreement with such a policy. This is certainly a common practice in countries where medicine is practiced without undue legal harassment. Even when such a policy has been agreed to for an individual case the patient may still live for some years. However, the Data Bank study showed that of 94 patients who were judged at *1 month* to be definitely or probably vegetative, 50 percent were dead within a year. Of those declared definitely vegetative at *3 months,* 60 percent were dead at 1 year after injury.

QUALITY OF LIFE

When life is saved (or prolonged) by intensive therapy, questions are sometimes asked, both within the health professions and by other observers, about the quality of survival. For example, doubts have been expressed about the wisdom of neonatal surgery for some major congenital abnormalities and about aggressive treatment for certain kinds of malignant disease. This debate most often arises, however, in relation to brain damaged patients, in particular survivors after head injury or major stroke. Some sensitive observers, including members of the families of victims, sometimes even express the view that the degree of disability has proved to be so great that it might have been better if the patient had not been rescued in the first place. Such individual comments may seem no more persuasive than anecdotal accounts of remarkable recovery supposedly occurring unexpectedly after severe head injuries. But as with these there is need to respond positively by providing an analysis of what facts can be ascertained, so as to construct a framework within which to conduct further discussion.

In attempting to give guidelines for assessing the quality of life, discussion will be limited to the severely disabled or vegetative. This is not to deny the significance to many patients of moderate disability. And there are some patients who must be judged to have made a good recovery, but who have been restored to a kind of life that might not be considered, by certain standards, to be of a high quality; for example, a patient may be back in prison, or again living the life of a chronic alcoholic.

When assessing outcome, the level of ultimate social functioning may be gauged on a relatively coarse scale, such as the one described, which is applicable to the population in general; or by a finer measure that relates the post-traumatic condition to the particular patient's former state. For example, patients in the professional or managerial occupations may suffer mental deficit, which renders them less effective, and they may indeed be demoted; yet by comparison with the population in general, they may still be functioning at a superior level, socially, economically, and intellectually. Nonetheless, their family and close associates know that they are changed, perhaps quite profoundly, and for the worse. By contrast some patients live lives that make little demand on their capacity to solve problems or even to maintain complex interpersonal relationships, and in such circumstances even manifest brain damage may appear to cause little change in the patient's life style. What needs to be discussed now is a more general issue, namely, the quality of life when there is impairment of mental and physical function of such severity that the patient's plight can be discussed without regard to his pretraumatic psychosocial status. That discussion will revolve around the limits of life as a human being, rather than as a certain kind of social person.[18]

Vegetative State

The definition of the vegetative state should be strictly adhered to, and a clear distinction made between this and both the locked-in syndrome and akinetic mutism. It may then be questioned whether this state is, for the patient, any different than death. Indeed, the popular press has dubbed it a "living death"; and an annotation in the Lancet, which referred to the prolonged survival of two patients in this state after cardiac arrest, wrote of it as "the death of a human being."[17] The mother of a teenager who lived for 6 years in the vegetative state after head injury said, in a British television documentary, that her son had died at the roadside, but that the funeral was 6 years later. The Karen Quinlan case has provoked wide discussion of this issue on both sides of the Atlantic.[3]

In an attempt to confirm that there was a consensus view about the quality of life in the vegetative state, the question was put to a group of health professionals and lawyers in San Francisco, and to a group of medical students in Glasgow.[9] Over 90 percent of both groups indicated, in a written anonymous questionnaire, that they regarded the vegetative state as worse than death; this view has since been found to hold also for groups of general practitioners and of nurses in Britain. Further evidence of this view comes from statements of theologians, including Pope Pius XII and the Archbishop of Canterbury.[10,20] It may be concluded that patients in this state are widely held to be no different from those who are dead, from the patient's point of view; but that for the family and those attending the patient, vegetative survival may be regarded as worse than death, in humanitarian and also in economic terms. Analysis of outcome for head injured cases in the Data Bank has usually classified the dead and vegetative patients 6 months after injury as a single outcome category. The vegetative state is regarded as death temporarily postponed.

Severe Disability

It is about these patients, particularly the worst affected of them, that there is most concern and argument. Those who have written about formal measurement of outcome after illness in general have stressed the need to take account not only of the intensity or degree of disability, but also of its duration. In this respect brain damage at 25 years of age is more devastating in its emotional impact on those who witness it, than is the same condition at the age of 65. It is also more significant in measurable terms, because these patients may be facing many years of continuing disablement. This has implications for the quality of life as well as for the economic consequences of the injury. In estimating quality of life, it is helpful to consider the following six aspects of living.

1. *Activities of daily life (ADL)* are frequently used as an index of dependence for stroke victims. Activities listed usually include feeding, dressing, toileting, and ability to get out of bed and move around the room. It may be that the patient can do some but not others of these, or that he needs only minimal help for some of them; or he may be completely dependent for one or more of these activities.

2. *Mobility and life organization* take the patient out of his room and, hopefully, out of the house. Is he able to get from one room to another whenever he wants to; or only when it is all set up for him to walk; or does he need actual help, step by step? Can he be left to organize a day or two on his own; will he be able to plan his meals, cook them at the right time, deal with visitors or callers on the telephone? Or must each separate piece of the day be arranged for him, lest he forget to start, or be distracted from finishing, the various separate activities that make up the day?

3. *Social relationships* are two-way affairs, dependent on initiative and response on both sides. Whatever the reasons, however, it is fair to find out whether a disabled person has visitors (or goes visiting) beyond the immediate family, who are bound by duty to be around him. Does he have any continuing relationship with others, or even with those looking after him?

4. *Work or leisure activities* are important for most people's sense of purpose,

once the acute stage of struggling for survival is over and the period of initial rehabilitation is underway. Does the patient have on-going activities, whether in open or sheltered employment, or in the way of leisure or voluntary activity, which enable him to feel that he is contributing in some measure to the community or to the lives of others?

5. *Present satisfaction* will depend much on the pretraumatic personality traits of the patient, as well as on the degree of disability. Pain is not an important component of disability after head injury, and if insight is very blunted, there may be no obvious distress for the patient himself. But many patients are well aware of their plight and are frustrated by their limited capacity; sometimes they become depressed and are occasionally aggressive. A level of recovery that may satisfy doctors and nurses, or even the family, all of whom knew how bad the patient was at his worst (a period of which the patient remains unaware for the rest of his life), may well seem devastating and awful to the patient himself. Some satisfaction may be derived from meeting short-term goals within a rehabilitation program, but that can be only for a finite time.

6. *Future prospects* are a matter of concern to younger patients, who make up the bulk of brain damaged survivors after head injury. Many are on the threshold of their careers, unlike the older stroke patients, many of whom have already achieved something in life, perhaps having children and an established home. For teenagers their career choice may be suddenly restricted, with no hope of fulfilling ambitions formerly cherished. For their parents there is the worry of what will happen when they are no longer there to provide support. For those in their twenties or thirties there is concern for the financial future of their wives and young families, as they see themselves either unemployable or, at best, unlikely to gain the position they once expected. Also there is the prospect of many years of coping with disability. These factors are what make severe brain damage in the young more difficult as well as different than it is in the elderly, when most strokes occur.

There is no formula by which to calculate the quality of life, even when all the factors mentioned have been considered; in the end it must depend largely on the personality and resources of the patient and his family. But sober consideration of all these factors may at least enable doctors to guard against glib judgments, such as "worthwhile survival," "practical recovery," and "fairly good result"— terms that usually prove to be euphemisms for severe disability. Rejection and denial of disability is a well-recognized psychological strategy used at certain stages in the recovery process both by the patient and often by his family. There is, however, no excuse for the doctor being drawn into this—he will best serve his individual patient, and his own understanding of the complex problem of brain damage, if he tries always to make a realistic yet sympathetic appraisal of the effect that an injury has had (or is likely to have) on the quality of life of those affected.

The groups of people who had been asked about the vegetative state were also asked whether they considered that survival in severe disability might be judged worse than the vegetative state. About 40 percent of each audience thought it would be worse for the patient himself; but rather less than 20 percent considered that the family would feel this way. This seemed a perceptive judgment, because it is well known that families can derive satisfaction, sometimes even renewed cohesion, from the need to care for a dependent relative. More often, however, as Bond's investigation has shown, the effect on the family is disruptive.[4]

315

REFERENCES

1. ADAMS, G. F.: *Prospects for patients with strokes.* Br. Med. J. 2:253–259, 1963.
2. BATES, D., CARONNA, J. J., CARTLIDGE, N. E. F., ET AL.: *A prospective study of non-traumatic coma: methods and results in 310 patients.* Ann. Neurol. 2:211–220, 1977.
3. BERESFORD, H. R.: *The Quinlan decision: problems and legislative alternatives.* Ann. Neurol. 2:74–81, 1977.
4. BOND, M. R.: *Assessment of the psychosocial outcome of severe head injury.* Acta Neurochir. 34:57–70, 1976.
5. Bond, M. R., and Brooks, D. N.: *Understanding the process of recovery as a basis for the investigation of rehabilitation for the brain injured.* Scand. J. Rehab. 8:127–133, 1976.
6. BROCKLEHURST, J. C.: "Alternatives to geriatric care." In Phillips, C. I., and Wolfe, J. N. (eds.): *Clinical Practice and Economics.* Pitman Medical Publishing Co., London, 1977, pp. 81–88.
7. CULYER, A. F., LAVERS, R. J., AND WILLIAMS, A.: In Shonfield, A., and Shaw, S. (eds.): *Indicators and Social Policy.* London, 1972, p. 94.
8. HIGASHI, K., SAKATA, Y., HATANO, M., ET AL.: *Epidemiological studies on patients with a persistent vegetative state.* J. Neurol. Neurosurg. Psychiatry 40:876–885, 1977.
9. JENNET, B.: *Resource allocation for the severely brain damaged.* Arch. Neurol. 33:595–597, 1976.
10. JENNETT, B.: *The Archbishop and the neurosurgeon.* Br. Med. J. 1:45, 1977.
11. JENNETT, B., AND BOND, M.: *Assessment of outcome after severe brain damage.* Lancet i:480, 1975.
12. JENNETT, B., AND PLUM, F.: *Persistent vegetative state after brain damage.* Lancet i:734–737, 1972.
13. JENNETT, B., SNOEK, J., BOND, M. R., AND BROOKS, N.: *Disability after severe head injury: Observations on the use of the Glasgow Outcome Scale.* J. Neurol. Neurosurg. Psychiat. 44:285–293, 1981.
14. JENNETT, B., TEASDALE, G., GALBRAITH, S., ET AL.: *Severe head injuries in three countries.* J. Neurol. Neurosurg. Psychiatry 40:291–298, 1977.
15. JENNETT, B., AND ADAMS, H.: *The apallic syndrome* [*book review*]. Brain 102:434–437, 1979.
16. KARNOFSKY, D. A., BURCHENAL, J. H., ARMISTEAD, G. C., ET AL.: *Triethylene melamine in the treatment of neoplastic disease.* Arch. Int. Med. 87:477, 1951.
17. LANCET: *Death of a human being.* ii:590–591, 1971.
18. PLUM, F., AND LEVY, D. E.: "Outcome from severe neurological illness: should it influence medical decisions?" In *Brain and Mind.* CIBA Symposium 69 [new series]. Excerpta Medica, Amsterdam, 1979.
19. LEVY, D. E., KNILL-JONES, R. P., AND PLUM, F.: *The vegetative state and its prognosis following non-traumatic coma.* N.Y. Acad. Sci. 35:293–306, 1978.
20. LONDON TIMES: *The last taboo.* 14th December, 1976.
21. MILNER, B.: "Residual intellectual and memory deficits after head injury." In Walker, A. E., Caveness, W. F., and Critchley, M. (eds.): *The Late Effects of Head Injury.* Charles C Thomas, Springfield, 1969, pp. 84–97.
22. NAJENSON, T., MENDELSON, L., SCHECHTER, I., ET AL.: *Rehabilitation after severe head injury.* Scand. J. Rehab. Med. 5:1–10, 1974.
23. RANKIN, J.: *Cerebral vascular accidents in patients over the age of 60.* Scot. Med. J. 2:200–255, 1957.
24. ROBERTS, A. H.: *Long term prognosis of severe accidental head injury.* Proc. R. Soc. Med. 69:137–140, 1976.
25. SMITH, E.: *Influence of site of impact on cognitive impairment persisting long after severe closed head injury.* J. Neurol. Neurosurg. Psychiatry 37:719–726, 1974.
26. STOVER, S. L., AND ZEIGER, H. E.: *Head injury in children and teenagers: functional recovery correlated with the duration of coma.* Arch. Phys. Med. Rehabil. 57:201–205, 1976.

CHAPTER 14

Prognosis after Severe Head Injury

When patients are in coma after head injury it can be difficult to know what the future holds, because so many factors may be considered likely to influence the outcome. Moreover, in the early stages the situation is dynamic, with new factors developing hour by hour or day by day. Because of the complexity of the situation it is impossible for clinicians to match in their minds any patient in front of them with their previous personal experience; even a busy neurosurgeon is unlikely to have encountered more than a few patients before who resembled the present case, and his recollection of these is seldom accurate enough to form a reliable basis for comparison and for decision-making. This is where formal predictive systems prove their worth. But the effort required to evolve such a system should not be underestimated. The computerized Data Bank of 1500 severe head injuries, which will be described later, took 12 years to collect; it is still being expanded, and its potential has not yet been fully exploited. Reference to it in this chapter will emphasize the principles involved, rather than giving conclusive findings, because these will have been developed further by the time this book is published. In establishing a data bank two questions have to be answered: What data should be collected and on what kind of patients?

SELECTION OF DATA

Until it is known what factors do influence outcome, and which will therefore be useful as predictive criteria, it might seem prudent to collect all information possible. But the lack of success of previous attempts to define prognostic criteria, or to devise a practical predictive system, was largely because too many kinds of data were amassed, with assessment made too soon and too often. For a method to be useful, it should be applicable in the wide range of hospitals where head injuries, even when severe, may now be treated; many of these hospitals do not have the full range of specialist staff and investigational facilities associated with university neurosurgical units. It is not only because of clinical limitations that the number of observations on which prediction is based should be limited, but also because, even with the capacity of modern computers to deal with data, the statistical evaluation of the predictive power of various criteria becomes difficult if too many are simultaneously considered. There is a need, therefore, to concentrate on data about the patient that can be reliably observed and readily recorded; and the extent of the data considered should reflect what it is realistic for the practicing clinician and nurse to collect on a routine basis, rather than what is only possible for a research fellow on a head injury project. During the evolution of a system, however, it is necessary to analyze an excess of data, until the minimum required for predictions of various kinds is known. Studies of this kind in several fields of medicine have consistently shown that the information required to make a diagnosis or prognosis is contained within a small fraction of the data that are traditionally collected. This possibility of "test reduction" is one of the advantages that comes from the more efficient manipulation of data that a formal statistical approach makes possible.[1,11]

What matters for prognosis is the amount of brain damage as a whole, whether primary, secondary, or a combination of both; this is most consistently reflected in general brain dysfunction, that is, in the various aspects of coma, its depth, and duration. These aspects of brain dysfunction are dynamic, often changing dramatically in the first few days after injury. In the Data Bank a profile of this changing situation was captured by recording, during each epoch, both the best and the worst state of the patient on various hierarchical scales of responsiveness. This enabled the depth and duration of coma to be measured, using the various aspects of coma previously described. These dynamic aspects of general brain dysfunction prove to be powerful predictors. Clinical details of focal brain damage are of less significance for outcome, and that is why a predictive system need not be encumbered with all the associated facets of the traditional neurological examination. Similarly, many investigations that are important for diagnosis and management prove to be of limited prognostic value; most tend only to confirm what is already evident from clinical observations, as far as severity of brain damage is concerned. In certain circumstances, however, some may give added discrimination over clinical criteria (p. 326). In addition to various facets of the changing picture, which reflect the brain damage suffered by the patients, there are other factors that may affect the outcome after severe injury. These kinds of data are unchanging, and serial records are therefore not required; they include the age of the patient, the cause and type of the injury, whether there is a skull fracture, and whether major extracranial injuries have been sustained. Of these, age is the only powerful predictor.

SELECTION OF PATIENTS

What Is a "Severe" Head Injury?

Patients with injuries covering a range of severity can be entered into a data bank, because they can be subsequently subclassified by the computer according to relative severity. But it is advisable to define a minimum degree of brain damage in order to avoid the system's becoming impractical owing to the dispersion of effort on collecting cases about which the prognosis is never seriously in doubt. Indeed, it seems likely that problems with previous computerized collection of data on head injuries may have been due to the attempt to construct an all-embracing system, which would include all cases, whatever their severity.

There can be no absolute definition of "severe head injury"; the alternative ways and means of assessing and scaling the severity of injury are discussed elsewhere (p. 334). For the purposes of the collaborative Data Bank of cases in coma, we defined a severe injury as one that was followed by at least 6 hours of coma, either immediately after impact, or after an interval of complete or relative lucidity. Coma was defined as not opening the eyes, not obeying commands, and not uttering any recognizable words (p. 80). A lucid interval, defined as a period after injury when the patient was reported to have talked, occurred in more than a quarter of cases in the Data Bank.

The requirement that coma must persist for 6 hours was made in order to exclude patients who might regain consciousness during this period, and who would be judged by most as therefore having every chance of a good recovery. It is, however, a matter of some dispute whether there are many head injured patients who are in coma (by this definition) by the time they reach hospital care (say 1 to 2 hours after injury), and who will come out of coma by the sixth hour. There are certainly some children who look very sick, indeed, in the early stages, but who recover rapidly; and among adults with multiple injuries associated with hypotension, hypoxia, and partial respiratory obstruction, there are some whose neurological status may improve dramatically once initial resuscitation is carried out (p. 97). Another factor that may affect initial assessment of brain damage is drugs, in particular alcohol; the combined effect of drugs and recent trauma on cerebral function is impossible to calculate, and time alone can tell.

It is not suggested that 6 hours represents a time interval of crucial biological significance, but it does provide an interval during which initial resuscitation can be completed. Moreover, it has been our rule to exclude patients who died (or became brain dead) during this period, as their prognosis is not long in doubt. Although it might seem a more appropriate definition to specify "still in coma after initial resuscitation," this would allow a considerable variation in the interval since injury, according to local geographical and administrative arrangements.

When to Begin Assessment

Many previous attempts at defining prognostic criteria have been based on the patient's state "on admission." This is clearly unsatisfactory because it is seldom stated whether reference is made to initial admission to any hospital or to an emergency room, or whether it is "admission" by transfer to a neurosurgical or intensive care unit. The interval between injury and the assessment of the patient may therefore vary widely, while due allowance may not be made for the temporary influence on brain function of extracranial factors, such as those described above. Even in the patients entered into the Data Bank, because their coma did exceed 6 hours, many improved rapidly after admission. The *best* coma sum during the first 24 hours was higher than that recorded on admission in a quarter of all patients, and in a half of those whose admission score was 3 or 4 (deepest coma). The frequency of occurrence of signs of severe brain dysfunction in the first 24 hours is much higher if it is based on the worst rather than the best state during that period (Table 1).

Table 1. Frequency of severe dysfunction at 24 hours

	Best State		Worst State	
Coma sum 3/4	176	19%	467	49%
Nonreacting pupils	226	23%	424	44%
Absent/bad eye movements	186	23%	268	34%
Abnormal motor pattern	393	41%	600	62%

(From Jennett, Teasdale, Braakman, et al.,[5] with permission)

Table 2. Comparison of features of head injury in three countries

	Glasgow n=593	Netherlands n=239	Los Angeles n=168
Mean age	35 yr	32 yr	35 yr
Lucid interval	32%	25%	23%
Intracranial hematoma	54%	28%	56%
Extracranial injury	32%	51%	51%
Responsiveness			
(24 hours, best)	21%	21%	21%
Coma sum 3/4	65%	58%	66%
Coma sum 5/6/7			
Pupils not reacting	19%	29%	31%
Eye movements			
absent/impaired	45%	37%	40%

(From Jennett, Teasdale, Braakman, et al.,[5] with permission)

Characteristics of Patients in the Data Bank

Having defined a head injury as "severe," on the basis of a specified depth and duration of coma rather than by administrative or outcome criteria, the population of patients collected from three countries proved to be remarkably similar.[6] Yet socioeconomic and cultural differences between these three countries are considerable, and they have different methods of delivering health care. Not only was the initial severity of the patient populations similar (Table 2), but so also was their outcome (Table 3). This Data Bank, therefore, provides a sound basis for exploring the influence on outcome of various factors.

SINGLE FACTORS WITH PREDICTIVE POWER

Several factors have been long recognized to have an influence on outcome, such as the patient's age and the depth and duration of coma. To some extent, therefore, the international Data Bank has only confirmed these previous findings; but because it consists of a well-defined set of patients, it has been possible to establish the relative predictive power of different factors and to explore the interactions between some of them when other aspects of severity are relatively constant. In this section we are concerned with single factors, considering each on its own. We shall refer to the main previous publications on each of them as they are discussed.

Table 3. Outcome at 6 months in three countries

	Glasgow n=593 (%)	Netherlands n=239 (%)	Los Angeles n=168 (%)
Dead	48	50	50
Vegetative	2	2	5
Severe disability	10	7	14
Moderate disability	18	15	19
Good recovery	23	26	12

(From Jennett, Teasdale, Braakman, et al.,[5] with permission)

320

Factors Strongly Related to Outcome

Age

This is perhaps the most widely acknowledged influence on outcome, reported to influence both mortality rate and, in survivors, the degree of recovery. The age at which the prognosis is recorded as changing has varied widely between different reports; but it is not clear whether the particular ages at which authors have chosen to divide their series were reached arbitrarily, or by examination of the outcome of a number of alternative ranges. In our Data Bank series, there was a continuous relationship between increasing age and a bad outcome (death or vegetative state); there was a corresponding decline in the proportion making a good recovery[14] (Figs. 1 and 2). Young children (less than 5 years) had a higher mortality than that for the 5 to 19 group; they are omitted from the figure because the numbers were too small for reliable analysis. Otherwise, younger patients can make a better recovery after deeper or more prolonged coma, as previously ob-

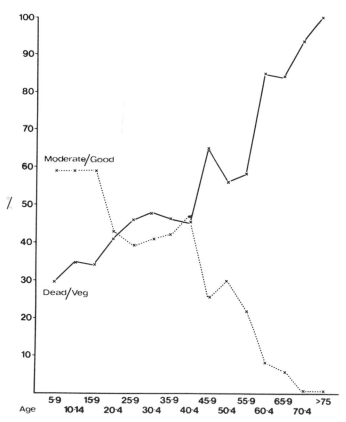

Figure 1. Outcome at 6 months of patients in different 5-year age groups.

321

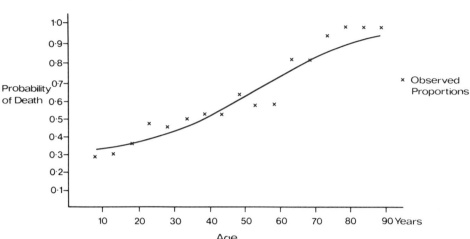

Figure 2. Probability of death as a function of age. The fitted curve is an exponential, where
$$\frac{\text{Probability of death}}{\text{Probability of survival}} = \text{exponential} (C_0 + C_1 \text{ age } + C_2 \text{ age}^2)$$
(From Teasdale, Skene, Parker, et al.,[14] with permission)

served by Carlsson and associates[2] and by Heiskanen and Sipponen.[3] Age has an effect on outcome that is independent of the state of coma, eye movements, and pupil reactions, but its effect is less apparent in the most severely injured patients (who do badly whatever their age). Compared with other predictive factors in the Data Bank, particularly the reliable measures of the severity of brain damage that have been evolved, age proved to be less influential than might have been expected.

Aspects of Coma

It would be generally acknowledged that the most important factor in determining prognosis is the degree of brain damage, as reflected in impaired responsiveness. Others have reported that the depth or duration of coma is related to outcome,[2,3,7] but have not defined coma and its various components in generally recognizable and reliable terms. In Chapter 4, we have described hierarchical scales by which responsiveness, pupils, and eye movements can be ranked. Each of these aspects of brain function, when assessed in any of the epochs of the first week, is related to outcome (Table 4 and Fig. 3). By using the coma score rather than the individual levels of response in the eye, motor, and verbal components, there is a loss of predictive power (Fig. 4A); among these components, some are more powerful than others (Fig. 4B).[11] Outcome is better in relation to a given level of brain dysfunction when this was the patient's worst state during an epoch, than if it was his best level of responsiveness (Table 5). Estimated mortality will therefore be lower in a series of patients with a given degree of severity if this has been based on assessment when they were at their worst (in any epoch). This can account for discrepancies between the outcome distribution in series of patients

322

Table 4. Outcomes associated with best level of responsiveness in first 24 hours after coma

	n	Dead or Vegetative (%)	Moderate Disability Good Recovery (%)
Coma Response Sum			
>11	57	12	87
8/9/10	190	27	68
5/6/7	525	53	34
3/4	176	87	7
Pupils			
Reacting	748	39	50
Nonreacting	226	91	4
Eye Movements			
Intact	463	33	56
Impaired	143	62	25
Absent/bad	186	90	5
Motor Response Pattern (any limb)			
Normal or weak	568	36	54
Abnormal	393	74	16
Motor Response Pattern (best limb)			
Obeys/localizes	395	31	58
Withdraws/flexes	402	54	35
Extensor/nil	191	85	8

(From Jennett, Teasdale, Braakman, et al.,[5] with permission)

who appear to have had injuries of comparable severity, because a patient's worst state is often only temporary (p. 319).

In survivors, PTA provides a permanent marker of the duration of altered consciousness (p. 89). As would be expected, outcome is closely correlated with the duration of PTA, although there are some patients who make a satisfactory recovery even after a month or more of PTA (Table 6).

Factors Less Strongly Related to Outcome

Autonomic Abnormalities

In that abnormalities of respiration, cardiovascular function, and control of body temperature are possible indicators of brain stem dysfunction, they have from time to time been considered as of prognostic significance after head injury. In particular, respiratory abnormalities[9] and also systolic hypertension[10] have been regarded as bad signs. In our experience these abnormalities occurred only in a minority of even the severely injured patients whom we studied (p. 146); moreover, many other factors, including extracranial injuries and complications, may affect these functions, and this reduces their value as indicators of the severity of brain damage. The relationship between respiratory abnormalities and outcome after various kinds of brain damage (including trauma) has been explored

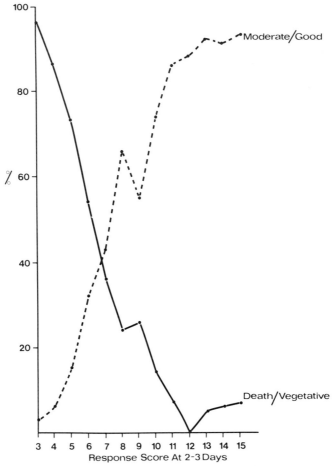

Figure 3. Outcome at 6 months for patients with different Glasgow Coma (response) Scores—best in 2–3 day epoch.

Table 5. Outcome at 6 months for patients with different coma scores as best or worst in 2–3 day epoch

	Coma Sum				
	3/4 *(%)*	*5* *(%)*	*6* *(%)*	*7* *(%)*	*8* *(%)*
Proportion dead or vegetative					
Best state	97	79	61	41	28
Worst state	75	48	30	21	5
Proportion good recovery or moderately disabled					
Best state	0	11	21	38	61
Worst state	13	39	56	65	82

(From Jennett, Teasdale, Braakman, et al.,[5] with permission)

324

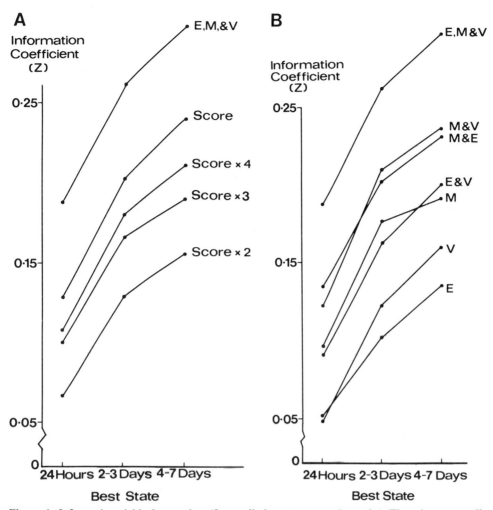

Figure 4. Information yield of coma data (for predicting outcome at 6 months). There is more predictive power as time passes; at all times data about all three components yield the most information (E = eye, M = motor, V = verbal score).

A, The score contains less information than does the knowledge of its actual composition. Knowing the actual score is better than knowing only the band (e.g., 3–5, 6–8). **B,** Different combinations of E, M, and V have lesser power; the value of M is clear—it is as good as E and V together. Z (outcome/data) = H [outcome − H (outcome/data)] − H (outcome). (From Jennett, B.: *Defining brain damage after head njury*. J. R. Coll. Physicians Lond. 13:197–200, 1979.)

in detail by North and Jennett,[9] who found the relationship much less close than previously reported. Patients with autonomic abnormalities tend to have a worse outcome (Table 7), but they are also more brain damaged, as evidenced by reduced responsiveness (p. 84).

Intracranial Hematoma

In Carlsson's study,[2] patients with intracranial hematoma were excluded, presumably because this was considered to be a confusing factor. However, this

Table 6. PTA and outcome at 6 months

PTA	n	Severely Disabled (%)	Moderately Disabled (%)	Good Recovery (%)
< 14 days	101	0	17	83
15–28 days	96	3	31	66
>28 days	289	30	43	27

complication occurred in about half the patients in the Data Bank, and such a common occurrence cannot be ignored in a predictive system. Miller has reported that intracranial hematoma makes for a worse outcome;[8] this could be regarded as somewhat unexpected, in that the chances of recovery for the patient in coma might be considered to be improved by the presence of a potentially treatable lesion. In the Data Bank series also those patients with a hematoma did less well; however, this proved to be partly because patients with hematoma were older.[5] When adjusted for age, hematoma proved to increase the likelihood of a worse outcome markedly only when under the age of 20 years, and not at all over 40 years (Table 8). Many patients with operated hematoma in the collecting centers did not remain in coma long enough to qualify for inclusion in the Data Bank, because they recovered rapidly after evacuation of the clot. A valid comparison cannot therefore be drawn between these and series of hematomas in general.

Special Investigations

On the whole these have proved disappointing as predictors. Patients with severe brain damage tend to include a larger proportion with abnormal findings in various investigations, so that an overall relation between radiological and laboratory abnormalities and a bad outcome will be inevitable. However, it will almost always be obvious from clinical assessment of responsiveness that these patients

Table 7. Outcome related to autonomic abnormalities in first week

	n	Dead or Vegetative (%)	Moderate Disability or Good Recovery (%)
Periodic respiration	181	62	30
Not periodic	676	47	45
Respiration>30	298	65	28
Not tachypneic	618	44	46
Pulse>120	334	60	31
Not tachycardic	640	47	43
BP>160	213	58	31
Not hypertensive	755	50	40
Temperature>39°C	222	59	29
Not pyrexial	739	48	45

(From Jennett, Teasdale, Braakman, et al.,[5] with permission)

Table 8. Influence of acute intracranial hematoma on outcome

Age	Frequency of Occurrence of Hematoma		Dead or Vegetative at 6 Months			
	n	%	No Hematoma		Hematoma	
<20 yr	337	30	62	26	36	36
20–39 yr	309	45	61	36	69	49
40–59 yr	268	65	49	53	98	56
>60 yr	170	71	42	86	102	84

(From Jennett, Teasdale, Braakman, et al.,[5] with permission)

are badly brain damaged, and investigations may not provide additional predictive information. Moreover, not all severely brain damaged patients show abnormalities; a normal intracranial pressure, or cerebral blood flow, or CT scan is therefore of little predictive value. For example, in severely injured patients without an intracranial hematoma, the level of responsiveness gave a good indication of outcome, but whether or not the CT scan was normal or abnormal added little discrimination (p. 115).

Investigations may, however, prove vital when routine examination of responsiveness is not possible, usually because relaxant or depressant drugs are being therapeutically administered. A promising investigation is the evoked cortical response to visual, auditory, and somatosensory stimuli. Not only may this indicate the degree of cortical responsiveness, but it may distinguish between dysfunction that is mainly in the brain stem or in the cerebral hemisphere (p. 137). It is a more direct measure of responsiveness than other intermediary factors (such as cerebral blood flow or intracranial pressure), abnormalities of which may be either the cause of or the result of brain dysfunction. Biochemical markers of severity are less reliable, indicating as they do the amount of structural brain damage sustained rather than the functional state of the brain as a whole. These include brain antigens and enzymes (p. 139) released into the circulating blood, the level of which can be estimated at various stages after injury.

Factors Showing Little Relation to Outcome

A number of features that might have been expected to relate to outcome have been found, at least in the severe injuries of the Data Bank, to be of little significance (Table 9). When it comes to considering a series of patients that may be limited to patients either with or without one of these features, it is useful to know that comparison will not be invalidated by such a restriction.

CALCULATING PROBABILITIES FOR OUTCOME IN INDIVIDUAL PATIENTS

It is seldom realized how little help it is to the clinician to know that an individual patient under his care has one or more features known to be associated with a bad or a good outcome. Only when the brain damage is at one extreme or the other of severity, in a category in which *all* patients die or *all* will recover, does the clinician have a useful guide; but only a small minority of patients have such distinctive characteristics. For the rest it is of limited value in decision-making to

Table 9. Factors having little influence on outcome

Cause of Injury	n	Dead or Vegetative (%)	Moderate Disability or Good Recovery (%)
Road accident	578	47	42
Alcoholic fall	134	56	34
Work	61	51	26
Assault	56	50	36
Skull fracture	632	54	38
No fracture	337	43	43
Hemiparesis	234	32	55
Normal motor pattern	232	29	65
Right hemisphere damage	293	47	41
Left hemisphere damage	317	48	41
Chest injury—major	40	58	33
None or minor	562	49	39
Extracranial injury	399	52	40
None	598	50	38

(From Jennett, Teasdale, Braakman, et al.,[5] with permission)

know that a given fraction of patients with certain characteristics will die (or recover). For the care of individuals the doctor needs to know for a given patient what the probabilities of alternative outcomes are.

Having identified which factors do in fact influence outcome, it is therefore necessary to consider the effect of various combinations of adverse or favorable factors. This can be done by a number of different statistical methods. We have described how several factors can be combined, using an independence model to make estimates of the probability of certain outcomes in individual patients in the first week after injury.[4,11] Although several of the predictors used in this system (responsiveness, pupil reactions, and eye movements) can be shown statistically to be related to each other, they each prove also to be independently related to outcome. This dependence between different factors makes it possible to reduce the amount of data required to make a prediction. This can be of value to the clinician in two ways: it limits the amount of data that needs to be collected for predictive purposes; and it makes it possible to calculate a prediction even when some data is missing—as it inevitably is under some circumstances. It is, however, not wise to reduce the data collected to the absolute minimum; some redundancy is useful as a check against data that are atypical, or in which there has been an error in collection.

We have explored the feasibility of making individual predictions, and the preliminary results, which we have published on the first 600 cases, will serve to indicate the principles and practicalities involved.[4,11] More than 100 items of data were available for each patient and the outcome at 6 months was known. The patients were randomly divided into a training set of 400, and a set of 200 whose outcome was to be "predicted" on the basis of the conditional probabilities derived from the 400. We arbitrarily decided to consider a prediction confident only when the probability of one outcome was greater than 0.97. The way in which uncertainty is reduced as additional items of data are added can be seen from a graphical presentation (Fig. 5). The predicted outcome can be compared with the actual outcome, in order to assess the reliability of the system. When the actual and predicted outcomes coincided, the prediction was termed "correct."

This method of studying the possibility of prediction on a large series of patients for whom the outcome was already known enabled us to explore the effect on prediction of varying certain aspects of the system. As might have been expected, the number of patients confidently predicted to reach one of two outcomes (dead or vegetative, as compared with surviving) increased from one epoch to the next during the first week (Table 10). If the number of outcomes was increased, the performance of the system became less good.[13] At an early stage after injury it seems practical to ask for outcome only into these two large categories, but as time passes it becomes more important to distinguish between the quality of recovery likely to occur in survivors. The outcomes of more patients can be predicted if the confidence level is reduced (below 0.97), but inevitably this

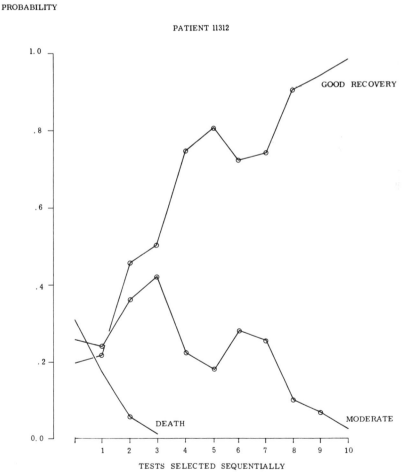

Figure 5. Change in probability of each of three outcomes (at 6 months) for one patient as items of data are sequentially added by computer.

Table 10. Time after injury and predictive yield

	Prediction	
Epoch	Confident (%)	Correct (%)
24 hours	45	94
2–3 days	60	94
4–7 days	68	93

(From Teasdale, Parker, Murray, et al.,[13] with permission)

brings more errors (Table 11). There could, however, be circumstances in which the clinician would be willing to accept this.

Although the computer had access to some 300 items of data, it soon became clear that when a confident prediction was made, the probability reached 0.97 after a relatively small number of data items. This proved to be around 17, and they were identified and listed in rank order in respect to the contribution that each made to reducing uncertainty of outcome. When this was reduced to only 8 indicants, the system performed almost as well. Using such a reduced data set it is possible to transfer the system to a pocket calculator, using tables derived from the training set; we have found this to be a practical means of making individual predictions for newly arriving patients. Looking back at the accumulation of the Data Bank, it became clear that the optimum level of predictive power, using the present statistical method, was reached when some 400 cases were available in the training set (Table 12). However, the larger bank makes it possible to include patients in categories that occur relatively seldom, about which even a series of 400 does not provide a sufficiently large set of cases with known outcome.

Although few erroneous predictions are made, there are some. When the actual and predicted outcomes were compared, most errors proved to have been overly optimistic predictions—patients who were calculated to survive but who actually died. This was usually because of newly developing complications, which the system was not designed to predict, such as pulmonary embolism. What we aimed to predict was the potential for recovery—the possibility that, given adequate treatment, the patient could regain consciousness and become independent. When we predicted the outcome to be death or the vegetative state, we were asserting that the brain damage was so extensive that, no matter how much was done, the patient would not recover. Only an occasional patient predicted not to recover did survive; such patients were all severely disabled and dependent.

Table 11. Probability level and predictive yield

Level of Probability	Confident (%)	Correct (%)
.90	76	92
.95	67	96
.97	61	98
.99	49	99

(From Teasdale, Parker, Murray, et al.,[13] with permission)

Table 12. Size of training set and predictive yield

Training Set Size	Predictions for Same Sample	
	Confident (%)	Correct (%)
100	41	97
200	54	98
300	57	99
400	58	99

FUTURE DEVELOPMENTS

The establishment of data banks is now recognized as a useful means of accumulating information about patients at a greater rate and in a more efficient way than is possible for an individual clinician or a single hospital. Because initial severity and ultimate outcome are assessed in a standardized way, data banks make it possible to compare different head injury populations, in order to detect changes over time that are a result of deliberate interventions (therapeutic or organizational) or outside events (e.g., amount of road traffic, or motoring legislation). If comparisons are to be made it is important to ensure that patient populations are sufficiently closely matched for severity[12] (p. 337). Once a bank has been accumulated, subsets of varying severity may be abstracted for comparative purposes. In this way it may be possible to carry out trials of new therapeutic regimens, using previously collected cases as a control group. This may obviate the need for a "no treatment" series—always an ethically difficult problem when dealing with a condition that carries a high mortality rate. However, an even more effective way of assessing the efficacy of a new management regimen would be to make predictions for individual patients and then to find out whether a significant number of those managed with "new" treatment had a better outcome than had been predicted, on the basis of patients conventionally treated.

REFERENCES

1. CARD, W.: "Parsimony in clinical medicine." In Phillips, C. I., and Wolfe, J. N. (eds.): *Clinical Practice Publishing Co., London, 1977, pp. 120–132.*

2. CARLSSON, C. A., VON ESSEN, C., AND LOFGREN, J.: *Factors affecting the clinical course of patients with severe head injuries. Part 1: influence of biological factors. Part 2: significance of post-traumatic coma.* J. Neurosurg. 29:242–251, 1968.

3. HEISKANEN, O., AND SIPPONEN, P.: *Prognosis of severe brain injury.* Acta Neurol. Scand. 46:343–348, 1970.

4. JENNETT, B., TEASDALE, G., BRAAKMAN, R., ET AL.: *Predicting outcome in individual patients after severe head injury.* Lancet i:1031–1034, 1976.

5. JENNETT, B., TEASDALE, G., BRAAKMAN, R., ET AL.: *Prognosis in series of patients with severe head injury.* Neurosurgery 4:283, 1979.

6. JENNETT, B., TEASDALE, G., GALBRAITH, S., ET AL.: *Severe head injuries in three countries.* J. Neurol. Neurosurg. Psychiatry 40:291–298, 1977.

7. LECUIRE, J., DECHAUME, J. P., AND DERUTY, R.: "Long term prognosis of the prolonged and serious traumatic comas." In *Head Injuries.* Proceedings of an International Symposium held in Edinburgh and Madrid, 2nd to 10th April, 1970. Churchill Livingstone, Edinburgh, 1971, pp. 141–144.

8. MILLER, J. D., BECKER, D. P., WARD, J. D., ET AL.: *Significance of intracranial hypertension in severe head injury.* J. Neurosurg. 47:503–516, 1977.

9. NORTH, J. B., AND JENNETT, S.: *Abnormal breathing patterns associated with acute brain injury.* Arch. Neurol. 31:338–344, 1974.

10. OVERGAARD, J., CHRISTENSEN, S., HVID-JANSEN, O., ET AL.: *Prognosis after head injury based on early clinical examination.* Lancet ii:631–635, 1973.

11. TEASDALE, G., MURRAY, G., PARKER, L., ET AL.: *Adding up the Glasgow Coma Score.* Acta Neurochir. Suppl. 28:13–16, 1979.

12. TEASDALE, G., PARKER, L., MURRAY, G., ET AL.: *On comparing series of head injured patients.* Acta Neurochir. Suppl. 28:205–208, 1979.

13. TEASDALE, G., PARKER, L., MURRAY, G., ET AL.: *Predicting the outcome of individual patients in the first week after severe head injury.* Acta Neurochir. Suppl. 28:161–164, 1979.

14. TEASDALE, G., SKENE, A., PARKER, L., ET AL.: *Age and outcome of severe head injury.* Acta Neurochir. Suppl. 28:140–143, 1979.

CHAPTER 15

Objectives, Organization, and Audit of Care for Head Injured Patients

Head injuries seem likely to continue to be common in all countries, though their numbers may be contained or even reduced by preventive and protective measures. They will certainly remain too frequent and too dispersed to consider centralizing their care to the degree that has been possible in many countries for spinal cord trauma. Some form of two-tier system of care seems likely to remain the rule in most places, the milder injuries being cared for in community hospitals near to where the accident occurs, and the more severe sent to centers equipped to investigate and treat intracranial complications.

Views will differ as to what degree of severity will warrant sending a patient to a special center, perhaps many miles away; whatever the policy there is likely to be a need for initial care in peripheral hospitals, even for some of the serious cases. Opinions will also vary about the size of the community that justifies the establishment of certain special facilities—remembering that expensive equipment that is seldom used is unlikely to be skillfully handled when the occasion arises. Arguments about the distribution of neurosurgeons, about the choice of sites for CT scanners, and about which patients should have the supposed benefits of one or of both will continue until the objectives of head injury care are more clearly defined, and there is more general agreement as to how these are best met.

In general terms the central objective is to minimize the occurrence of avoidable factors that could either aggravate the brain damage already sustained or impede the process of recovery. In practice, the risks associated with mild injuries are largely different from those that predominate after severe injuries. No systems for dealing with head injured patients, nor any method of auditing their efficacy, can ignore the influence of severity of injury—a theme to which reference has already been made in various contexts in every chapter of this book. The need now is to bring together these separate strands and to review the alternative (and over-lapping) ways and means of assessing severity. Another reason why this is so important is the fact that most disparities between recommendations for the care of head injuries, and discrepancies between reports about the results of treatment, stem from the failure clearly to define what range of severity was under consideration in different contexts.

The avoidable factors that it is the aim of management to reduce are considered next. Against this background the therapeutic possibilities are discussed, dealing separately with the logistics of coping with the large numbers of mild injuries and with the different problem of ensuring continuity of care for the minority of patients who have severe brain damage.

The chapter concludes with a discussion of organizational and ethical issues that have arisen in recent years, particularly with the evolution of expensive and elaborate methods of treating badly brain damaged patients. This leads to consideration of the need for a more rigorous approach to the establishment of the efficacy of alternative methods of management, both at the organizational level and also with respect to specific therapeutic techniques. Finally, we stress the need for more intensive biomedical research into mechanisms of secondary brain damage and of the recovery process, as a basis for evolving new approaches to therapy.

ASSESSMENT OF SEVERITY OF INJURY

This is central to many aspects of head injury: for the definition of populations for epidemiological review, for early management decisions and for prognosis, and for later review of the efficacy of treatment. For most purposes the implication is that *brain* damage is what matters, although apparent discrepancies will arise in assessing severity in the occasional case with extensive scalp or skull damage associated with little or no involvement of the brain.

A more common difficulty is to distinguish clinically between the severity of *impact* damage and the consequences of various *secondary* events. While it is the combined effects of these that determine the ultimate outcome, there are situations in which it is vital to distinguish between impact and secondary damage. In particular it is important to avoid classifying early severity retrospectively, that is, deciding that the patient did not originally have a certain degree of damage, because he has now made a good recovery. The fallacy of this argument has been exposed by neuropathological data, which show that even mild concussion can leave a permanent mark on the brain, and that patients who have died many years after making an apparently complete recovery from a more severe head injury may be found to have the scars of extensive contusions and lacerations (p. 39). It would be equally misleading to assume, because a patient had developed serious complications resulting in permanent disability, that the original injury must therefore have been severe. It cannot even be assumed that those who die after injury necessarily had more *impact* brain damage than those who lived; careful autopsy commonly reveals minor impact damage associated with major secondary complications, either intracranial or extracranial or both.

Administrative Classification

This classification is usually based on what happened to the patient—whether he came to hospital, was admitted, and if so for how long. Most national statistics depend on such measures, but unless definitions and the customs of local practice are known, such figures may be deceptive. For example, in the United Kingdom a road accident casualty is recorded as "serious" if admitted to hospital, although most such patients with head injury are discharged the next day. In the report by Field,[2] a useful distinction was made between head injured patients who stayed in hospital only a day or two, those staying more than 7 days, and those more than 14 days; however, prolonged stay frequently proves to be due to associated extracranial injuries, and in such cases duration of stay is an unreliable guide to the severity of the head injury.[8]

Another administrative index of severity is the ICD Classification (p. 1), but this does not provide a ready means of ranking severity on *clinical* grounds, because the basis of the rubrics is pathological. The best that can be done is to assume that certain codes usually represent more serious injuries than others; for example, Field's report[2] allocated as "less severe" the codes N802, N805, and N854. However, it is well known that local custom rather than clinical severity often determines which code is used (p. 1). It is hoped that the tenth revision of the report will provide for using a fifth digit to record duration of unconsciousness (Table 1). If this is properly and widely used, then ICD statistics could become a more useful source of data about severity than they are at present.

Table 1. Proposed severity digit for head injury rubrics of ICD

4th digit for: 850
and 5th digit for: 851-854
                       800.0.1; 801.0.1; 803.0.1; 804.0.1
Duration of loss of consciousness
.0   none
.1   brief, <1 hour
.2   moderate, 1–24 hours
.3   prolonged, >24 hours with complete recovery
.4   prolonged, >24 hours with residual deficit
.5   other or unspecified

Clinical Grading

What the clinician needs is an operational definition of severity grades, based on clinical observation alone, and capable of encompassing both impact and secondary brain damage. Initial assessment usually relies on alteration of consciousness, and on the presence of a skull fracture—the first being indicative of brain damage, the second of injury to bone. Although many patients have both, one or other often happens alone; the occurrence of either is usually taken as an indication for admission to hospital and therefore influences certain administrative classifications.

A practical definition of a *mild injury* is that the patient is already talking when he reaches first medical contact (p. 96). In those who have a period of altered consciousness, the duration of this (p. 89) and of the subsequent post-traumatic amnesia (p. 90) provides a useful guide to the severity of the diffuse brain damage, caused by acceleration/deceleration injury, which is the mechanism of most civilian head injuries. The value of PTA in individual patients is that it affords a measure of severity for the doctor who first sees the patient long after injury, and who has no access to records made in the acute stage. Even when case notes are available, data about altered consciousness can seldom be gleaned from them unless a standardized method of recording responsiveness has been used.

Focal neurological signs are not infrequently included in the initial assessment of severity. For example, the traditional distinction between commotio and contusio cerebri is usually made on the basis that contusio is assumed if the patient has been "unconscious" for a time *or* if he has focal neurological signs. But what are focal neurological signs—a cranial nerve paralysis, dysphasia or hemiplegia, abnormalities of the pupils, or irregularities of autonomic function? Many severe injuries never have focal signs, while patients with frank contusion of the brain (e.g., compound depressed fracture) frequently have neither unconsciousness nor focal signs. As for the duration of coma that determines classification as contusio, this can vary from 1 or 2 minutes to 12 hours; it is usually rather loosely defined as "several hours."

Open injuries of the vault can be relatively simply classified. In military missile wounds, whether or not the dura was penetrated, and if so whether the ventricle was reached by the missile or the brain was totally traversed, gives a practical guide to the degree of brain damage. Civilian depressed fractures can usefully be graded into closed, compound with dura intact, and compound with dura penetration.

There have been attempts to introduce comprehensive *injury scales,* applicable to trauma anywhere in the body. These have included many aspects of trauma, including the supposed force of the original injury, the prognosis, and the frequency of occurrence, each of which is scaled on a one to five basis. The abbreviated injury scale, subsequently derived, is based primarily on initial prognosis.[13] This did not take account of the fact that head injuries differ from most other types of trauma, in that secondary events frequently dominate the clinical condition and also the prognosis, in those who survive the first half hour; this contrasts with fractures of the limbs or of the spine, for example, when the impact injury alone more often determines the prognosis. However, the 1980 revision[15] makes it possible to record separate scales for skull injury (fracture), for anatomic lesions demonstrated by CT scan, surgery, or autopsy, and for level and duration of altered consciousness. This promises to be useful, particularly when there are multiple injuries, as occur so often with traffic accidents—for which the AIS was specifically designed.

Complications and Outcome as Severity Measures

Injuries can be severe without being complicated, in the sense of developing a specific secondary condition such as intracranial hematoma, meningitis, or epilepsy. The former two constitute life-threatening conditions that can occur after relatively mild injuries; even if the patient recovers completely following successful treatment, it must be conceded that he has had a serious illness, if not a severe injury. Epilepsy may constitute a life-long disability, and it can occur in patients who have otherwise made a good recovery; it is more common in patients whose initial injury was severe, but it can also affect those whose injury would be judged mild but for this complication. That recovery may not be as complete as appears at first sight has already been emphasized, and this should be remembered when an injury is regarded as less severe than another on the grounds that recovery has been "satisfactory." It is worth remembering that half the patients with a PTA of 2 to 4 weeks, who would be judged by more observers as having been severely injured, make a good recovery on the outcome scale.

Describing Severity in Individual Patients

No one method of assessing severity is suitable for all kinds of injury, nor for the many different circumstances for which a measure of severity is required. It is suggested that as many as possible of the measures listed in Table 2 should be

Table 2. Measures of severity

Initial features	conscious state fracture CNS signs
Complications	epilepsy hematoma meningitis
Duration	coma PTA
Sequelae	physical mental

(From Jennett, B.: *Assessment of severity of head injury.* J. Neurol. Neurosurg. Psychiatry 39:647–655, 1976, with permission.)

used, making it clear which are considered to relate to the initial injury, and which to secondary events. It is unwise to try to encapsulate the entire chain of events that may follow violence to the head in a single adjective of quality, such as mild or severe. Where possible the duration of coma and of PTA should be quoted, and individual patients might be then described in this way:

1. Severe impact injury without skull fracture; survival in the vegetative state.
2. Compound depressed fracture with 5 minutes PTA; complicated by abscess and by persisting epilepsy.
3. Acute intradural hematoma, coma for 5 days from time of injury; PTA 3 weeks, good recovery.

Describing Severity in a Series of Patients

It is frequently necessary to compare successive groups of patients in one center, or series of patients in different places, especially when alternative therapeutic regimens for severely injured patients are being evaluated. Whether this is done retrospectively, or as a formal randomized trial, the requirements are similar—to decide how closely the two populations of patients should be matched for the comparison to be valid. One method is to require that there is a minimum severity, and that no patients are accepted who are less severely affected than this. Definition will usually be by duration of coma, or of PTA; but notice that an *average* (or mean) duration of coma (or of PTA) cannot be accepted as an adequate description of severity in a group of patients. The selection criteria for entry to the international study of severe head injuries based on Glasgow was 6 hours in coma.[6] While all these patients had more than 24 hours of PTA, which was Russell's definition of "severe injury," 94 percent of them had more than a week's PTA—so they were considerably more severe (as a group) than a series defined only by PTA duration of 24 hours or more.

Selection of patients by a single level of severity does nothing to ensure that groups of patients so chosen will have a similar distribution of various other features, including those that indicate degrees of severity worse than the upper cut-off level. In comparing series of severely injured patients, it would therefore

337

Table 3. Effect of age distribution on expected mortality in series of severely head injured patients

Age Group	Mortality*	Proportion of Patients		
		Series I	Series II†	Series III
10–29 years	35%	62.5%	50%	25%
30–49 years	40%	0	25%	75%
50–69 years	80%	37.5%	25%	0
Mean age for series		35 yr	35 yr	35 yr
Expected mortality for series		52%	48%	38%

* Estimates from data bank.
† Approximates to 1000 cases in data bank.
(From Teasdale, Parker, Murray, et al.,[14] with permission)

be necessary to see that they were not significantly different with respect to various features known to be of prognostic significance, and therefore to be valid as indicators of "severity." However, matching for severity factors is not as simple as it seems.[14] For example, two series of patients might have the same *mean* age, yet their age distribution might be sufficiently different for the expected outcome to be dissimilar (Table 3). When two factors are taken into account, there is even more opportunity for error. An example is shown in Table 4, admittedly highly contrived, of two populations that are matched perfectly for age and for coma score separately; but because of the way that these two factors are combined, the expected outcomes are quite different.

Some severity features have several points on a scale (e.g., the motor response of the coma scale has six), and even a limited number of features can give rise to a large number of combinations. This would be over 18,000 for the eight features that form the basis of the predictive system we have so far evolved. It is therefore unrealistic to require that series of patients that are to be compared should be matched exactly, even for this small number of characteristics.

Table 4. Mortality of two series with different distribution of age and coma score*

Number of Patients	Age	Coma Score (Best in 1st Day)	Mortality†	
			Subset	Whole Series
Series A				
100	0–19 years	3–4	66%	
				80%
100	>60 years	5–7	94%	
Series B				
100	0–19 years	5–7	31%	
				63%
100	>60 years	3–4	96%	

* Each series has half its patients in youngest and oldest age groups, and half in each coma score category.
† Estimates from data bank.
(From Teasdale, Parker, Murray, et al.,[14] with permission)

There is an alternative approach, if a large data bank of cases is available for comparison. It could then be determined whether the distribution of severity factors was "similar" in the new series, and in particular whether there was internal consistency in the data when the relationships between severity factors were analyzed. It would then be possible to base predictions of outcome for the new series on the basis of the data bank, as we have previously described. If the patients had been treated similarly to those in the data bank, then their actual outcomes should not differ substantially from those predicted. If the outcomes are better than predicted, then either the cases were in fact less severe, or else some more effective treatment (whether recognized or not) may be the explanation. Similarity of severity needs to be carefully checked before accepting the latter; in particular, whether definitions and time of assessment were in fact the same in the two series (e.g., was severity based on admission data, or on data at some later stage? was the best or worst state used as an index?).

The most frequent source of error, whether in comparing initial severity or ultimate outcome, is sample size. Small samples are liable to large statistical variation: a small series may appear to have a different mortality rate, when this is not (yet) of statistical significance.[14]

AVOIDABLE FACTORS CONTRIBUTING TO MORTALITY AND MORBIDITY

Without a postmortem examination it is all too easy to assume, especially if death occurs in the first few hours, that the initial damage has been irrecoverable. If such damage is not found at autopsy, then it is appropriate to consider what pathological processes have led to the patient's death and then to review the clinical course in order to detect factors that might have contributed to these processes and that might have been avoided.

Some years ago we postulated that patients who had talked at some stage after injury, but had subsequently died, might include many whose lives could have been saved—on the premise that to have talked indicates that irrecoverable impact brain damage did not occur.[10] We have subsequently extended our clinical and pathological studies on patients who "talk and die" to a larger series of patients in Glasgow, and we also set out to identify avoidable factors.[11] Over 90 percent of patients who talked and died had evidence at autopsy of raised intracranial pressure, and 75 percent had an intracranial hematoma. Lesions in those without hematoma included brain swelling in relation to contusions and lacerations, hypoxic brain damage, meningitis, and occasionally fat embolism.

Factors in patient care that were regarded as avoidable included delay in recognizing or in initiating action for the management of those injuries or complications that without timely intervention are known to have serious implications. Some of these factors were intracranial, such as hematoma, open injuries, or status epilepticus; the commonest extracranial factors that adversely affected the brain included hypoxia and hypotension. For each avoidable factor in each patient the significance of the contribution to death was judged to be either certain or only probable, taking account of both clinical and neuropathological evidence (all patients in these studies had an autopsy).

Patients quite often had more than one avoidable factor; 120 factors were considered to have had a certain effect on the deaths of 78 patients. Two thirds of these certain factors were intracranial; by far the commonest intracranial avoidable factor was delayed treatment of an intracranial hematoma. Avoidable factors were not confined to patients who died, although it was much easier to identify them with confidence at autopsy. In a series of patients who survived evacuation of an intracranial hematoma, and who had been in coma at the time of operation, avoidable factors similar to those in fatal cases were found in 60 percent.

The circumstances that may lead to delayed diagnosis and treatment of intracranial hematoma are discussed fully elsewhere (p. 170). In a fifth of the cases, delay was due to the patient not having come to hospital soon after injury, but only after deterioration had developed. Delay was more frequent with intradural than extradural hematoma; and recent alcohol ingestion was recorded twice as often in patients with delay as in those without.

Epilepsy was frequently recorded as inadequately managed, but not often as a certain contributor to death; when it was, it was because status epilepticus and hypoxic brain damage, usually in young children, had followed a mild injury (p. 237). Meningitis, caused by overlooked open injury, was not common, but when it occurred it could be the undoubted cause of a fatal outcome in otherwise recoverable patients. Extracranial factors were equally divided between airway obstruction, hypotension, and a miscellaneous group of problems. About a third of incidents of airway obstruction and of hypotension were judged to be significant in contributing to death.

Airway obstruction most often arose during an ambulance journey between one hospital and another; we confirmed the findings of other studies that airway obstruction was rarely a factor contributing to death before the patient reached hospital. Although it is widely acknowledged that every effort should be made to ensure a clear airway in unconscious patients, there is evidence from several studies that patients are quite frequently transported in the supine position, and without an oral or endotracheal airway.

Hypotension is usually associated with either an extracranial injury, which, because of the head injury, has been overlooked or inadequately treated, or with general anesthesia and surgery, either for the head injury or for other injuries. The need to be alert to the possibility of extracranial injury, whenever there is any hypotension, has already been emphasized (p. 109). When surgery is needed soon after injury, hypotension should always be anticipated—it may result from added blood loss during surgery, or because compensating mechanisms that are maintaining an adequate blood pressure are affected by relaxant or anesthetic drugs or by the sudden relief of intracranial pressure when the hematoma is removed.

The frequency of avoidable factors, and the proportion that are due to various causes, differ according to local organizational factors and with the type of injury. Where secondary referral from a distance to neurosurgeons is common, delayed treatment of intracranial hematoma tends to predominate. When there is rapid admission to neurosurgery, a more frequent avoidable factor is an overlooked extracranial injury. Extracranial insults are particularly common after road accidents, because they are usually associated with multiple trauma. It has been shown in one American study that hypotension and hypoxia are equally common in patients transported directly to the neurosurgical unit as in those making a short stop in the emergency room of another hospital.[9] The detour does not result in effective first aid, only in delay in starting adequate resuscitation.

If avoidable factors are to be minimized, then regular review of all head injury deaths should be routine; and if avoidable factors are to be recognized at such reviews, then a high autopsy rate and good quality neuropathology are essential.

340

Therapeutic Possibilities

Some clinicians are sceptical of the value of active intervention in all but a minority of head injuries. They believe that mild injuries get better, however little is done for them, and that severe ones do badly, no matter how much is done. This is a curious inversion of the aphorism of Hippocrates about head injuries: "No injury is too trivial to ignore nor too serious to despair of."

It is certainly true that nothing can be done to repair the impact damage, but it is at least probable that the secondary processes of swelling, edema, and ischemia could be limited if not always prevented. Likewise there is probably no way to prevent the development of an intracranial hematoma, but early evacuation will minimize the harm a clot can do. Perhaps nothing can be done to accelerate the recovery process, but good management will reduce reactions that can impede the restoration of function.

While not agreeing with as negative an approach as has been caricatured above, there are probably many surgeons who would consider that the care of the majority of head injuries is satisfactory, and that there is no call for a radical reappraisal of attitudes or of organization. Such complacency is readily explained by the dispersion of head injury problems among so many individual doctors, and so many different disciplines. This makes it difficult for anyone to see the problem as a whole, or to view separate parts of it in perspective. There is now evidence from several countries, which will be briefly reviewed, to suggest that all is not well; it seems likely that an appreciable amount of mortality and morbidity that is accepted as an inevitable aftermath of head injury, is potentially preventable by better medical treatment of the head injured victim, both in the early and in the late stages.

It seems that more lives are likely to be saved, and brain function in survivors more likely to be preserved, by measures designed to minimize avoidable factors that cause secondary brain damage, than by ever more energetic treatment of patients who are already severely brain damaged. More effort should be put into preventing patients from going secondarily into deep coma than into the attempted rescue of those already suffering from a degree of irreversible damage. This means better organization of care in the early stages, and more concentration on the mildly and moderately injured, who may get worse, than on those already severely affected. This calls for nice judgment, for sound policies, and for good clinical assessment. What is appropriate in one place may not be the best for another, and no overall rules can be proposed.

Perhaps the most hopeful development for the less severely affected is the CT scan, which makes possible the earlier detection of intracranial hematomas. An important advance in the management of the more severely brain damaged is the evolution of reliable, widely accepted methods of measurement, both of the initial severity and of the ultimate outcome. The combination of standardized clinical assessment with the use of the CT scanner should make the selection of cases for treatment more rational, and the assessment of the results of alternative methods more valid.

LOGISTICS OF CARE FOR MINOR INJURIES

So numerous are these injuries, the great majority of which will make an uninterrupted recovery no matter what is done for them, that the need is to

341

decide what is the minimum care that is safe. Some among these patients will develop symptoms of the post-traumatic syndrome, and a few will have serious complications such as intracranial hematoma or infection. There is still no general agreement as to whether the post-traumatic syndrome can be predicted from the previous personality traits and other characteristics of the patient, or from the circumstances of the accident. But there seems little doubt that prolonged disability from these symptoms can be reduced in the majority of patients by more sympathetic, formal, early management, with follow-up of mild injuries in the first few weeks after injury (p. 263). It is doubtful whether admission to hospital is beneficial in this respect, provided that circumstances at home are reasonable.

The anticipation of intracranial hematoma is the reason most commonly given for the policy of admitting large numbers of mild injuries to hospital for 24 hours or more of "observation." There is good evidence that this policy is not particularly effective, perhaps for the very reason that this complication is so unusual. Therefore, few of those responsible for observing head injured patients in community hospitals or in primary surgical wards ever see a patient who develops the dramatic deterioration that is so familiar to neurosurgeons who work in large centers. Not surprisingly, vigilance becomes blunted, and patients are then less carefully observed than they might be, with the result that when a complication does develop it may not be recognized as soon as it should be. If fewer patients were admitted, and those that came in were known really to be at risk, then there might be a higher standard of observation; moreover, many hospital beds would be freed for more cost-effective use, and fewer patients would be unnecessarily inconvenienced.

Such a policy could be pursued only if it was agreed that patients at risk could be identified, and if those sent home, in whom the risk had been judged to be low but could obviously not be entirely excluded, were known to have a relative or friend who could accept responsibility for reporting any unusual developments over the succeeding 24 to 48 hours. Review of patients who suffered undue delay in the detection of hematoma[3] revealed that in most cases a fracture had been overlooked, or there had been inaccurate assessment of the state of consciousness, or a mistaken diagnosis of the cause of unconsciousness. Inadequate observation rather than the caprice of nature was the most common reason for the apparently unsuspected development of this complication.

Unsatisfactory treatment of scalp lacerations, and failure to diagnose underlying depressed fractures of the vault, account for most instances of intracranial infection; some patients, however, suffer meningitis because a fracture of the base has been overlooked. There is clearly need for a higher index of suspicion of open injuries; it should be recognized that such patients may appear deceptively well in the early stages, seeming to have been only mildly injured (p. 195).

All patients with traumatic intracranial infection and 90 percent of adults with extradural hematomas have a skull fracture; and up to 75 percent of those with only intradural hematomas have a fracture. Although only a small proportion of patients with skull fracture will develop complications, most patients who do develop serious secondary events after injuries that were initially mild do have a skull fracture. It therefore makes good sense to admit all patients who have a skull fracture seen on x-ray, whether linear or depressed, or who have clinical signs of a fractured skull base (p. 99). This rule should apply whether or not consciousness is, or has been, impaired. All patients who have any impairment of consciousness in the accident department, those who have neurological signs, and those who have marked headache or vomiting should be admitted, no matter whether they have a fracture or not. When there is doubt about the case, as with young children or when alcohol is confusing the assessment of an adult, it may be necessary to admit patients outside of these criteria. With children it is wise to admit whenever there is doubt, because intracranial hematoma not infrequently develops in them without a skull fracture.

Reducing avoidable morbidity (and mortality) after milder injuries, while avoiding the unnecessary admission of large numbers of patients, depends largely on making appropriate arrangements for securing adequate skull x-rays in the accident department and on having a standardized method of assessing level of consciousness and of dealing with scalp lacerations. An admission policy needs to be agreed to in advance, and its foundation and objectives clearly understood. Observation of patients taken into hospital should likewise conform to a system that is reliable, and criteria for taking further action should be agreed to in advance. Action may consist of investigation or intervention, either of which may require removing the patient to a specially equipped center. Distance and availability will naturally influence these decisions, as may the presence of other major injuries that limit the transportation of the patient.

There is now abundant evidence that it is unsafe to wait until there is such obvious evidence of any deterioration that the likelihood of finding an intracranial complication is high. If a patient does not rapidly regain consciousness, or if there is any evidence of deterioration at all (and this will usually be in the level of consciousness, rather than the development of focal signs), there is need for urgent appraisal of the situation. What is the time factor (rather than the distance) in moving the patient to where he can have a CT scan or an angiogram? And if these investigations should show a lesion that needs surgical intervention or intensive medical therapy, where and how soon can this be available? It may be wise to consider moving the patient to where both investigation and intervention are possible. If deterioration is rapid, intervention without investigation may be called for; also, if anesthesia is needed for investigation, it will be wise to be able to proceed to operation under the same anesthetic. Local circumstances must dictate how the interaction between the various needs of individual patients will determine the appropriate course of action. However, an outline can be given within which local variations can be accommodated.

Primary Hospital
    Assess
        brain damage
            diffuse—altered consciousness
            focal—signs
        skull damage
            fracture
            ? open injury
        extracranial factors
            drugs
            injuries
            complications
    Treat
        hypotension

hypoxia
hemoglobin loss

Admit

adults with brain damage or skull fracture and those in whom these injuries cannot be properly assessed

children, if in any doubt, even without fracture, unless convinced that sensible, caring parents will maintain observation

Transfer to neurosurgery—previously agreed criteria

Neurosurgical Service

Advise

on criteria for transfer

on individual cases by consultation

Accept—all patients with

coma persisting after resuscitation and stabilization of cardiorespiratory state

or confusion lasting more than a few hours, sooner if there is a skull fracture or focal signs

or deterioration of level of consciousness, as soon as this is recognized

or open injuries of skull, proven or suspect

CONTINUITY OF CARE FOR THE SEVERELY INJURED

It is by no means easy, in these days of specialization in medicine, to be sure that the care of the severely injured patient is as well coordinated as it should be, especially for those with multiple injuries. Much benefit has come in recent years from intensive care, but there is now a risk that the responsibility for the overall care of the head injured patient may pass to a specialist whose primary concern is not the brain, and who does not have training or skills in the management of intracranial conditions. No one would dispute the importance of maintaining normoxia and normotension, of preventing serious chest complications, and of ensuring adequate fluid and caloric intake. However, it is a mistake to underestimate the powers of natural recovery, and for the physician to react to every deviation from physiological norms by instituting elaborate therapeutic interventions, without first considering the possible disadvantages. Few interventions are free of risk—whether it be the administration of drugs, the use of mechanical ventilators, or the performance of tracheostomy. Each may be life-saving when appropriately used, but the widespread application of methods of management without prior agreement about the objectives, and therefore the specific indications, is bad medicine. Not only may treatment be used for patients who are not sufficiently badly affected to justify the risks associated with that therapy, but it becomes impossible to judge the efficacy of these particular regimens if they are applied to patients with a wide spectrum of severity of injury—including many who would recover without such treatment.

Some methods currently advocated deprive the clinician of most of the signs by which he normally assesses brain dysfunction, in particular the responsiveness of the limbs, eye movements, and pupils. If such a treatment regimen is applied very soon after injury, it may not be possible adequately to assess even the initial severity of brain damage. And once the treatment has been instituted, it is difficult to judge the patient's reaction to treatment, and to know whether there is a continuing need for it. There is no ready answer to this dilemma. It is, however, vital to insist on adequate initial assessment, without which it becomes impossible to establish the efficacy or the necessity for various methods of management. The indications for various levels of therapy should be defined, and these should be conditional on the failure of simpler methods to control the situation within a specific time period. After the institution of techniques of treatment that inevitably interfere with clinical assessment, there should be re-examination at planned regular intervals, when drugs are withdrawn for this particular purpose; this might be at 24 hours, 3, and 6 days after the institution of therapy. In such circumstances, methods of monitoring that depend on machine measurements rather than on the evaluation of responsiveness may be useful, such as the CT scan, ICP measurements, and evoked electrical responses.

In the acute stage of management of multiply injured patients there is need for a fine balance between the priorities for intervention with respect to the different injuries. It may be wise to defer, at least for a day or two, definitive treatment of facial or limb fractures, so as to avoid the risks to the brain of anesthesia and possible hypotension. But life-threatening crises such as pneumothorax, ruptured spleen, or leaking gut must be dealt with—not regardless of the brain, but taking due account of the possibility of brain damage during surgery, and modifying techniques of anesthesia and surgery in order to minimize these risks.

Continuity of care is also important at the stage of rehabilitation, when many different skills must again be assembled and coordinated. And again there are aspects of management that can prevent complications. In particular, psychosocial counseling of the family to prepare them for the changed relative returning from hospital, and to enlist their help in the adjustment of the patient to his new life, may pay dividends.

PROBLEMS OF ORGANIZATION AND ETHICS

It used to be enough that doctors did their best. If the patient recovered they were thanked, while if he died or remained disabled that was regarded as the work of fate. When there was little that doctors could do, as often seemed to be the case after severe head injury, this may have been a reasonable philosophy. But it is altogether too passive in the light of present knowledge, because we now know that many of the events that follow head injury are either preventable or they can be controlled; therefore, if mortality and morbidity are to be reduced, active intervention may be required. Because of this there is concern that there should be sufficient effort to avoid secondary damage, especially after less severe injuries.

Recognition of the problem posed by the continued occurrence of avoidable factors evokes from neurosurgeons in different places a variety of responses, by way of solution. Inevitably these reflect, as they rightly should, local differences in available facilities, in the organization of medicine, and in the relationship between doctors and the public. In the United States, in most of which there is an abundance of neurosurgeons, and where the threat of malpractice suits influences strongly the way in which medicine is practiced, awareness of avoidable factors tends to confirm the view that as many head injured patients as possible should be seen by neurosurgeons. In some institutions a neurosurgical resident may even be called to the emergency room to confirm a decision to send home a mildly injured patient. Those who are admitted to hospital usually go to the neurosurgical

345

service, if there is one; consequently, neurosurgical wards have a high turn-over of mild injuries of the kind that in Britain are managed in primary surgical wards. Indeed, a comparative study has shown that the proportion of head injured patients discharged within 48 hours of admission was the same (about 70%) in a university neurosurgical clinic in Texas as in primary surgical wards in Scotland.[5] In regard to the more severe injuries, again the American response is to emphasize the need for rapid transport to a neurosurgeon, avoiding stopping off at another hospital if possible,[9] and using helicopter evacuation when appropriate.[5]

The opposing view, held by some British neurosurgeons, is that the availability of CT scanners in community hospitals should make it possible for head injured patients to be dealt with locally—even those requiring evacuation of an intracranial hematoma. This presupposes a sufficient number of head injuries coming to a general hospital to maintain skills in CT scanning (and its interpretation), and also a willingness on the part of primary surgeons to operate on the head, as they used to do 30 years ago, before regional neurosurgical services became generally available.

It is not only the advent of CT scanning that is changing the background against which a policy of head injury care has to be developed. The development of intensive care units, under the supervision of specialists in that discipline, and the emergence in some places of doctors devoted to accident surgery or emergency medicine, make it no longer a simple question to decide who should care for head injuries. Considering the prevalence of head injuries, their dispersion over wide areas, and the fact that most are mild and uncomplicated, it seems unrealistic to expect the majority to be looked after (or even to be seen) by a neurosurgeon. But the complexity of the problems associated with severe head injury, and the need for special investigative and monitoring techniques, even if no intracranial surgery is required, make it difficult to expect anyone other than a neurosurgeon to take on this responsibility.

The initial question is one of patient selection. Views will differ as to what degree of severity will merit transfer to a neurosurgical facility, but whatever is decided, there is need for good liaison between neurosurgeons and those personnel who are concerned with the early care of accident victims. Policies should be agreed upon regarding roadside care, transportation, initial resuscitation, and clinical observations, and about continuing monitoring. All this may seem obvious for the severely injured, but the majority of injuries are mild, and it is even more important to have agreed procedures for these patients—who to x-ray, who to admit, what to observe, and when to consider CT scanning or transfer to a neurosurgical unit. There can be little doubt that mortality and morbidity could be significantly reduced by better organization, and one example of how to do this comes from the University of Virginia at Charlottesville. Policies there have been reproduced in two booklets, and wall charts on head injury care and monitoring have been made available for every emergency room in the state. Unless policies are made explicit by the neurosurgeons in this way, there will inevitably be ambiguities and doubts about what to do, even about what the local neurosurgeons recommend.

Comparative international studies suggest that the optimal care of head injuries is likely to come from a compromise between the systems currently most prevalent in Europe and in the United States. In Britain a larger proportion of head injuries would benefit from going to neurosurgery and going there sooner than currently is the case; in the United States fewer mild injuries than at present need to go to neurosurgeons. In both countries better organization of early care in severe cases en route to the neurosurgeon should reduce secondary brain damage. When policies are changed there should be an audit to discover how effective the new system is, not only for dealing with patients referred to neurosurgeons, but for head injuries in the whole community; this should include reliable autopsy data.

Discussions about the management of patients who already have sustained severe brain damage, whether this be primary or secondary, now often focuses on a new concern: whether doctors might at times be doing too much, rather than not enough, for patients with severe irreversible brain damage. It is suggested that prolonging the survival of some patients who can never recover may be against their best interests as well as those of their families and of society. Such concern is most often voiced by theologians, philosophers, and other commentators who are not themselves involved in the decision-making that they are implicitly criticizing. However, this concern is now spreading to doctors and nurses, who not only see the problem at close quarters, but are themselves responsible for it. The problem arises from the possibility, with modern methods of resuscitation and of continued intensive care, of securing the survival, for a time at least, of patients so badly brain damaged that they would previously have died.

The most obvious problem might seem to be that of brain death; however, this is short-lived at the worst, and in any event a consensus is emerging both about criteria for its recognition (p. 86) and about the propriety of discontinuing ventilation as soon as brain death is diagnosed. The vegetative state is now regarded by many as worse than death, while there are some who are now prepared to concede that to regain consciousness, but to remain very severely physically and also mentally crippled, may be even worse (p. 315).

At the same time there is evidence that an undue proportion of the resources available for resuscitation and intensive care are being expended on those who do not recover. Without limitless resources it is inevitable that there is a risk that other patients who do have a reasonable chance for recovery, provided they are given sufficiently intensive treatment for long enough, may be denied that opportunity because all the beds or all the machines are already committed—some of them to the continuous support of patients whose conditions are irrecoverable. This is most readily apparent when there is direct competition between patients with the same or similar basic condition (e.g., head injury and stroke), but there is also the drain on overall resources, not only of money and machines, but more importantly of skilled personnel. Not only does the expenditure of an undue proportion on the irrecoverable patients deny facilities to other brain damaged patients, but there is less available for alternative activities such as elective, cost-effective surgery, whether in the same or other disciplines. Severe head injury is only one among several conditions to which this applies—similar dilemmas apply to renal dialysis, severe congenital abnormalities, malignant disease, and general intensive care. While it is the responsibility of both the medical world and the rest of society to decide upon these issues in principle, the onus of efficient decision-making in the individual case will always lie with the doctor.

Doctors whose work frequently involves conditions with a high mortality and morbidity are now facing up to these issues. Selection of patients is becoming an essential part of their decision-making. This selection may be whether or not to admit a patient to special facilities, such as an intensive care or a neurosurgical unit, or in deciding in advance which circumstances demand that a patient be

347

resuscitated, and even more important, which patients should have continued life-support therapy and for how long. These decisions will depend upon the general principle that all patients must have all possible treatment as long as they have a reasonable chance of recovery. The word "reasonable" is used advisedly, because how it is interpreted will naturally and rightly vary from place to place and from person to person. It will also vary from patient to patient, in that the potential recovery depends upon the underlying pathology, the severity of brain damage, and the amount of treatment already applied. Thus it is almost always reasonable to resuscitate a recently head injured patient, because until this is done, assessment of severity can be fallacious. There is a need to recognize that the decision to stop treatment once it has been started is, in principle, no different than to decide not to treat initially—although it will seldom appear to be as straightforward. Severe head injury presents a sudden crisis and there is seldom the opportunity to consider alternative managements after discussion between different doctors or between the physician and the family, as can occur with less immediate conditions. Rescue procedures must be initiated immediately if they are going to be effective. The question that is crucial is when they should be discontinued, once there is evidence that there is no chance of reasonable recovery. Prior consensus is the only way to ensure that the individual doctor with a given patient will be able to act wisely when a crisis occurs, and in a way that he knows will command respect and will justify the support of his colleagues, should it be subsequently questioned. The need to accept (and to define) limits to the extent and duration of intensive care in certain circumstances has been acknowledged recently by several American anesthesiologists.[1,4,12] Unless clear criteria for such decisions are agreed upon, there is likely sooner or later to be a reluctance to initiate rescue procedures, and some patients will suffer from that.

Until recently doctors could avoid making the decision to discontinue treatment on the grounds that prediction was not possible, and that therefore every patient must have all possible treatment (or life-support) until the outcome declared itself. That situation is now changing. One reason is the real possibility of making reliable predictions of outcome relatively soon after injury, at least in some patients. It is now becoming accepted in several fields of medicine that calculations of the probability of outcome, with and without a given course of action, is a reasonable basis for deciding what action is appropriate. What action should follow would depend on many circumstances, including how medicine is practiced locally and the attitudes of the individual physician and family.

It is likely that knowledge of probabilities of different events will, in the near future, play an increasingly important part in decision-making about many aspects of the care of head injured patients. Probabilities can be applied to the prediction, soon after injury, that complications such as epilepsy or intracranial hematoma will develop; this will provide a basis for rational decisions about who should be treated or investigated prophylactically. Probabilities will also indicate the likelihood of finding abnormalities with certain investigations, such as a skull x-ray or a CT scan, and they are also involved in deciding what action should follow the demonstration of an abnormality in these investigations. There is nothing new or sinister in choosing who to investigate, or who to treat and how, or whose treatment should be continued. Such selection has always been common practice in medicine, but it was previously concealed beneath comfortable words, such as the "experience" or "intuition" of the clinician. Providing the clinician with calculated probabilities should help him make decisions, but will never make a decision for him.

THE FUTURE

Whether there has been any material change in the outcome after head injury in the last 50 years was a question posed in a recent editorial.[7] Its conclusion was that there had not been much change, at least until very recently—but it is doubtful whether either of these views was justified. It is difficult enough to make valid comparisons between contemporary series of patients, let alone to feel confident about reports of many years ago. What is certain is that we now know much more about the pathophysiological consequences of acute brain damage—processes that are not unique to trauma but are similar (in varying degrees) to those that occur following ischemia and in association with tumors and infection. Much of the experimental research on which this new-found knowledge is based was not directed specifically to solving the problems of traumatic brain damage. Experimental work aimed at producing models of human head trauma is fraught with difficulty, but much has been learned about the mechanical aspects of impact damage from such experiments (p. 20).

Better understanding of the clinical problems posed by head injuries seems likely to depend largely on research directly on patients. This can be of three main kinds: epidemiological, clinical, and neuropathological. It is surprising that so few competent and comprehensive studies have been reported in any of these fields, although there are reasons for this. The dispersion of head injuries through many hospitals and disciplines makes it difficult for the epidemiologist, or for clinicians in any one specialty, to focus on the problem; and the pathologist is often frustrated by forensic considerations. Whether these are explanations or excuses, most of those who might contribute to knowledge in this field prefer to devote their skills to other, easier subjects. However, a number of recent studies in each of these three areas of research reveals them to be rich fields, ripe to yield data that are both of considerable scientific interest and that are also likely to improve the care of head injured patients—if the lessons are learned and translated into practical action.

Clinical and pathological studies reveal the sources of preventable mortality and morbidity, which largely lie in suboptimal management in the acute stage. Epidemiological studies indicate the scale of these problems, and what the implications would be of providing better care for a greater proportion of head injured patients in terms of facilities. But effective change will come only when attitudes alter, when head injuries are no longer regarded as an unfortunate nuisance, preventing those who have to deal with them from getting on with more interesting matters. Head injuries should be regarded as an unusually challenging group of problems, and of particular importance because they are so common, and because they affect primarily the young—so that many years of life are lost if death or permanent disablement results.

In the clinical field there is a need for well-conducted therapeutic trials, both soon after injury and at the later stage of rehabilitation. Doctors dealing with the acute stage need to question new techniques and also the continuing use of methods whose adoption owes more to custom than to proven worth. Psychologists need to find out more about how the diffusely damaged brain works, and to do less reiterative studies of localized brain lesions. They might relate their findings to the restructuring of rehabilitation programs, most of which remain empirical in design and anecdotal in report.

The increasing awareness in many countries of the importance of the problem of head injuries is hopeful, as is the evolution of more standardized methods of assessment of severity and outcome, and the recognition of the need for large scale data collection and the application of rigorous statistical methods. The stage is now set for the discerning clinician to recognize with alacrity the value of any new method of treatment that may be evolved. It should also be possible to discover which existing therapeutic techniques should continue to be used.

New investigative techniques have given clinicians an opportunity to advance knowledge of the processes that occur in the early stages after more severe injury. Three-dimensional isotope scanning, biochemical investigations, measurement of blood flow and intracranial pressure, and CT scanning have each provided data not previously available. The first 5-year's use of CT scanning was naturally dominated by establishing its value as a diagnostic tool, as a basis for informing the clinician concerned with making immediate decisions. It is time now to conduct studies beyond the needs of clinical practice, to correlate serial scanning with other observations—changes in clinical state and intracranial pressure, electrical potentials, blood flow, and autonomic functions. It is also important to correlate CT scans with neuropathological findings in fatal cases, so that we can know better how to interpret what is seen in the CT scan in life. Additional techniques may now make it possible to calculate the changes in cerebral blood flow, water content, and metabolism on a regional basis. These may make it possible to distinguish between the relative contributions of engorgement, edema, and ischemia to secondary events soon after injury and to monitor the effects of therapeutic interventions on these. CT scanning months after injury may lead to better understanding of the mechanisms underlying persisting disability; again this will come only from systematic investigation of large series, rather than from the random scanning of interesting cases.

Neuropathologists should not overlook the amount to be learned from careful mapping of the topographical distribution of lesions, plotting their time course and elucidating the relationship between what is found at autopsy and what happens in life—what events the clinicians recorded, and what the CT scan and other dynamic investigations showed. Autopsy is an essential part of the audit of fatalities and thus of the success or failure of various methods of management. Means must be found of ensuring that forensic considerations do not limit the access of skilled pathologists to adequately fixed brains.

As knowledge from all these sources accumulates, so the organizational arrangements that are deemed appropriate are likely to evolve and to change. These should always aim to ensure that as many patients as possible have access with as little delay as possible to whatever investigations and treatment are regarded as necessary. One useful guide to the adequacy of arrangements for the care of head injuries is to review all patients admitted to all hospitals in a community, and to record the incidence of intracranial hematoma, together with the death and disability rate. In addition, every dead or disabled patient (with or without a hematoma) should be reviewed to identify avoidable factors in management that might have contributed to the unfavorable outcome. Such a process of continuing audit is informative to local clinicians and should lead to continuous updating of their policy and practice. But it also can add to the sum of knowledge about head injuries if the results of such investigations are periodically published.

The only value of recriminating about the past is to improve the future. Clinicians concerned with head injury face a particular challenge, in that there is now abundant evidence that much of the mortality and morbidity associated with this common condition are potentially preventable. Moreover, the means of prevention are in their hands, because prevention depends largely on the adequacy of the arrangements made for the medical care of these injured patients.

REFERENCES

1. CULLEN, D. J., FERRARA, L. C., BURTON, R. N., ET AL.: *Survival, hospitalization charges and follow-up results in critically ill patients.* N. Engl. J. Med. 294:982–987, 1976.

2. FIELD, J. H.: *Epidemiology of head injuries in England and Wales.* Her Majesty's Stationery Office, London, 1976.

3. GALBRAITH, S.: *Misdiagnosis and delayed diagnosis in traumatic intracranial hematoma.* Br. Med. J. 1:1438–1439, 1976.

4. GRENVIK, A., POWNER, D. J., SNYDER, J. V., ET AL.: *Cessation of therapy in terminal illness and brain death.* Crit. Care Med. 6:284–291, 1978.

5. JENNETT, B., AND GROSSMAN, R.: *Head injuries in Glasgow and Galveston* (unpublished observations).

6. JENNETT, B., TEASDALE, G., BRAAKMAN, R., ET AL.: *Prognosis in series of patients with severe head injury.* Neurosurgery 4:283, 1979.

7. LANGFITT, T. W.: *Measuring the outcome from head injuries.* J. Neurosurg. 48:673–678, 1978.

8. MACMILLAN, R., STRANG, I., AND JENNETT, B.: *Head injuries in primary surgical wards in Scottish hospitals.* Health Bull. (Edinb.) 37:75–81, 1979.

9. MILLER, J. D., SWEET, R. C., NARAYAN, R., ET AL.: *Early insults to the injured brain.* J.A.M.A. 240:439–442, 1978.

10. REILLY, P. L., ADAMS, J. H., GRAHAM, D. I., ET AL.: *Patients with head injury who talk and die.* Lancet ii:375–377, 1975.

11. ROSE, J., VALTONEN, S., AND JENNETT, B.: *Avoidable factors contributing to death after head injury.* Br. Med. J. 2:615–618, 1977.

12. SKILLMAN, J. J.: *Ethical dilemmas in the care of the critically ill.* Lancet ii:634–636, 1974.

13. STATES, J. D., HUELKE, D. F., AND HAMES, L. H.: *Revision of the abbreviated injury scale (AIS).* Proceedings of the American Association for Automotive Medicine, 1974.

14. TEASDALE, G., PARKER, L., MURRAY, G., ET AL.: *On comparing series of head injured patients.* Acta Neurochir. 28:205–208, 1979.

15. *The abbreviated injury scale. 1980 Revision.* American Association for Automotive Medicine, 1980.

Index